Epidemic Disease and Society in the Premodern Low Countries

In this book, evidence from a long-run history of epidemic-society interaction in the Low Countries shows that most recurring outbreaks were accommodated by communities, and most reactions, responses, and changes seen were the product of frequent and incremental adaptations, sometimes in periods outside of epidemics.

Epidemics blur the distinction between the normal and the sub-normal. Accordingly, although histories tend to emphasise epidemics' capacity to create sharp changes, deviations, or transitions within societies and economies, this book develops an alternative argument that the most relevant questions are not "how and why change", but given the substantial pressures of raised mortality, why was change often so modest? It brings together around five centuries' worth of existing and new evidence on epidemics and societal resistance, wealth redistribution, and women's experiences to support this interpretation.

Challenging conventional narratives about epidemics as agents of dramatic change, this book will be of interest to researchers examining historiographical debates about crisis and continuity in European history.

Daniel R. Curtis works at Erasmus University Rotterdam, the Netherlands, and has published three previous books, namely, *Coping with Crisis: The Resilience and Vulnerability of Pre-Industrial Settlements* (2014), *Disasters and History: The Vulnerability and Resilience of Past Societies* (2020), and *Infectious Inequalities: Epidemics, Trust, and Social Vulnerabilities in Cinema* (2022).

Disaster Studies

Throughout history disasters such as floods, famines, earthquakes, and epidemics have affected human experience in myriad ways. Disasters are given historical meaning through the impact of socioeconomic and political conditions, trauma support on a regional and national scale, and how transnational ties between global communities have ignited relief campaigns. Furthermore, for centuries, news about catastrophic events has been disseminated via media such as documentary, pamphlets, chronicles, newspapers, poems, illustrations and prints. As such, disasters have also been mediated through recurring cultural repertoires of representations.

This series seeks to address the ways in which communities in and beyond Europe have intervened in, coped with or given meaning to disasters that occurred close by or far away, in terms of both time and space. We invite submissions (both monographs and edited collections) in the fields of (political, socioeconomic and cultural) history, cultural studies, religious studies, art history, memory studies, gender studies, literary studies, and media studies.

Titles in this series:
Epidemic Disease and Society in the Premodern Low Countries
Inequality and Community
Daniel Curtis

For more information about this series, please visit: www.routledge.com/series-title/book-series/DISST

Epidemic Disease and Society in the Premodern Low Countries

Inequality and Community

Daniel R. Curtis

Routledge
Taylor & Francis Group
LONDON AND NEW YORK

First published 2026
by Routledge
4 Park Square, Milton Park, Abingdon, Oxon OX14 4RN

and by Routledge
605 Third Avenue, New York, NY 10158

Routledge is an imprint of the Taylor & Francis Group, an informa business

British Library Cataloguing-in-Publication Data
A catalogue record for this book is available from the British Library

ISBN: 978-9-048-56285-5 (hbk)
ISBN: 978-1-041-17886-6 (pbk)
ISBN: 978-1-003-69490-8 (ebk)

DOI: 10.4324/9781003694908

Typeset in Sabon
by Deanta Global Publishing Services, Chennai, India

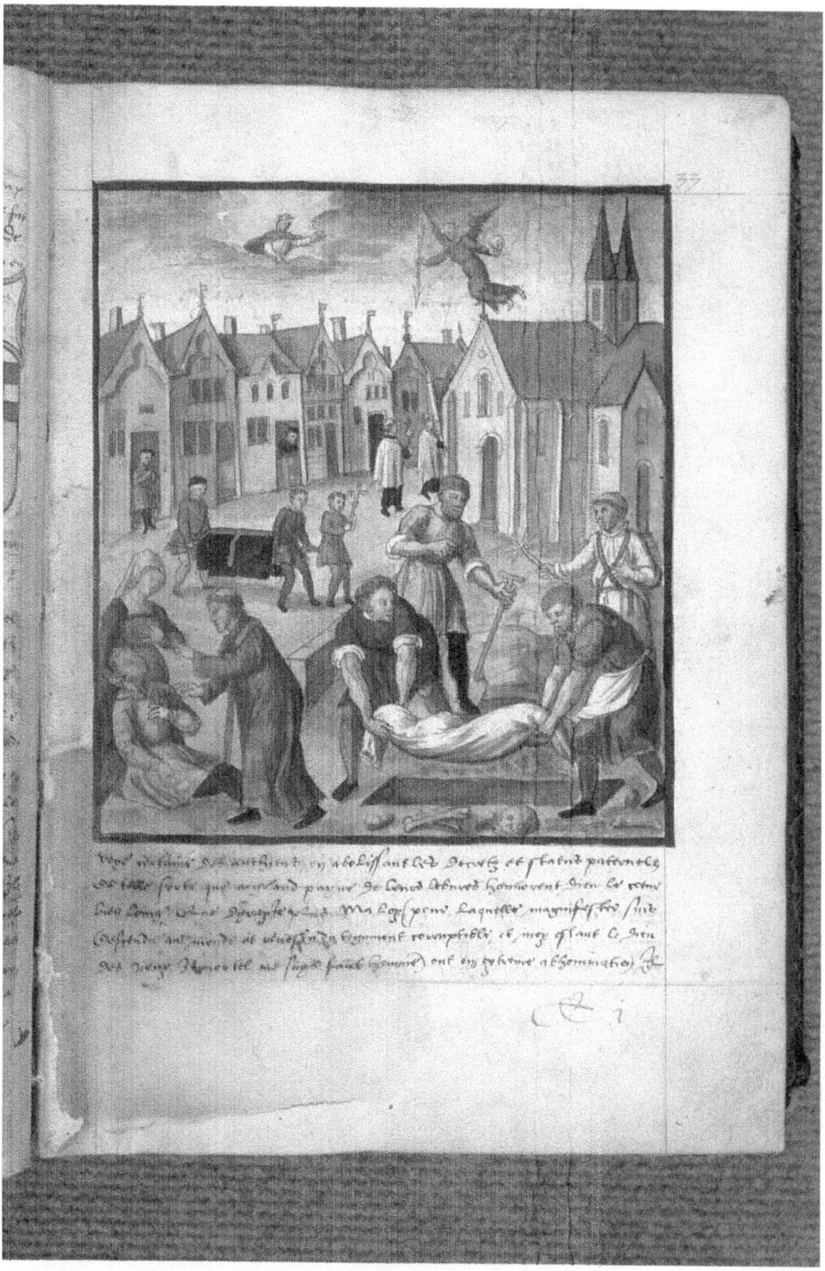

Source: Front image taken from: Hubert Cailleau, Peste à Valenciennes en 1515. In: Louis de la Fontaine, ed., *Recueil des antiquités de Valenciennes*, fo. 33r. http://initiale.irht.cnrs.fr/decor/56276 (manuscript composed between 1551 and 1554).

In memory of my Nan, Jean

Contents

Figures

Tables

Acknowledgements

This book is the product of numerous helpful collaborations and exchanges over the years, supported financially by two consecutive grants funded by the *Nederlandse Organisatie voor Wetenschappelijk Onderzoek* (*NWO*). My first three-year grant (*VENI*) was carried out under the title "Why do some epidemic diseases lead to hatred? An investigation into the impact of economic inequality on the extent of blame, persecution, hatred, and violence after early modern plagues in the Northern Low Countries" in the period 2016–18, and my second five-year grant (*VIDI*) was carried out under the title "Positively shocking! The redistributive impact of mass mortality through epidemic diseases and violent conflict in early modern northwest Europe" in the period 2019–24. Such an extended period of financial support for research is a privilege that I recognise—particularly in the context of meagre funds available for humanities disciplines. The open access version of the book has been supported by the Erasmus University Library's "*Open Access Book Fund*".

My closest collaborations and intellectual stimulation have been with my own talented *VIDI* team members—the sharp quantitative skills and critical sounding-board of Bram van Besouw and the independent and creative thinking of Bram Hilkens. Several of the figures used in this book have been created or refined by Bram van Besouw based on my own or shared data and are reproduced with his permission. I also have had fruitful collaborations with Joris Roosen and Roos van Oosten. Remi van Schaïk has pointed me to specific sources in Guelders and Groningen and provided useful advice. In an earlier phase of my career, I am grateful for the friendly and inspiring working conditions shown by Bas van Bavel, and then the late Peter Hoppenbrouwers—his passing a great loss for medieval history in the Low Countries. I was personally supported by Maria Grever and Paul van de Laar in my current job. Many of the lines of argumentation in this book have been developed through inspiration by academic influences, some recent, some longstanding, and some direct, some indirect—the work of Samuel Cohn, Chris Dyer, Tim Soens, Janna Coomans, Guy Geltner, Bruce Campbell, and more.

My greatest gratitude goes to my partner, Qijun Han, who has always been a source of inspiration and encouragement.

Notes on terminology and measurements

The Low Countries is a region roughly comprising the modern-day countries of the Netherlands, Belgium, Luxembourg, and parts of northern France, which is the geographical confines of the book. Historical terminology, however, is more complicated. The transformation of the political landscape in the Low Countries across five centuries makes for some difficult choices regarding terminology, and it is difficult to maintain absolute consistency. Up until the late fifteenth century we could refer to the area as the Burgundian Netherlands, and thereafter the Habsburg Netherlands, and then the Seventeen Provinces—with many of these provinces originally fiefs of the Holy Roman Empire or France. After the political succession of the autonomous Dutch Republic to the north in 1581, the southern parts of the Low Countries remained under the political control of the Spanish and Austrian courts. The separate Kingdoms of Belgium and the Netherlands only came into being in 1830. In this book, I try to use terminology as appropriate for the political context of the time but also use phrases such as "northern parts of the Low Countries" and "southern parts of the Low Countries" when precision is not necessarily needed. Distinctions in political terms do not necessarily translate into distinctions in economic, cultural, or environmental terms, and of course although epidemic diseases could be affected by political institutions and the legislation enacted, they did not necessarily neatly respect political boundaries.

Archival sources are referenced according to their location in physical archives, although if the reference ends with the abbreviation [AO] for "accessed online", then I have accessed the original manuscript digitally via the archive's website. Widespread and increasing levels of digitisation in the Low Countries of both manuscript sources kept in archives and printed sources in repositories have made this book possible, especially during COVID-19.

In the endnotes I use a contracted form of citation with page numbers and folios, but the full reference is consultable in the bibliography. Folio numbers of manuscripts are often noted with v (*verso*) for the left-hand or back side and r (*recto*) for the right-hand or front side.

Money

Many different currencies circulated in the Low Countries in the medieval and early modern periods. Usually scribes used "units of account" as a form of conversion (i.e., not real coins). The diversity over time and place makes it difficult to account for the different localised variations. Nevertheless, a basic principle to apply, as elsewhere in western Europe, is the standard unit of a pound, being divided into 20 *solidi* (*schellingen*), or 240 *denarii* (*penningen*). A frequent expression of currency was the guilder (or *florin*) which was the equivalent of 20 stuivers (*sous*).

Measures (with local variations mentioned in the text where appropriate)

In the text, I have attempted to make all conversions of surface areas into modern metrics of hectares, and distances in kilometres.

For measurement specifics according to localities and period, an excellent resource is *De oude Nederlandse maten en gewichten* provided by the Meertens Instituut, collected in a database by Ritzo Holtman, and adapted from a 1982 print version by J.M. Verhoeff. Localised translations into modern metric measures are found in the text as and when appropriate.

1 Epidemics as windows into society

In comparison with other parts of Eurasia, where substantial books have long discussed plague's role in shaping divergent economic fortunes, the contagion of rebellion that followed in the wake of the Black Death, or the impact of cholera on instigating social conflict down class lines in nineteenth-century cities, the historical literature on epidemic disease in the Low Countries is much more restricted.[1] Moreover, it has not always played a key or perhaps obvious role in the biggest discussions about political, economic, societal, and cultural developments in the region. For instance, in examining the economic and cultural florescence of the so-called Dutch Golden Age, and its subsequent or relative decline, we find few considerations of epidemic disease as a factor of relevance.[2] Even in Johan Huizinga's classic account of the changing sense and understanding of mortality in the late Middle Ages, and the symbolism and cultural background behind it, epidemic diseases were peripheral to the narrative developed.[3] Take a look at some of the most prominent general syntheses of economy and society in the Dutch Republic and one will find barely any mention of epidemic disease at all—in some cases in books of more than 1,000 pages.[4] Curiously, even the more recent environmental histories of the Dutch Republic do not devote considerable attention to disease outbreaks—despite discussing at length related topics of warfare and climate change.[5]

In fact, the only synthesis of information we have on epidemic disease outbreaks in the northern part of the Low Countries is a short monograph on plague written in Dutch and originally published almost 40 years ago, and while *De gave Gods* (the Gift from God) remains a valuable source of information, most of the evidence corresponds mainly to the County of Holland in the sixteenth and seventeenth centuries.[6] In more recent times, a new work has appeared, mainly focusing on the administrative attempts to manage the threat of epidemic disease in the Dutch Republic, and mainly focusing on the last two plague outbreaks of the 1650s and 1660s and the period thereafter once plague disappears from the region.[7] For the southern parts of the Low Countries, no such book-format synthesis exists—we have, instead, important regional or city-based reconstructions of epidemic diseases for particular periods.[8]

DOI: 10.4324/9781003694908-1

In other parts of western Europe, disease has featured prominently in narratives for long-term historical developments, often by focusing specifically on the Black Death of the mid-fourteenth century. This might explain why epidemic disease has not shared the same prominence in histories of the Low Countries. First, several relevant developments in the Low Countries predated the Black Death. In parts of Flanders, for example, "an extraordinary number of rebellions and revolts" occurred already in the thirteenth and first half of the fourteenth century in pursuit of political representation and economic controls,[9] while in the countryside in the northern Low Countries, rural insurrections against (sometimes self-proclaimed) authorities proliferated in the same period in the pursuit of freedoms and rights to self-organisation.[10] The foundations of "communal emancipation" (Dumolyn and Haemers' term) already preceded the great mortality effects of this outbreak. We might draw similar parallels with concepts such as manors and serfdom. In other parts of western Europe, scholars have often shown how the Black Death helped unravel seigneurial institutions and customary extra-economic practices,[11] while in many parts of the Low Countries, and especially in the coastal areas, these same kinds of institutions and practices had already either dissolved well before 1350 or had never been of any importance.[12] Meanwhile, institutions for corporate collective action (commons, guilds, and beguinages, for example) had started to proliferate in the Low Countries centuries before the Black Death.[13]

Another factor, even more fundamental, is that the basic evidence for the impact of epidemics in the late-medieval Low Countries has for a long time been very sparse. Indeed, so sparse that initial scholarship from the 1950s tended to suggest that the Black Death of the mid-fourteenth century did not even occur in the Low Countries—a notion reproduced in well-known maps of plague spread in Europe.[14] This argument was subsequently debunked—most famously in an important paper from 1980, which showed the presence of the Black Death all across different parts of the southern Low Countries, and in some parts of the north.[15] Yet still, to this day, we do not have strong evidence for the impact of the Black Death in Holland, notwithstanding some plausible indirect indicators in a pioneering doctoral thesis from 1978.[16] Of course, it would be curious if the Black Death did not appear in Holland given that we have direct evidence for its significant impact on agricultural production around nearby Utrecht, but at present the case remains unresolved.[17] Accordingly, some economic historians have seen the purported "light touch" of the plague in Holland as a key component behind its so-called developmental jump-start, where mild disease interacted with pre-existing tendencies towards capital-intensive production, a frontier economy with low population pressures on resources, and freedoms from many elements of feudalism, which created strong population recovery and set the base for convergence of nominal and real wages.[18] While not disputing the broad economy and population lines set out in that narrative, it seems unlikely that a mild experience of epidemic disease can be part of this explanation, however. Just as for the southern parts of the Low Countries,[19] recurring epidemics in Holland have been shown to be very severe.[20] Only in very recent years has the appearance (rather than absence) of the Black Death and other recurring epidemics started to become a more explicitly considered variable in understanding changes and divergences in development in the Low Countries, although, still, mainly for the southern areas such as Flanders and Hainaut.[21]

The relative scarcity of epidemic disease in central narratives for the early modern period and beyond is more complicated since the issue does not lie in a lack of source material. Probably it could be said that the rise of the Dutch Republic, especially in the period 1581–1650, fed into a Golden Age narrative that was very distinct and different from the narratives of the "seventeenth-century crisis" seen elsewhere around the world and characterised by serious environmental challenges and pressures.[22] International demand for products, rather than domestic population developments, has often been given greater primacy in the narratives of economic development and decline, and this is reflected in the interaction between shifting "urban cores" across the Low Countries.[23] Hence, epidemic disease was hidden in the background, especially when we consider that much of the economic and demographic boom seen in the cities and towns of Holland in the late sixteenth and seventeenth centuries was derived from inward migration streams. Population growth in Amsterdam and Leiden was seen as detached from internal demographic mechanisms guiding fertility and mortality, and hence not explainable through the usual preindustrial Malthusian frameworks of a population and resources equilibrium.[24] Indeed, despite losing more than a third of its inhabitants in the epidemic of 1635, ten years later Leiden had already achieved a larger population than seen before the outbreak.[25] Wars helped seed epidemics that reduced populations, but these populations were replenished by those fleeing wars elsewhere, especially if this conflict had characteristics of religious persecution.[26] The notion that the Dutch Republic had escaped the scourge of famine by the seventeenth century likely only entrenched this tendency towards minimising epidemics in the historiography.[27] In fact, rather than conditions producing disease, some scholars have even foregrounded high levels of hygiene in early modern Holland—as a posited side-effect of the proliferation of a highly capital-intensive dairy farming sector producing butter and cheese.[28]

A second related factor is likely the dominance, especially from the late 1990s onwards, of the more institutionalist types of explanation for the economic rise and decline of different parts of the Low Countries from the Middle Ages to the nineteenth century, and thus marginalising any explanations connected to "exogenous" forces associated with the environment or demography.[29] In fact, rather than population developments (potentially affected by epidemics) impacting upon societal and economic institutions, there has been a reverse tendency to see how different institutional settings supported different sizes of populations.[30] Furthermore, although historical demography of the preindustrial period gained some traction in the Netherlands and Belgium in the 1960s and 1970s,[31] much of the significant demographic literature on epidemic diseases in the Low Countries has tended to focus mainly on developments during the nineteenth and twentieth centuries, exploiting the luxury of modern censuses, and in more recent times focusing on issues such as selectivity of mortality and knock-on health implications of diseases.[32] Often, we see the goal of providing more evidence for epidemics killing selectively among the poor, often framed as "health inequalities" research—but at present not really challenging our prior expectations.[33] Demographic approaches to mortality in the preindustrial Low Countries have been left mainly to those trained in social and economic history.[34] And for those explaining economic outcomes in the Low Countries through demographic behaviour, in the process developing complex explanatory frameworks, this is often on the back of remarkably few original demographic indicators.[35] Thus, in sum, although we are increasingly knowing a lot more about the implications of developments such as germ theory, vaccination, pasteurisation, and sanitisation of water supplies on the potential damping down of epidemic impact in the Low Countries since industrialisation, we often miss refined demographic analyses of how epidemics play out in a "historical laboratory" of conditions without modern hygienic interventions—i.e., what has been the norm in the past.

This book brings epidemic disease back into the major historical narratives of the Low Countries and does so by bringing together scattered (and sometimes difficult-to-find or very old) pre-existing evidence into one coherent place, but more than that adds further substantial original empirical evidence. Compared to pre-existing work, this book examines the interaction between society and epidemic disease across a long time period—from the beginning of the fourteenth century (and sometimes fragments from before 1300) up to the end of the nineteenth, and thus allowing us to trace long-term impacts and the role of disease in provoking change (or not, as the case often is) over time.[36] Similarly, the book also eschews a tendency in the Low Countries epidemic disease literature to focus on individual case studies (regions or cities) in isolation—providing instead quantitative demographic and economic information across a wide area (for example, employing a mortality database comprising millions of burials from hundreds of localities), and combining quantitative and qualitative information on impact and experiences of epidemics through illuminating examples from all kinds of urban and rural contexts across the Low Countries.[37] Much more so than other public health literature from both within the Low Countries and in other places around the world, this book gives far greater attention to the impact of disease in the countryside—making a case for the necessity to look at how society-epidemic interaction worked at scales other than the usual global, national, or urban.[38] And as mentioned in the "notes on terminology section", the book has benefitted considerably from the widespread digitalisation of archival material in the Netherlands especially, but also Belgium, and to a lesser extent, Luxembourg and northern France.

Most fundamentally, the approach of the book is to provide an integrated history of epidemic disease, bringing together economic, demographic, and social issues with cultural, medical, and environmental concerns—in the process trying to avoid sub-discipline-driven myopia. Indeed, while there was a small growth of historical literature discussing medical and public health aspects of epidemic diseases in the Low Countries from a socio-cultural angle during the 1990s,[39] this has also seen recent fertile reemergence through new methodologies and theoretical frameworks connected to environmental history.[40] Using this integrated approach, my book moves away from well-worn topics such as "how administrations managed epidemics to exert social controls over populations" or "how epidemics affected real wages of urban workers" to link up with new debates discussed in the wider literature such as the extent to which epidemics impacted upon community cohesion and either cooperation or resistance to authority,[41] whether epidemics led to redistribution of resources and whether that left societies more equitable or unequal than before,[42] and whether, how, and why epidemics affected women and men differently—a subject that has not had that much systematic treatment beyond a focus on selective mortality outcomes.[43]

A substantial literature on the connection between epidemics and societies in the past has tended to present these diseases as massive breaking points that pushed societies down new paths—sometimes said to be influential in establishing geographically divergent economic developments or sharp economic transitions, establishing demographic changes such as new patterns of marriage behaviour, or invoking cultural changes such as new attitudes to health, religion, and death.[44] Likely this is a legacy of a historiographical emphasis on the Black Death, hardly a representative epidemic outbreak of the past 1,000 years. Yet similar narratives have recently featured for explaining the decline of different areas of the ancient Roman Empire—suggested to be connected to the impact of epidemics such as the Antonine Plague, the Cyprianic Plague, and the Justinianic Plague, although also in interaction with other environmental and climatic pressures.[45] Even more explicitly, one significant recent overview of epidemic and society interaction throughout history has suggested that "epidemics are not an esoteric subfield for the interested specialist but instead are a major part of the 'big picture' of historical change and development. [They are] as important to understanding societal development, as powerful forces in societal change as wars and revolutions".[46] In a way, this echoes the words of the famous *Plagues and Peoples*, written nearly half a century ago now, where "infectious disease…has been hitherto, one of the fundamental parameters and determinants of human history".[47]

Nevertheless, although stories of disease shaping the world are easier to market to audiences willing to be convinced about epidemics' transformative powers through grandiose historical narratives, or even the idea of entire societal collapses (with plenty of scholarly disagreement about what this constitutes), the position of my book is more in line with the broader literature surrounding a "historical disaster studies" field which has grown over the past decade or so.[48] Here, my point of departure is that most epidemics in the Low Countries were not sudden unexpected shocks, as used incorrectly in the economics and economic history lexicon,[49] but entirely accommodated recurring hazards that were absorbed fully into the rhythms of everyday life.[50] Accordingly, these outbreaks were so frequently recurring and so anticipated that even the conceptual lines between what we can categorise as epidemic and endemic become somewhat blurred—especially if taking epidemic to mean something broader than epidemiological parameters and referring to the capacity for a disease to present a "societal problem".[51]

In fact, what we see during many of the epidemic outbreaks in the Low Countries from the fourteenth to the nineteenth century is that rather than being a mechanism for change within society, or a modernist preoccupation, people from all different backgrounds and statuses instead came together to try and preserve the status quo or "the ordinary" under threat or pressure.[52] People came to terms with these frequent challenges by employing and reinforcing old or known structures and frameworks.[53] Indeed, epidemic diseases became accommodated or acclimatised to rather than "dealt with" or "managed" as distinct crises (Chapters 2 and 3).[54] Thus, during these epidemics, people protected their customary time-honoured social and cultural practices, sometimes with passive foot-dragging and sometimes resorting to direct violent resistance (Chapter 4), and discovered different ways to shield economic assets from being redistributed (Chapter 5). If epidemics did redistribute economic resources, it was often a temporary deviation from the norm and barely resembled a structural reorganisation of hierarchies and strata within and across communities. It meant little for ordinary people and their economic fortunes in the longer term. Cities and towns saw temporary reductions in their populations but frequently saw these replenished very quickly through inward migration from the countryside and outside the Low Countries—often within a matter of less than a decade—although the rebound rates of rural populations were more variable and depended on institutional arrangements. Indeed, what the long-term historical experience of the Low Countries with epidemics shows is that rather than stimulators of massive changes within society or watershed moments creating divergences or transitions, the impact of these recurring diseases tended to be played out incrementally over the long term with slow onset forms of almost imperceptible adaptation. Older literature on slow incremental movements across long timespans—Le Roy Ladurie, Braudel, Delumeau, and others—remains highly relevant.[55]

All this is not to say people did not fear disease outbreaks, nor suffer burdens and hardships—they clearly did, and we have direct evidence to show that people could be afraid or impoverished. But instead of seeing epidemic diseases as explanatory variables capable of causing sharp developmental changes—one of the hallmarks of positivist and teleological thinking on the subject—the view taken in this book is that these outbreaks can be seen as a useful window to reveal obscured inequalities or vulnerabilities within societies and communities, or inequalities or vulnerabilities that cannot be straightforwardly classified as such. The focus on the specific epidemic experiences of women vis-à-vis men in the Low Countries (Chapter 6) brings that point sharply into view—although, again, female experiences were neither wholly about adaptive agency nor about forced (patriarchal) coercion.[56] Overall, and in line with the recent work of Tim Soens, I suggest that what all this shows is that the "resilience" of particular institutional frameworks in certain historical settings over time is not necessarily something to be championed, but in fact occurred simultaneously with, and perhaps contributed to, the vulnerabilities experienced (and agency exerted) by certain individuals within unequal communities.[57]

The book's chapter-by-chapter argumentation can be summarised as follows. In Chapter 2, focusing on the long-term dimensions of how communities interpreted and understood epidemic disease in the Low Countries, I show that there was some change over time—in particular, the idea that disease becomes a product of external dangers rather than internal moral corruptions starts to take place around the sixteenth century. Over time, there are also developments in the types of social groups identified as connected with epidemic disease. In the sixteenth century, we see the first signs of the links (consistently) being made between plague and poverty, but in the seventeenth century, we see a more coherent "outbreak narrative", where women and physical outsiders are more explicitly condemned and restricted.[58] Nevertheless, there were also strong continuities in understanding epidemic disease in the Low Countries. During the late Middle Ages, we find a complicated mix of providential, miasmatical, and contagionist ideas where it was impossible to separate the three from one another, and they tended to work in tandem rather than in opposition. Religious interpretations of disease response and impact remained present in communities well into the late nineteenth century, even when germ theory was taking hold. Most fundamentally, and in accordance with other recent historical scholarship on medieval public health,[59] epidemics were rarely instigators for massive changes or developments in public health institutions, and infrastructure—adaptations were small and incremental and built upon practices already seen outside of epidemics.

While Chapter 2 is more concerned about how preindustrial societies were recognising, classifying, interpreting, and explaining epidemic diseases, Chapter 3 is about identifying and distinguishing between epidemics based on more standardised measurements—bringing together a new wealth of quantitative information on epidemic mortality to draw broad conclusions. The Black Death of 1349–51 had a severe impact in some (but perhaps not all) parts of the Low Countries—although evidence suggests that other outbreaks, both before (in the thirteenth century) and after the Black Death (in the second half of the fourteenth and fifteenth centuries), might have been worse. Usually, late-medieval epidemics tended to precede grain price spikes rather than vice-versa and hence point to these outbreaks having a causal role in creating production and distribution problems rather than being a product of these problems. Nevertheless, the outbreak of 1439, probably the worst in Low Countries history in terms of combined severity and territorial pervasiveness, was one of the rare ones to coincide very closely with weather-induced harvest failures. Severe epidemic outbreaks continued into the early modern period—and the exceptional severity and spread of the 1636 plague shows that there was no clear linear teleological path towards an obvious escape from epidemic disease. The frequent recurring nature of these epidemics is one of the basic preconditions behind societal acclimatisation to these anticipated hazards. My view is that other studies arguing for the exceptional nature of certain outbreaks in other parts of Europe—such as northern Italy—are overstating the case.[60] Another finding developed in Chapter 3 is the complete rejection of a narrative that accentuates the urban character of epidemic disease in the transition from the late Middle Ages to the early modern period—no evidence supports this contention, and moreover, still in the seventeenth century, epidemics caused by plague, dysentery, and malaria, for example, tended to be *more damaging* for areas away from the urbanised and commercial cores of the Low Countries. Finally, while we need to remain cautious, especially with explanatory mechanisms, most epidemics were selective down the lines of age, sex, and socio-economic status. Indeed, a wide variety of evidence shows that adult women tended to be more severely afflicted by epidemics compared to men (relative to normal patterns of mortality)—although contextual social, economic, and cultural conditions did create key exceptions.

In Chapter 4, by analysing societal responses to epidemic disease over the long term, I argue that most anxieties were not connected to fears of falling sick or dying, but more connected to the authorities' restrictions and infringements. Rather than an instrument of control—a so-called Foucauldian framework—epidemics in the Low Countries were instrumentalised by ordinary people to resist elites actively or passively. Perceived agents of the administration or those involved in the "disease economy" were most likely to be subject to (sometimes violent) pushback—even if those on the receiving end of this resistance, abuse, or violence were sometimes hardly representatives of the elite but vulnerable people themselves. Epidemic disease did not bring about revolutionary ideals or structural change—quite the opposite, these outbreaks stimulated conservative and reactionary tendencies based around maintaining a kind of lifestyle under threat. Ordinary people, then, did not "manage" epidemic disease outbreaks in the same way that authorities might—they acclimatised themselves to these repeat anticipated hazards, which stuck in the collective memory for long periods—as they were not massive departures from the norm but part of the norm, and in the process blurred the conceptual lines between epidemic and endemic status.

In Chapter 5, by bringing together a substantial amount of new quantitative information linking epidemic outbreaks and wealth or asset indicators, I shine new light on mortality-induced redistribution. Evidence from the

Low Countries suggests that while conditions were present for theoretical changes in wealth distribution within communities (increasing turnover of assets, for example), this often did not occur in practice. Indeed, although we often see small declines in Gini Coefficients in various wealth indicators after epidemics—mostly this was of a small magnitude and very temporary. Rather than the importance of the shielding mechanisms said to be vital in other literature, preventing asset dispersal or fragmentation,[61] my arguments are more philosophically grounded. Any downward flickers of the aggregate distribution hardly represented greater egalitarianism in principle. Thus, post-epidemic household redistribution in the city of Leiden tended to be in sectors of poor housing owned by wealthy investors, which ended up in the hands of similar investors. In rural areas, after spiked mortality, households often got access to land that they either did not want or was depreciating in social or economic value. In fact, while the appearance of *The Great Leveler* in 2017 might have been the high point for a general view linking epidemics and equitable distribution outcomes,[62] I suggest that any epidemic-induced redistribution tended to simply entrench or crystallise existing inequalities. Initial insights into the direct economic damages that epidemics could create at the micro level potentially affirm that—given that it is highly plausible that the direct economic damages disproportionately bore a toll on the poorest within society.

Finally, in Chapter 6, in the process of making a call for more systematic attention to the subject of how female epidemic impacts differed across context, time, and status of women, I make an initial assessment for the preindustrial Low Countries that female experiences of epidemic disease were often harsh, burdensome, and painful, and could combine a variety of imposed restrictions or losses of fortune—some of which were of course shared with men, but others were slightly more accentuated or distinctive. Although women could adapt to new conditions presented by significantly raised mortality, it is unclear whether new roles or the opening of access to untapped resources truly benefitted women, or rather, women were able to secure and keep hold of this wealth or status. Interestingly, however, and mirroring more general observations about social resistance in Chapter 4, women in the preindustrial Low Countries often used epidemic disease as a vehicle for pushing back against perceived restrictions—and were at the forefront of most violent epidemic protests across history. Such an observation is important when we consider the spikes in domestic abuse and violence towards women seen during our recent experiences of COVID-19—and reminds us that all developments need to be contextually explained and temporally compared rather than assumed to be inevitable expressions of a form of behaviour.

The book concludes with some reservations about some current trends in historical research connected to epidemics—questioning three aspects in particular: (i) the focus on the capacity to cause divergences or structural changes within societies, (ii) the modernist preoccupation with viewing epidemics as "sub-normal" or "crisis" conditions to be "managed", and (iii) the broader trend towards using historical epidemics as a template to draw "lessons" from the past.

Notes

1 On plague and economic divergences: Bailey, *After the Black Death*, 283–325; Alfani, *Calamities*; Belich, *The World the Plague Made*. On the Black Death and rebellion, with emphasis on the Jacquerie uprising in northern France in 1358, the Ciompi Revolt of unrepresented labourers in Florence in 1378, and the Peasants' Revolt in parts of England in 1381: Cohn, *Popular Protest*; Cohn, *Lust for Liberty*. On cholera and class-based conflict: Evans, *Death*; Cohn, *Epidemics*, 163–262.

2 A non-exhaustive range of literature that sets out the long-term economic dimensions of the rise and decline of areas of the Low Countries compared to other parts of the preindustrial world: Van Bavel, *The Invisible Hand?*; Van Zanden, *The Long Road*; De Vries and van der Woude, *The First Modern Economy*; Zanden and van Riel, *The Strictures*; Prak and van Zanden, *Pioneers*. On the rise and decline of areas within the Low Countries: Van Bavel, *Manors*; Gelderblom, *Cities*.

3 Huizinga, *The Waning*. Perhaps unsurprising given that many of the fears mentioned by Huizinga as intrinsic to late-medieval societies can be seen as backward projections, that "tell us as much about fear that hung over war-ravaged Europe in 1919 [when he was writing] as they do about the fourteenth and fifteenth centuries": Peckham, *Fear*, xvi. Likewise, future historians will make the same critique of myopic scholarship produced during the COVID-19 years: Curtis and van Besouw, Not Learning from History.

4 Two pages in Prak, *The Dutch Republic*; nowhere in Israel, *The Dutch Republic: Its Rise*; one page in Price, *The Dutch Republic*. Not just epidemics but also not disease or health offered as individual topics of interest in Helmers and Janssen, eds., *The Cambridge Companion*.

5 Degroot, *The Frigid Golden Age*. Also, Sundberg, *Natural Disaster*, which refers to ship worm epidemics and cattle plagues but not epidemics affecting humans. A recent Dutch-language synthesis of environmental history devotes only a few pages to epidemics: De Keyzer et al., eds., *Mens*.

6 Noordegraaf and Valk, *De gave Gods*.

7 Kerkhoff, *Per imperatief plakkaat*.

8 Bruneel, *La mortalité*; Charlier, *La peste*; Lemaire, *La peste*; Devos, *Allemaal beestjes*; Vermeersch, *1349*; Anon., ed., *Épidémies*. We also have the valuable conference proceedings: Anon., ed., *De pest*. Some important books focus on related topics such as warfare with epidemic mortality foregrounded: Gutmann, *War*, 133–73; Govaerts, *Armies*, 182–226. Of course, besides monographs, there are numerous individual articles and chapters too extensive to list here but appear cited throughout this book.

9 Dumolyn and Haemers, Patterns, 369.

10 Van Bavel, Rural Revolts, 266–7.

11 Bailey, *After the Black Death*, 313–15.

12 Van Bavel, *Manors*, 86–93. Although Van Bavel asserts that the relative importance of these feudal institutions differed sharply across regions of the Low Countries, even recent work that asserts the importance of seigneurial lordship in places such as inland Flanders still explicitly states, "seigneurial burdens were extremely limited when compared with those of other parts of Europe": Buylaert et al., The Political Economy, 12.

13 De Moor, The Silent Revolution, 186. In line with the chronology Reynolds applied to other parts of Europe: Reynolds, *Kingdoms*.
14 Van Werveke, *De Zwarte Dood*; Van Werveke, Nogmaals. One of the most important early maps is Carpentier, Autour, 1070. Reproduced in Slack, *Plague*, 19.
15 Blockmans, The Social and Economic Effects.
16 De Boer, *Graaf*, 64–5.
17 Huiting, *Domeinen*, 163. On the limited evidence for Holland: Curtis, Plague, 80–2. Of course, two features—a lack (but not absence) of seigneurial institutions and fewer direct pieces of evidence for the Black Death in Holland—might be related given that in other places, such as England or northern France, much of the evidence of plague impact comes from manorial administrations.
18 Van Bavel and van Zanden, The Jump-Start, 515. The connection between a mild plague impact and favourable economic and demographic growth outcomes is further asserted in Van Zanden, A Third Road, 90; Van Bavel, Medieval Origins, 67.
19 Roosen and Curtis, The "Light Touch".
20 All summarised in Curtis, Plague, 87–90; Curtis, From One Mortality Regime to Another? Even in recent important literature, there is a tendency to repeat the claims that the Low Countries experienced a "slightly milder impact of the plague": Coomans, *Community*, 25. Scholars tend to equate population rises between 1350 and 1500 in Holland as evidence for the "effects [of epidemics] were far less dramatic than elsewhere": Prak and van Zanden, *Pioneers*, 63. Surely this is an unwise interpretation since high epidemic mortality and population stability or increases were not mutually exclusive, as illustrated in the next paragraph on early modern urban population recoveries.
21 See the recent doctoral theses of Geens, *A Golden Age*; Roosen, *The Black Death*; Espeel, *Prices*.
22 On the Dutch Republic as a clear outlier to the crisis narrative: De Vries, The Economic Crisis; Degroot, *The Frigid Golden Age*. For the global crisis of the seventeenth century and epidemic disease's role within it: Parker, *Global Crisis*, 82–7.
23 For international demand arguments: Israel, *The Dutch Republic: Its Rise*; Brenner, The Low Countries, 229; for the domestic urban cores: Blockmans, *Metropolen*.
24 Prak and van Zanden, Demographic Change, 245.
25 Van Besouw et al., Epidemic Mortality.
26 Van Besouw and Curtis, Estimating.
27 On the absence of serious seventeenth-century famines noted in the literature: Curtis and Dijkman, The Escape; and on the related lack of serious food riots: Dekker, *Holland*. This was only a temporary escape as famine-related mortality returned to the Netherlands in the late eighteenth and nineteenth centuries: Curtis et al., Low Countries; Corporaal and Jensen, Famine.
28 Van Bavel and Gelderblom, The Economic Origins; a reaction to an earlier argument made about excessive desire for cleaning on the grounds of Calvinistic zeal in Schama, *The Embarrassment of Riches*, 375–97. Van Bavel and Gelderblom's argument is perhaps valid for certain parts of the Holland countryside, although unlikely to apply to the growing cities where public health infrastructure was pressurised: Van Oosten, The Dutch Great Stink.
29 For a limited selection of literature using explanations based around institutional arguments or asserting certain types or qualities of institutions: Van Bavel, *Manors*; Gelderblom, *Cities*; Prak et al., eds., *Craft Guilds*; De Vries and van der Woude, *The First Modern Economy*; Prak and van Zanden, *Pioneers*; De Moor, *The Dilemma*; with a focus on state formation, the qualities of fiscal institutions, or military finance: 't Hart, *The Making of a Bourgeois State*; Fritschy, *Public Finance*; Brandon, *War*; on the qualities of religious institutions: Semih Akçomak

et al., Why Did the Netherlands Develop So Early?; and on the impact of particular marriage patterns: Van Zanden et al., *Capital Women*. Also, a related literature using or leaning heavily on the concept of "social agrosystems", especially for the rural southern Low Countries: Thoen, Social Agrosystems; Thoen, A Commercial Survival Economy; Soens, *De spade*; De Keyzer, *Inclusive Commons*. In the text, exogenous is in scare quotes since, of course, no environmental or demographic factors were truly independent of human interaction: Campbell, *The Great Transition*, 397. The institutionalist approach pushed into the background a previous literature more likely to assert the primacy of political and military events: Israel, *The Dutch Republic: Its Rise*; Parker, *The Army*.

30 Van Bavel, People; Thoen and Soens, The Family; Curtis, The Impact; Roosen, The Black Death. Or in the context of the Dutch colonial regime in nineteenth-century Java, the impact of institutions on epidemic-induced mortality: De Zwart et al., The Demographic Effects. A new synthesising book on that topic takes a similar kind of route too by analysing the impact of different arrangements of institutions on disease outcomes (described as externalities), rather than how diseases shape institutions: Ogilvie, *Controlling Contagion*.

31 Summarising some of that literature: Van der Woude, Demografische ontwikkeling; Thoen, Historical Demography. In line with growing prevalence of quantitative approaches in the mainstream of the historical discipline in the 1960s and 1970s.

32 Muurling et al., The Last Nationwide Smallpox Epidemic; Rijpma et al., Unequal Excess Mortality; Murkens et al., Transitory Inequalities; Vervaeke and Devos, Much Ado About Nothing?; Devos et al., The Spanish Flu; Janssens and Riswick, What Was Killing Babies; Quanjer, Height; Thompson and van Ophem, Re-Examining. A recent post-COVID-19 overview of historical demography's contribution to epidemics considers only the nineteenth and twentieth centuries: Devos et al., Navigeren.

33 A promising avenue for challenging our expectations might be explicitly comparing those places with little social gradient in (epidemic) mortality: Antonio Luque de Haro, Social Inequalities.

34 As noted already some years ago in De Moor, Dare to Dig! In recent years, empirical work on preindustrial epidemic mortality in the Low Countries has mostly been carried out by me and colleagues.

35 For example, De Moor and van Zanden, Girl Power.

36 However, the major focus of the book is preindustrial. Nineteenth-century developments are only mentioned to emphasise similarities or deviations from what has occurred in the deeper past and hence should not be seen as exhaustive or comprehensive for the period post-1800.

37 The previous major work on epidemics and society in an area of the preindustrial Low Countries was produced during a strange time when historians started writing curious things such as the danger of "sacrificing history to quantification": Noordegraaf and Valk, Rotterdam, 115. In defence of: Noordegraaf and Valk, *De gave Gods*. To me, and surely uncontroversial, it seems impossible for convincing historical analysis to take place without integration of both quantitative and qualitative methodologies.

38 See a supporting recent case made in Waddington, In Constant Fear, 227.

39 Huisman, *Stadsbelang*; De Blécourt et al., eds., *Grenzen*; Binneveld and Dekker, eds., *Curing*; Steendijk-Kuypers, *Volksgezondheidszorg*; Vis, *650 jaar*; Van Hee, ed., *Ziek*; Various, Patiënt; Van der Korst, *Om lijf te leven*; Juch, *Voorkomen*; Zwart-Kramer and Zwart, *Van pest tot pokken*.

40 The most important work being Coomans, *Community*.

41 Cohn, *Epidemics*; Bowers, *Plague*.

42 Scheidel, *The Great Leveler*; Alfani and Di Tullio, *The Lion's Share*; Alfani, *As Gods Among Men*; Cristoferi, ed., *Socio-Economic Inequalities*.
43 I have a short book in preparation on this subject: Curtis, *The Impact*.
44 On the transformative powers of the Black Death, sometimes in tandem with other environmental hazards and interacting with different institutions, a small selection of the literature: Belich, *The World the Plague Made*; Herlihy, *The Black Death*; Aberth, *From the Brink*; Cantor, *In the Wake of the Plague*; Bailey, *After the Black Death*; Cohn, *The Black Death Transformed*; Cohn, *Cultures*; Campbell, *The Great Transition*.
45 Harper, *The Fate of Rome*.
46 Snowden, *Epidemics*, 2.
47 McNeill, *Plagues*, 295. Or see, Diamond, *Guns*, 197: "Because diseases have been the biggest killers of people, they have also been the decisive shapers of history".
48 In *The Economist* book of the year for 2022, it is immediately suggested that "society collapsed" in Siena, Tuscany, after the outbreak of the Black Death: Doig, *This Mortal Coil*, 2. The observations of tax collector and shoemaker, Agnolo di Tura are used, without any consideration of the rhetorical effect of the source material: see, Steinhoff, Artistic Working Relationships, 42. On the disagreements on the merits of the collapse concept: Curtis, Where's the Disaster in Disaster Studies?
49 A small selection of examples: Jedwab et al., Negative Shocks; Lagerlöf, From Malthus to Modern Growth; Cervellati et al., Epidemic Shocks; Karlsson et al., The Impact; Van Bavel and Scheffer, Historical Effects.
50 Expanding upon ideas partially developed in Curtis, Preserving; Curtis, Disasters; Curtis, Where's the Disaster in Disaster Studies?; Curtis, Trade; Curtis et al., Household; Hilkens et al., A Modern Rendition.
51 Pelling, "Bosom Vipers". And a distinction which makes little sense for preindustrial understandings of public health: Meloni, An Unproblematized Truth, 109–10.
52 For the critical remarks of the modernist assumptions at the heart of much of the literature on epidemic and society interaction: Geltner, The Path, 5.
53 Slack, *Plague*, 52.
54 For a pioneering statement on epidemic accommodation: Smail, Accommodating Plague, 38.
55 Le Roy Ladurie, Un concept; Braudel, *La Méditerranée*; Delumeau, *La peur*.
56 Munkhoff, Poor Women, 596.
57 Soens, Resilient Societies.
58 A concept developed originally in Wald, *Contagious*.
59 Coomans, *Community*.
60 Alfani, Plague.
61 Alfani and Di Tullio, *The Lion's Share*, 84–5.
62 Scheidel, *The Great Leveler*.

2 Dangers inside and outside the community

Community interpretations of epidemic disease over the long term

The trouble with retrospective diagnoses

The combination of bioarchaeological excavation and genetics research has revolutionised investigation into epidemic diseases of the past, and especially plague.[1] We now have the techniques available to know for a particular burial site whether plague was present in excavated skeletons through DNA evidence of the causal pathogen, the bacterium *Yersinia pestis*.[2] Advances in genetic sampling, and the reduced expense of the process, also mean that greater amounts of this DNA evidence can be formally analysed in the laboratory. On this basis, whole new debates are now taking place about the origins of the Black Death, and the timing, chronology, and direction of its spread across Eurasia and Africa.[3] Of relevance to this book, one of the major sources of *Yersinia pestis* extracted and analysed through a series of high-profile studies has come from the Low Countries—a mass burial connected to the cemetery of a medieval hospital in the town of Bergen op Zoom, west Brabant, which was likely, though still not definitively, dated to the outbreak after the Black Death often known as *pestis secunda* (1359/60).[4] More recently, further *Yersinia pestis* DNA has been sequenced from the St. Eusebius church cemetery (previously St. Martin) in Arnhem—yet, despite an improved "phylogenetically informed radiocarbon modelling" method for dating the samples, still could only attribute the DNA to any of three epidemic outbreaks occurring in the early fifteenth century.[5] Similarly, *Yersinia pestis* DNA has been extracted from an individual at the cemetery of the Onze-Lieve-Vrouwe church at Sint Truiden, but again supporting my point about the lack of temporal precision, the supporting documents from this study date it within a range of 120 years (1270–1390).[6]

As well as precise dating, one problem we have up to now is that our sample size is still very limited. We have uncovered *Yersinia pestis* DNA for several burial sites across Eurasia from late antiquity through to the nineteenth century, and then within this random sample of burial sites, only a select sub-sample of skeletons can provide evidence.[7] Furthermore, many of the excavated skeletons tend to be taken from so-called plague pits or mass burial sites, which also typically represent a very narrow fragment of the overall plague experience given that most victims of epidemic diseases were

DOI: 10.4324/9781003694908-2

still buried in ordinary churches and cemeteries alongside people who did not die from plague.[8] Put simply, and quite understandably, we do not have DNA evidence for all the plague outbreaks that occurred between the Middle Ages and the nineteenth century, we do not have DNA evidence for all localities across geographical space even when isolating one plague outbreak, we do not have DNA evidence for a large segment of the population when isolating one locality during one outbreak, and that DNA evidence which we do have at present is skewed towards atypical burial practices which are not wholly representative of people dying of plague.

Thus, although the only way to diagnose historical plagues definitively is through DNA evidence, the lack of systematic spatial and temporal scope to the evidence means that documentary (and, recently, epigraphical) evidence remains important.[9] However, the problems of relying on written sources for retrospective diagnosis of diseases have been discussed in a long historiography.[10] Indeed, the very suspicions that the Black Death was not plague but another disease—that is, before the twenty-first-century "laboratory revolution" proved this incorrect—were partially based on the very reasonable notion that we cannot always trust the observations and conclusions of contemporary observers from the Middle Ages or the early modern period in a literal or positivistic way.[11] Accordingly, scholars have claimed that in the preindustrial period, terms such as *peste* or *pestilentia*, or the variants thereof, were not specific references to plague per se (as caused by *Yersinia pestis*), but a catch-all general term used by these societies for many different afflictions.[12] Furthermore, terms such as *peste* did not have a universal translation but likely had subtle or significant differences in meaning across time and context.[13]

This problem was exacerbated by the fact that many of the diseases carried similar kinds of symptoms. Fevers, for example, could be one of the associated characteristics of plague, but also typhus, malaria, tuberculosis, and so on.[14] Probably the most reliable form of retrospective diagnosis using documentary sources is when buboes are mentioned in the groin or armpits—but the problem there is that this standard of evidence is hardly found systematically over time and space.[15] The same observation can be extended to visual culture. Paintings and illustrated manuscripts from western Europe rarely showed the precise symptoms of plague such as buboes from the Black Death and the recurring epidemics, instead focusing on the social impact of the outbreaks, whether experienced or for rhetorical effect, and it was not until the later phases of the fifteenth century onwards do we see more images showing these specific signs.[16] Perhaps surprisingly, Eurasian medical texts and treatises have very little to say about visible growths such as buboes before the seventeenth century.[17] Many of the warnings about retrospective diagnosis problems discussed frequently among historians of medicine and health are not heeded in fields less receptive to the cultural contexts of source production. Thus, natural science and social science scholars have attempted to understand the spatial and temporal distribution of plague outbreaks, making use of a digitisation of a large appendix of documentary references to plague produced by Jean-Noël Biraben back in the 1970s, fuelled by the desire to test new kinds of explanatory variables connected to economy such as trade networks and climate such as temperature and precipitation, and yet have left aside the issue of whether this represents an appropriate dataset for the task given the methodological issues involved.[18]

These issues are explicitly relevant in the Low Countries. Most of the time before 1450, we see general terms used in the written sources such as *peste* and *pestilentia*, sometimes vaguer such as *ex epydimia*, or even just general indicators of raised mortality, as for example, *magnas mortalitas* or *mortalitas dura*. Currently, to my knowledge the earliest potential medieval reference to a bubo was during the 1382 epidemic outbreak in Leiden, where the St. Pancras church "memory books" make a direct reference to visible symptoms such as a *nigra et venenosa pustula* (black poisonous blister).[19] And there are not many other medieval references to buboes in the Low Countries, with many occurring late in the period. In 1490, we see references in the miracle books of Amersfoort to the presence of large buboes on a woman—a sign of plague.[20] Written distinctions between potentially different types of diseases causing epidemics only tend to appear in documents in greater number towards the later parts of the fifteenth century, notwithstanding the odd references to contagious fevers.[21] Thus, during the drought of 1472/3 in different parts of Guelders and (what became) Limburg, terms such as *rode loop* and *rode melisoen* were used—likely in reference to the bloody excretion connected to the effects of dysentery.[22] Similarly, a known dysentery outbreak in 1492/3 in inland Flanders was referred to as the *rood mimzoen*.[23] In 1496–8, we see references in many places to *pokken* (pox)—another affliction with very distinctive outward symptoms.[24] Even with these finer distinctions, however, it was still likely the case that certain diseases were being recorded as *peste* or *pestilentia* when they were not plague. For example, at Groningen in 1529, an official plague ordinance was announced by the urban administration—one of the first in the Low Countries to explicitly connect plague, poverty, and begging—and yet based on timing and chronology from localities afflicted elsewhere, this was almost definitively an outbreak of sweating sickness.[25] Similarly, in the Catholic burial registers for the village of Oudenbosch, a reference is made to a pestilential disease (*morbo pestifero*) as late as 1715—roughly 45 years after plague had disappeared from the Low Countries.[26]

Recognising disease: Death descriptors in the early modern burial registers

Generalising terminology in the late-medieval period likely obscured a wide diversity of different afflictions occurring in the Low Countries—many of which might have been mistaken for plague—but we should also note that people had greater propensity over time to make (written) distinctions based on the symptoms or conditions they recognised or interpreted. As shown in Table 2.1, based on a collected database of church burial registers across more than 500 different localities (or parishes within localities) in the Low Countries, the number of different death descriptors could be quite wide

Table 2.1 Disease terms found in the seventeenth-century burial registers as cause of death

Term in burial records	*Potential meaning*	*Frequency found*	*Area found*
P / pest / peste / pestilentia / pestifero	Plague; general disease descriptor	Multiple people in many places	Everywhere
Haestige sieckte	Hasty sickness; plague	Several places	Dutch-language LC
Gave gods	Gift from God; plague	Infrequent	Usually, northern LC
De zwarigheid	The hardship; plague; famine-related sickness	Infrequent	Usually, Flanders
Febris / koorts / fièvre	Fever	Several places	Everywhere
Pokken / kinderpokken / variola	Smallpox; syphilis	Multiple people in several places	Everywhere
Brandziekte	Rash; burning skin ailment	Infrequent	Dutch-language LC
Dissenteria; rode loop; rode melisoen; buikloop; bloedgang	Dysentery; diarrhoea	Multiple people in several places	Everywhere
Hydropica	Dropsy	Several places	Usually, Flanders
Vallende Ziekte; epilepsia	Epilepsy	Infrequent	Everywhere
Phthysis	Tuberculosis	Several places	Usually, southern LC
Mazelen	Measles	Rare	Flanders
Gangraena	Gangrene	Rare	Coastal areas
Pleuritis	Pleurisy	Infrequent	Usually, Flanders
Totus exhaustus / uitgeput / misere	Famine-related sickness	Infrequent	Usually, southern LC
Contagion / ex contagione / maladie contagieuse / infection / morbo contagioso	Plague; contagious disease; general disease descriptor	Multiple people in several places	Everywhere
Lèpre / melaatsheid	Leprosy	Infrequent	Usually, southern LC

Sources: Similar sample of burial registers used in Curtis, Was Plague an Exclusively Urban Phenomenon?; Van Besouw and Curtis, Estimating. The geographical descriptors in the fourth column are very imprecise. The references to disease descriptors can be found in the burial registers dataset in Curtis, ed., Original Burials Data.

by the seventeenth century—although some terms were more frequent and widespread than others.

Of course, partially the diversity of terminology is simply a matter of language, with the Low Countries comprising Dutch and French-language areas, and between the religious denominations with Catholic areas more likely to use Latin. In general, the Catholic scribes made more attempts to classify and distinguish between causes of death, using a broader range of terminology, and thus we tend to have more detailed information from the southern Low Countries. Nevertheless, even within the same locality in the very same year, the variety of terms used could be diverse. At the village of Merchtem, Brabant, during the epidemic of 1646/7 at the end of the Thirty Years' War, we see references in the church burial registers to people having died of *peste*, *contagion*, *febris*, *variola*, *pokken*, *dissenteria*, *hydropica*, and *phytysis*.[27] Such diversity in the burial register entries was matched in other narrative and legal sources as well. In the chronicles from the Maria Wijngaard monastery in Weert, Limburg, in 1567, reference was made to the burning plague (*den brandt van de pest*), but also pox, diarrhoea, and an evil cough (*pocken, buijckloop, quaeden hoest*).[28] In a mid-sixteenth-century document outlining land use rights at two villages just outside Breda, explicit distinction was made between *pest* and another similar contagious infectious disease (*andere der gelijcke contagieuse besmettelicke sieckte*), which was an expression also shared in 1540 in an agreement between the Bishop of Liège and the urban administration of Den Bosch.[29]

Sometimes we have individual references in the burial records that provide a little more detail. In the village of Weiwerd, Groningen, for example, we learn of "a wretched plague, producing fire in the mouth" (*jammerlijke plaege, hebbende het vijer in den mondt*), and given the coastal environment a likely symptom of malaria or related ague.[30] In the likely plague outbreak of 1602 at Nieuwpoort, a small village on the south side of the Lek River in the central Dutch River area, we hear of someone dying with cold fingers, sweating arms, and impaired vision, while at Lottum in 1694, a period that coincided with widespread harvest failures, the fevers were so terrible that one woman was said to become the spectacle of the whole community (*spectaculum communitatis*).[31]

Terms that we might associate with plague in the burial registers include *P*, *pest(e)*, *pestilentia*, *haestige sieckte*, *de zwarigheid*, *de gave Gods*, and the various formations of *infection* and *contagione*, although we should recognise that (a) sometimes these were employed either deliberately or mistakenly for diseases that were not plague, and (b) there were plenty of times when people died of plague and did not receive an explicit cause of death marker. Indeed, we have four types of situations in the church burial registers—localities where perceived plague deaths were systematically recorded over time (rare);[32] localities where plague deaths were systematically recorded for some periods or years or outbreaks (quite common);[33] localities where plague deaths were recorded but unsystematically and apparently randomly (common); and those localities where plague deaths were never explicitly recorded (very common; and hence, evidence of an epidemic outbreak is only in the numbers of deaths above the norm—a form of measurement we address in Chapter 3). A reference to buboes is never found in the burial records to my knowledge.[34]

Of course, the disease diagnosis process was fraught with difficulties in the medieval and early modern Low Countries. While trained physicians could identify symptoms based on their knowledge and experience, not everyone had access to this kind of expertise. Even when available, some doctors refused to treat the poor during epidemic outbreaks, likely because of the greater financial rewards of just limiting themselves to wealthier urban citizens, as seen in a case from a plague at Namur in 1579.[35] Ordinary people could not afford the exorbitant costs of treating afflictions identified as plague by medics. A Rotterdam doctor noted in 1643 that during the plague of 1636, a brother and sister came to him to be cured of the *gave Gods*, and paid 60 guilders for treatment and 12 guilders for medication.[36] The total of 72 guilders was equivalent to more than four years' worth of rent for a modest residence in a Holland city in the first half of the seventeenth century.[37] And while professional medical provision became more accessible and commercialised over time in small towns of the Dutch Republic, this shift mainly occurred after the disappearance of plague from the Low Countries—i.e., from the final third of the seventeenth century onwards.[38] In rural areas, treatment of the sick often remained within family networks or the community, relying on remedies based on spices, herbs, and black poppy from Asia or concoctions of beer and sugar, rather than the involvement of physicians.[39] Even when the Low Countries start to industrialise after 1800, rural communities often resisted the advice and views of outsider medics, as elaborated upon more in Chapter 4.[40] Nevertheless, localised diagnoses should not be undervalued. Ordinary people with some medical capabilities sometimes received excellent reputations such as the Frisian farmer, Douwe Ales, and in certain contexts of eighteenth-century cattle plague in the Austrian Netherlands, governments were often reliant on local lay veterinary healers (*koeimeesters*) to carry out policy.[41]

The point being made here is that the diagnosis of a particular affliction was often not performed by a medic, whom themselves had limits to their understanding, but by an assortment of people with different levels of experience and different statuses, goals, and incentives—and the interest groups involved were not the same for each community across space and time.[42] The announcement of a death was often made by family or neighbours of the deceased based on what they could visually see, and then in the context of the burial registers, simply noted down by the local priest acting as a scribe.[43] Even when the relevant parties could diagnose the death, clearly it was not always in their interests to publicly announce this given that, first, disease was understood in moral terms (see later in this chapter on corruptions), second, this might then lead to a burial of the deceased within an anonymous mass grave (although this happened rarely), and third, local authorities tended to act in a restrictive way towards the surviving household. Households associated with plague, for example, were publicly marked out with a *P* and a bale of straw hung above the door, and then often could not perform economic activity such as trade or agricultural tasks for numerous weeks thereafter or participate in social or cultural rituals such as going to church.[44] It is unsurprising, then, that we see several times in the burial registers a reference to an unexplainable death, but also disagreements. In the Limburg village of Beek in 1652, one opinion was that a Jan Craechs had died with the *contagij* (contagion), but further consideration suggested he was "afflicted another way".[45]

Although the burial record death descriptors are insightful in a direct way, most social and cultural historians of medicine and public health tend to suggest that the more relevant insights taken from written interpretations of disease in the past are what that information can tell us about historical societies on their own terms.[46] Thus, a more relevant question might not be "what epidemic diseases were occurring in the Low Countries between the fourteenth and nineteenth centuries?" but instead "how did communities and different social groups of the Low Countries between the fourteenth and nineteenth centuries understand, interpret, and explain afflictions that were occurring?" In this sense, disease becomes a window to better understand how different people in the past viewed themselves in relation to others and the environment.[47] That is not, however, an instruction to completely disregard quantification. Even very basic acts of counting and comparison can help us show how societal perceptions of what was causing epidemic diseases changed or persisted over time. And we should be careful not to assume as we move into the nineteenth and early twentieth centuries that disease categorisation issues were entirely solved—the imperfections of the original source material in fact throwing up new concerns given the higher reliance on turning the information into standardisable digital datasets.[48] As illustrated in the following section, classifying and categorising different diseases rested on how communities understood disease to occur, spread, and disappear—and this was never straightforward.

Interrelated frameworks of providence, miasma, and contagion

In the Low Countries, as in many parts of western Europe, there were several overlapping and interrelated ideas on what caused people to fall sick or for diseases to take root within a community. In the medieval period, where religion was a fundamental building block of societal organisation, it is not a surprise to hear that one of the most important explanatory frameworks for disease was providential. Providence meant that disease outbreaks were seen as the work of God, and hence the description of plague as *de gave Gods* (the Gift from God).[49] Indeed, in a sketch from a mid-sixteenth-century manuscript depicting *peste* in Valenciennes in 1515, we see the visualisation of a burial with the "judgement from above", and an angel holding a skull and rod ready to spike down with apparent vengeance on the town (Figure 2.1). Famously, the well-known naval commander, Michiel de Ruyter, described in 1666 the death from plague of his daughter, Anna, as an example of God's will.[50]

Still, however, this was grounded in the worldly issues of human beings, as the providential affliction was also seen as a form of correction for poor morals or a lack of piety within a community or society. Accordingly, in the diaries of sixteenth-century Groningen farmer, Abel Eppens, we learn from him that the plagues were a punishment of the Popes and the dubious lifestyle of city folk.[51] The urban-rural dimension of this explanation contrasted with a plague ordinance written during 1636 in Utrecht, which directed its criticism *towards* the countryside and the papal practices (*Paapse praktijken*) that were going on.[52] Both were in agreement that Catholicism was to blame. Elsewhere, in a last testament written from the Limburg village of Geijsteren, also from 1636, it was noted that God Almighty (*Godt Almachtich*) looked to punish the wickedness of man (*de boosheit der mensch*), with the plagues of the pestilence (*mit die plaegen der pestelentij*).[53] Songs were written—such as one by Dutch Reformed minister, Franciscus Ridderus, of Rotterdam in 1658—which saw plague, the latest seen in 1655/6, like other recurring hazards such as storms, fires, and periods of dearth, as a Godly punishment for sins such as idolatry.[54] Further, many of the fears that emerged regarding shipworm

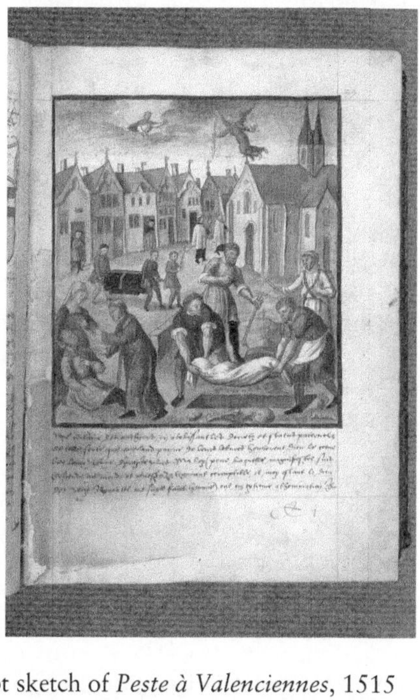

Figure 2.1 Manuscript sketch of *Peste à Valenciennes*, 1515

Source: Cailleau, Peste, fo. 33r.

epidemics or cattle plagues in the eighteenth-century Dutch Republic are recently argued to have been grounded in broader anxieties around societal decline.[55] At the same time, it should also be noted that God could be seen as merciful, especially with the intervention of religious figures. At Evergem, a Flemish village north of Ghent, a request was made (from 1667 but signed during a previous outbreak in 1635) to the Pope to save the people from the plague.[56] The Haarlem newspaper *Oprechte Haerlemse Courant* remarked in 1664 that the "Lord God had spared [the nearby town of Enkhuizen] the afflictions of the contagious disease".[57] In one depiction of the well-known plague saint in a painting found in the St. Martinuskerk, Aalst, Jesus is found explicitly appointing Rochus to this role (Figure 2.2), and those infected are portrayed as full of hope and expectation.[58]

Hence, during epidemics in the medieval and early modern Low Countries we see consistent references to observations of piety. One of the earliest processions, with some debate over the precise context of penance or thanksgiving, is said to have occurred in October 1349 during the Black Death at Mons and Soignies, where communities invoked St. Waudru and St. Vincent.[59] An official prayer and list of observances were written and proclaimed in Utrecht c.1440 in response to the severe epidemic of 1439 that coincided with exceptionally prolonged harvest failures.[60] In 1514, a procession was made

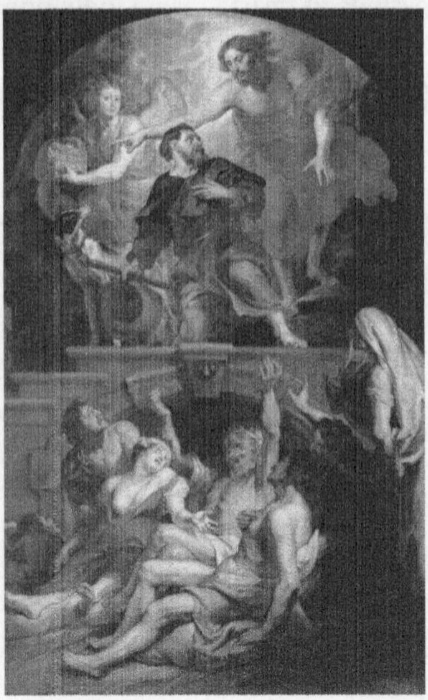

Figure 2.2 Christ Appointing St. Rochus as Patron Saint of Plague Victims painting, 1623–6

Source: https://en.wikipedia.org/wiki/Christ_Appointing_Saint_Roch_as_Patron_Saint_of_Plague_Victims.

in Luxembourg to honour the plague saint, Adrian, widely venerated for his protective force at an abbey in Geraardsbergen, Flanders, and repeated again in 1554.[61] In 1519, several pious street processions were organised during a disease outbreak at the town of Zutphen, and then again during an outbreak of 1529 in Deventer to "avert the wrath of God".[62] In 1553, we have a Carthusian reproduction, in Dutch, of a sermon addressing the ongoing plague—the original sermon of unknown date but potentially in the late fifteenth or early sixteenth century.[63] A well-known antiphon (a form of repeatable chant) from the late fifteenth century was repeated in processional hymns later down the line such as in 1556 at the Augustinian monastery of Mariënpoel to the north of Leiden.[64] During the seventeenth century, we see several calls for a general collective prayer day (*biddach*) during plagues—not just among the Catholics of Bruges in 1666, but in Dutch Reformed communities such as Wijk bij Duurstede, a village near Utrecht, in 1603, and in Delft during the plague of 1624, with an emphasis on collective piety.[65] We should also note that these kinds of processions or prayer days were sometimes so frequent that they did not necessarily represent reactions to epidemic outbreaks, but had more prophylactic qualities—collectively organised events that were ritualised within ordinary life to ward off the threat.[66] Local processions continued well after plague disappeared from the Low Countries—such as the one led around 1715 in Hamme, between Ghent and Antwerp, on the celebration day of Our Lady of the Rosary to remain free of the ongoing epidemic affliction.[67]

Providence was so important that some historians have suggested that by the latter part of the sixteenth century, influential clerics of the Calvinist Church in the Dutch Republic tended to argue against human acts of mitigation altogether, instead asserting the religious weapons of prayer, penitence, and repentance during epidemic outbreaks.[68] Indeed, even during smallpox outbreaks seen as late as the eighteenth and nineteenth centuries, similar theological rhetoric was used against those being inoculated—described by a medic from Middelburg, Arnoud Helvetius, in 1724 as "a provocation of God, unauthorised, and not an appropriately Christian practice".[69] In the mid-eighteenth century, similar attempts to inoculate cattle in the wake of ongoing outbreaks of rinderpest were also met with opposition from some farmers, and in some cases prompted a resort to prayer days instead.[70]

However, while some resistance to intervention might have been the case in theory or religious interpretation of scripture, it was not necessarily what always happened in practice—and certainly we do not often see too much deviation between Catholic, Calvinist, and mixed communities.[71] Thus, while panicked flight from the cities might be an over-exaggeration, as suggested for the case of Rotterdam, we do have evidence of 100 urban citizens purchasing safeguards (*sauvegarde*) for a fee of 6–20 stuivers per month to temporarily escape to the countryside for as long as half a year, as seen in Doesburg during the plague of 1624.[72] We also have numerous cases both in the medieval and early modern period of officials and administrators changing their travel plans on account of raging epidemics in a particular area.[73] Priests even wrote out elaborate instructions of advice on how to avoid infection, sometimes with nothing to do with piety, as what happened at the village of Didam, in the rural Achterhoek of Guelders, during the outbreak of 1556.[74] Children with smallpox were explicitly put in rooms together with the rationale of reducing the intensity of the symptoms.[75] These are hardly examples of societies acting passively and waiting for divine judgement.

More understandably, scholars have emphasised more strongly that the interpretation of and social responses to diseases were neither determined solely by the word of medics or the word of clerics and the Church, but instead the religious, natural, and supernatural were inextricably connected.[76] Recent systematic work with early modern chronicles has shown that although natural and supernatural explanations of epidemic disease became more complex across the Low Countries over time, still they remained in service to the divine.[77] Other work on cattle diseases in different parts of the coastal and inland Low Countries in the eighteenth century suggests similar seamless integration of providential and institutional responses.[78] Scouring through the useful collection of the numerous medical treatises and religious tractates written and printed in the early modern northern Low Countries, it is possible to trace the interrelated and interwoven interpretations used for disease outbreaks.[79] Thus, according to Joannes Heurnius, professor of medicine and rector magnificus at Leiden University, patience and prayer were as effective as any medicine, and moreover, such medicines only worked if God was not forsaken.[80] We have numerous cases of different remedies against *pest* being concocted using products such as herbs, flowers, and wine, but with qualifications that this was only effective with God's approval. For example, at the Drenthe *havezate* (fortified aristocratic house) located in the village of Dwingeloo, a recipe noted that red field roses would only rid the sickness with God's help (*met Godts hulp*).[81] Recipes were often found randomly inserted as individual pages within series of parish registers written by priests.[82] In line with a less passive interpretation of disease response, it should also be noted that many of these remedies were actively intended as preventative rather than cures per se—linking with the earlier point made about the prophylactic qualities of processions.[83]

Accordingly, more fundamentally, religious interpretations of the causes of diseases only made sense when working in tandem with other explanatory frameworks. One of the most important of these, informed by a Galenist health paradigm emphasising balance and imbalance of bodily humours interacting with several emotional, sensory, and environmental factors, was miasma theory.[84] Emphasis was placed on corrupted environments such as bad airs and smells, dampness, or poor light and atmospherics—conditions that created interacting pressures on human senses.[85] Thus, at Dordrecht in 1509, the *pestilentie* seen in the city was attributed to bad airs and smells coming from the canals.[86] Three years later, in 1512, an Antwerp medical treatise suggested that the causes of the *pestelencie* were twofold—the first universal and remote, and linked to the eclipse of the sun or moon, and the second as corrupt vapours mixed with the air.[87] Ghent chronicler, Philip van Campene, linked the plague of September 1568 to "bloody signs" seen in the night sky.[88] Later, in a letter of instruction about plague to the Franciscan (*minderbroeder*) order at Weert in 1644, signs of *pestis* and *mortis* are linked to the corruptions of the earth, the air, water, and fire.[89] Scribes in burial registers during epidemic years often drew doodles of people that appeared to be physically spewing matter out into the air (Figure 2.3).

Nevertheless, still, these corruptions were often seen as a product of moral or spiritual failings and thus relate closely to providential punishment for misdeeds. The links between the two (God and nature) can be seen in the two positions offered in the rhetorical play devised by bookseller and publisher, Zacharias Heyns, in his *Pest-spieghel*—written in Amsterdam during a plague in 1602.[90] Similarly, in the death-bed accounts of two children dying of plague in Leiden in 1664, one of the children, Susanna, explicitly started to critique the precise interrelationship: "What do people say, that it comes by the air? Is not God the creator of the air? If it came out of the earth, is it not done by God?"[91] Later, in the eighteenth century, as news of plague in Provence spread, one Dutch minister, Bernardus Smytegelt, noted to his congregation in 1721 that bad air, contamination, and unhealthy food were to blame, but only through God's origin as "the sword needs a hand".[92] It should be noted, however, it was not always socially accepted to publicly frame this in a negative light. Indeed, during an epidemic outbreak of 1669 in Leiden, potentially caused by an early form of cholera, one man was found guilty in the criminal records of describing the great death (*grote sterfte*) as a divine punishment (*goddelijke straf*) and was therefore banished from the city.[93]

Miasmatical concerns were seen in some of the epidemic-related regulations announced by urban administrations. Although these were clearly seen in early modern plague ordinances all over the Low Countries, many of the environmental infringements had already been made punishable in the fourteenth century in some places—especially with the maintenance of public

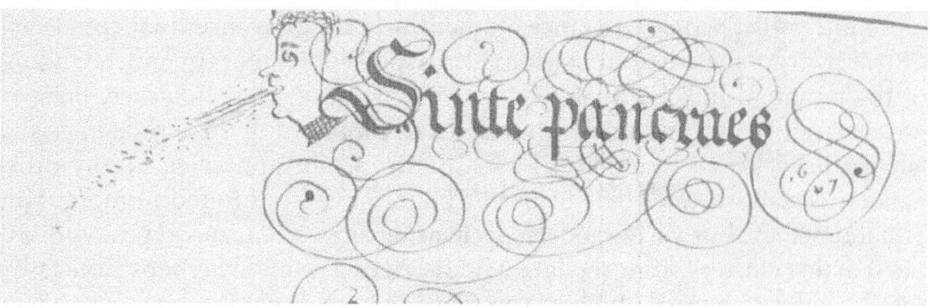

Figure 2.3 "Agent of death" doodle, St. Pancras Church, Leiden, 1605

Source: Leiden manuscripts cited in Curtis, ed., Original Burials Data.

spaces.[94] Objects that led to foul odours were most stringently addressed—thus, tar, gin, and beechwood were used to purify the air, and on occasion materials said to have come in contact with the infected were burned and then buried deep underground.[95] *Schrobbers* and *schrobsters* (plague cleaners) were instructed to deposit the waste of infected domestic households in which they worked as far as they could away from the streets at the end of the yard or garden.[96] Certain goods were restricted, especially cloth, and the same went for many foods that could spoil, and therefore give off bad smells, such as soft fruits and vegetables, fish and shellfish, and buttermilk.[97] Under the conception of the body politic, corrupted foodstuffs exposed the collective body of the community itself to the threat of disease outbreaks—and the poor were often seen as particularly vulnerable—thus, late-medieval and early modern administrations intervened in the name of maintaining the common good.[98]

Anxieties also tended to revolve around free-roaming animals that could cause mess and stench, although the levels of response could differ widely. It is known that certain animals were sometimes killed en masse during epidemics—for example, during the severe plague outbreak of 1400/1, 252 dogs were slaughtered by the local administration of Walcheren, Zeeland and 169 dogs in Courtrai.[99] In Courtrai, we see that the peaks in dog killing tended to track with the major epidemics—in 1439, 1466, 1481, and 1487/8, for example.[100] Emphasis should be put on "free-roaming", however—vagrant animals were persecuted in similar ways to mobile humans. For domestic animals, mostly the response was more moderate and tried to allow continuity in ownership by identifying animal threats and trying to ensure distancing. Thus, in one plague ordinance from late-fifteenth-century Ghent, pigs had to be locked in sties far from streets, and could be herded for sale or slaughter, but only in certain time-slots in order to reduce the chances of miasmatical odours mixing with people.[101] In the seventeenth century, in places such as Liège, Namur, and Huy, common strategies included keeping a separate enclosed compound for one's animals; locking or tying animals up; keeping the animals outside the city walls; or having the animals moved from domestic sites to common flocks or herds.[102] Clearly, this made sense given their economic value, people's reliance on them, and the grievances that could easily follow from mass exterminations.[103] Despite contemporary understanding of the potential link between rats and plague outbreaks, however, there is no reference to any coordinated attempts to catch or kill these rodents in the late-medieval or early modern Low Countries, not appearing in any ordinances, despite the fact that black rat bones have been found in more than 70 late-medieval or early modern excavation sites of various types (with 30 rat remains clusters from the late Middle Ages alone).[104] Perhaps ironically, the slaughter of animals such as cats removed one usual predator for rodent populations in urban environments.

Such concerns extended towards anxieties over corrupted sociability as well. On the grounds of lingering plague deaths in Utrecht in 1658, after the major outbreak of 1655/6, city authorities decided to cut the frequency of the neighbourhood collective meals (*buurmaaltijden*), which could also only last for two days—to avoid the morally repugnant effects of scandal, excess, and drinking.[105] Indeed, the seventeenth-century Nijmegen medic, IJsbrand van Diemerbroek, frequently mentioned in his plague tractate the infectious qualities of both fear and arguments.[106] Authorities did not need much incentive to attempt to restrict these events, as social disorder in the aftermath of funerals was a constantly recurring theme in the early modern period.[107] Women were banned from funerals repeatedly during epidemic outbreaks in the sixteenth and seventeenth centuries (an issue expanded upon in greater depth in Chapter 6), and in one case from Amsterdam during the plague of 1602 with the miasmatical rationale that "their presence increased the danger of contaminated air rising from the graves".[108] Church bells had a curious role within this framework as part of the "epidemic soundscape".[109] On the one hand, the tolling of the bells moved, and therefore were seen by some to improve the air within a community, and hence provide a form of protection against diseases and storms—see, for example, the inscription of a fifteenth-century bell in Louvain that noted "I call to the living, I mourn the dead, I break up lightning" (*vivos voco, mortuos plango, fulgura frango*) or the fire and emergency bells of 1455 in the tower of the Grote Kerk in Schiedam that read "I mourn the dead, I hunt the plague, I grace the feasts" (*defunctos ploro, fugo pestem, festa decoro*).[110] Yet, at the same time, there are many examples of regulations created during epidemic outbreaks that prohibited the ringing of bells, sometimes for certain groups such as children. Was this simply because too many were dying or a moral statement against those that had died? In Dordrecht during an epidemic in 1450, it was explicitly stated that bells could only be tolled once a day to not "depress people even more by the many deaths daily brought into the church, and to avoid plague".[111] This kind of rationale was visible almost 400 years later. Thus, in Montfort, a village near Utrecht, during the typhus outbreak of 1817/18 [after the famous Year Without a Summer (1816), the coldest European summer on record] it was noted that the sounding of the church bells was stopped on the grounds that it "makes a very discouraging, and therefore fatal, impression on the already depressed minds of the sick".[112]

Water sources were often seen as corrupted—of relevance in many parts of the Low Countries due to the exceptional prevalence of water—and could create bad smells when flows were disrupted and especially in tandem with hot weather. Waste that fouled the water sources endangered the communal wellbeing (*welvaert*) of the city collective, it was announced in Amsterdam in 1504—on the back of a series of by-laws throughout the fifteenth century referring to the pollution of the canals.[113] Parasite samples from cesspits in use across the fourteenth to seventeenth centuries in Leiden, Brussels, Nivelles, Aalst, and Namur suggest that diarrhoea-related sicknesses were commonplace through faeces contaminating food and drink via water sources.[114] In that way, we can understand how just before the terrible epidemic outbreak of 1635 in Leiden, where more than a third of the population died, the surveyor Jan Pietersz Dou had already written to the city administration arguing against the creation of a new polder that would prevent water from freely running through the city, leading to a foul stink (*vuijl stinck nest*) and the likelihood of diseases.[115] In the same year, authorities noted the hot weather, the poorly flowing stinking water, and the appearance of pestilence in Rotterdam.[116] In Leeuwarden, a plague ordinance in 1636 contained an article which asked for all water to be drained from the graves before burying the corpses of the infected.[117] Residents noted with concern the putrid stagnant water on the River Zaan, north of Amsterdam, which together with an exceptionally hot summer in 1679 and lack of wind, created fever-related deaths from August to October.[118] One cliché statement often made is that urban elites, especially in the seventeenth century, started to build country houses (*buitenplaatsen*) to escape the bad odours that were associated with epidemics in the summer.[119] Conversely, water noted for its purity was sometimes even seen to have protective qualities against disease—see, for example, the rush of residents to a water fountain during an outbreak in 1626 in the Hainaut village of Châtelet.[120]

Another explanatory framework for understanding and interpreting epidemic diseases in the preindustrial Low Countries was the theory of contagion. According to this view, physical proximity to a particular object, animal, environment, or person could lead to the spread of sickness. It still linked up coherently with the other frameworks—indeed, a person could be fearful of being physically close (contagion) to a corrupted site (miasma), impacting upon the body's sensory experiences, which in turn was corrupted through God's punishment of lack of piety (providence).[121] There has, however, been some debate about the timing and spread of contagionist ideas in the Low Countries. One recent work has suggested that the ineffective and uncoordinated attempts to manage disease in the Dutch Republic, usually ad hoc by individual urban administrations in isolation, were a product of an under-appreciation of contagionist principles.[122] According to this view, it was only during the final plague outbreak, apparently seeded in Amsterdam in 1663 via a ship that docked there from the eastern Mediterranean, that this started to change, and more coordination across larger areas came into action—and hence, after the 1660s, the plague no longer featured in the Republic.[123] Certainly, this late movement towards coordination fits within a broader literature that has emphasised the delayed creation of elaborate quarantine infrastructure in northwest Europe—perhaps only coming into full fruition in the eighteenth century and linked to more paternalistic understandings of the relationship between state and the populace.[124] According to some recent scholarship, it was not until the great plague of Provence in 1720–2 that there was a move towards centralising principles of "disaster management" in France, for example.[125]

Nevertheless, while it is undoubtedly correct that the Dutch Republic only set in motion territorially pervasive coordinated strategies from the mid-seventeenth century onwards, which stood out when compared to places such as Italy which implemented these techniques much earlier, it is unclear what the causes or the consequences were.[126] For example, can we really say that the move towards an integrated strategy in the Republic led to the disappearance of the plague, when in the southern Low Countries, already using some coordinated strategies since the sixteenth century (although the extent to which they were coordinated is exaggerated in *Per imperatief plakkaat*), similarly saw their final plague in the 1660s, just as it was the last plague in England, northern and central France, and northern Germany?[127] In fact, the southern Low Countries in the seventeenth century tended to temporarily mirror epidemic activity seen in the Republic—and even experienced some severe outbreaks that the Republic did not such as in 1645–7.[128] Furthermore, can we really say that the late move towards an integrated strategy in the Republic was connected to a lack of adherence to contagionist ideas, when it is clear that basic principles of contagion were seen all across the Low Countries (both north and south) even going back to the late-medieval period?[129] Already in the fifteenth century we learn from the notes of one Arnold van Goer in 1449/50, a Guelders land agent, that a forester's wife was so sick from the *pestilencien* that no one would dare touch one of his books.[130] People were already afraid of being physically close to certain objects or people. One potential reason posited might be not the lack of adherence to contagionist thinking, but more connected to the fact that politics and commerce were closely entwined in the Republic—with many public office holders also merchants—and hence perhaps reluctant to fully implement restrictions on trade and mobility.[131] Even this argument is not wholly complete, however, as we should also recognise that regardless of the restrictions enacted by decentralised governance, authorities were incapable of or ineffective in stopping those producers and traders (and in fact all kinds of people) that circumvented the rules—an aspect elaborated upon more in Chapter 4. Indeed, inland river and waterway transportation was not reduced during epidemic outbreaks in the Dutch Republic.[132]

From internal corruptions to external dangers

Recent literature on the interpretation of plague in other parts of western Europe such as in late-medieval Valencia has suggested a more nuanced chronology comprising two phases—one connected to concerns with corruptions from within communities (i.e., likely to be more miasmatic) slowly giving way to concerns with dangers external to communities (i.e., likely to be more contagionist).[133] While such a neat chronology might be more difficult to discern from a larger and more diverse territory such as the Low Countries when compared to an individual city such as Valencia, we do see by the middle of the fifteenth century a more visible identification of outside forces as potential sources of infectious vulnerabilities for communities—in other literature linked to an emerging "biopolitics of movement".[134] Thus, at Gouda in 1448, the city government put restrictions on farmers coming into the city from the surrounding countryside through fears of bringing disease—something that we did not see before the mid-fifteenth century.[135] By the time of a plague ordinance from Breda in 1515, reference was made to how plague was brought to the city by people from outside.[136] Even then, however, the lines between spiritual, moral, miasmatic, sensory, and contagionist forces continued to be quite blurred. In the Holland village of Den Briel in 1564, for example, the ongoing *peste* was said to have been caused at the same time by the presence of angry spirits (*boose geesten*), evil people (*quaede menschen*), and vagrants (*landlopers*)—vagrants, in turn, described as infecting houses deliberately with a venom (*fenijn*) prepared for that very purpose.[137]

By the seventeenth century, the dangers from outside view was stronger, as plague ordinances started to frequently instruct those supervising the gates of cities and towns to be more rigorous in their checks of people coming from other potentially infected places.[138] At Tilburg in 1616, an outbreak was blamed on a man who came into the city from outside and had brought plague with him. He was arrested, paid a large fine of 36 guilders—the equivalent of around 15 weeks' worth of wages for an unskilled male day labourer in a small provincial town in seventeenth-century Brabant—and had all his goods confiscated.[139] People coming into a locality were subject to restriction, but at the same time, residents of localities were also sometimes prevented from travelling out to other places. At the Campine village of Gierle in 1617, residents were told not to visit infected surroundings and were fined 25 guilders for doing so.[140] In nearby Herk-de-Stad in 1624, even people in uninfected houses were told not to go walking in cities, streets, and fields.[141] Still, however, we should recognise the interaction of outside and inside community interpretations of epidemic outbreaks in the Low Countries, even as late as the seventeenth century. Thus, for example, during the plague at Sluis in 1605, the urban authorities decided that it was the moral improprieties of the town's own "loose women and whores" (*lichte vrouwen en hoeren*) that had caused the ongoing infection, and yet an associated reason was that these sex workers had taken in men from outside the town.[142]

The interacting frameworks for interpreting and managing epidemic diseases connected to inward morality and outward dangers came to be reflected eventually in the spatial approach to treating the sick and burying the dead. In the late-medieval period those infected with plague and other afflictions were taken into all-purpose hospitals that had a number of functions, or sometimes designated rooms connected to monasteries, and in some cases certain structures such as orphanages or fortifications were converted into pest houses temporarily—see the foundling home of Delft acting in this way in 1537.[143] The plague afflicted were still being admitted into an ordinary hospital in the small Betuwe town of Culemborg in 1600—simply placed into a part of the institution known as the pox room (*pockkamer*).[144] Indeed, in Culemborg, it seems that a separate pest house was never created. Eventually though, in most places, new and more permanent pest houses were built in greater numbers which had the explicit role of taking in those infected during an epidemic or those infected with a kind of disease that could end up causing an epidemic. A clear separation of epidemic-related treatment and other types of healthcare started to emerge as the sixteenth century went on, and especially separating those that were seen as temporarily sick and those likely to stay in an institution for long periods.[145]

Some pest houses were initially founded in the fifteenth century, but their numbers really took off in the middle part of the sixteenth century (Figure 2.4)—which has parallels with what has been recently shown from France and to a lesser extent England.[146] These were funded through a combination of city budgeting (usually noted in the extraordinary expenditures section of the urban financial accounts), poor relief, donations, rents from landed estates, and the incorporation of goods and property from those that died there.[147] In Leeuwarden, the pest house built in 1611 was funded through contributions from three places—the orphanage, the poor table, and the St. Anthonygasthuis, and thus reveals an awareness that separation of the infected was something to benefit the functioning of existing institutions.[148]

Disputes, at times, broke out over whose financial responsibility it was to maintain the institutions—especially during the worst outbreaks when resources were overstretched.[149] In Amersfoort during the plague of 1636, for example, a conflict arose between the St. Elisabeth hospital and De Armen de Poth (a brotherhood that broadly cared for different categories of sick and the poor, and which included a pest house) over who had to take over exceptional costs connected to the midwives who ended up being infected in the institution.[150] Not all institutions descended into conflict though. A fraternity in Groningen borrowed 100 guilders from the women's (Ludeke Jarges) *gasthuis* after the *pest* of 1570 which had left many of the institution's stewards dead.[151]

The process of pest house creation, nevertheless, was not always straightforward and moving in a linear direction. In Leiden, a plan was in place in 1596 to convert the existing St. Cecilia hospital into a full pest house but was not realised due to a lack of funding.[152] The process of constructing new buildings was often slow and incremental—wooden emergency pest houses were still in operation in Leiden as late as the 1635 and 1655 outbreaks, and a stone one planned in 1557 was only finished in 1661, just in time for the final plague outbreak from 1664.[153] Such cases reveal the distance between what was desired and what was achievable. Generally, over time, and in a process that gathered speed only in the seventeenth century, these institutions were spatially oriented away from the city centres to peripheral neighbourhoods, and then outside the walls of the city.[154] In some cases, however, an alternative was to construct isolated temporary huts out in the countryside in order to take in the infected, who, if they survived, had to stay there a number of weeks.[155] This process was often forcible and rapid—in one case so quick that the afflicted from Tilburg moved to the rural huts had no clothes and had to buy new ones for 22 stuivers.[156] While a recent discussion

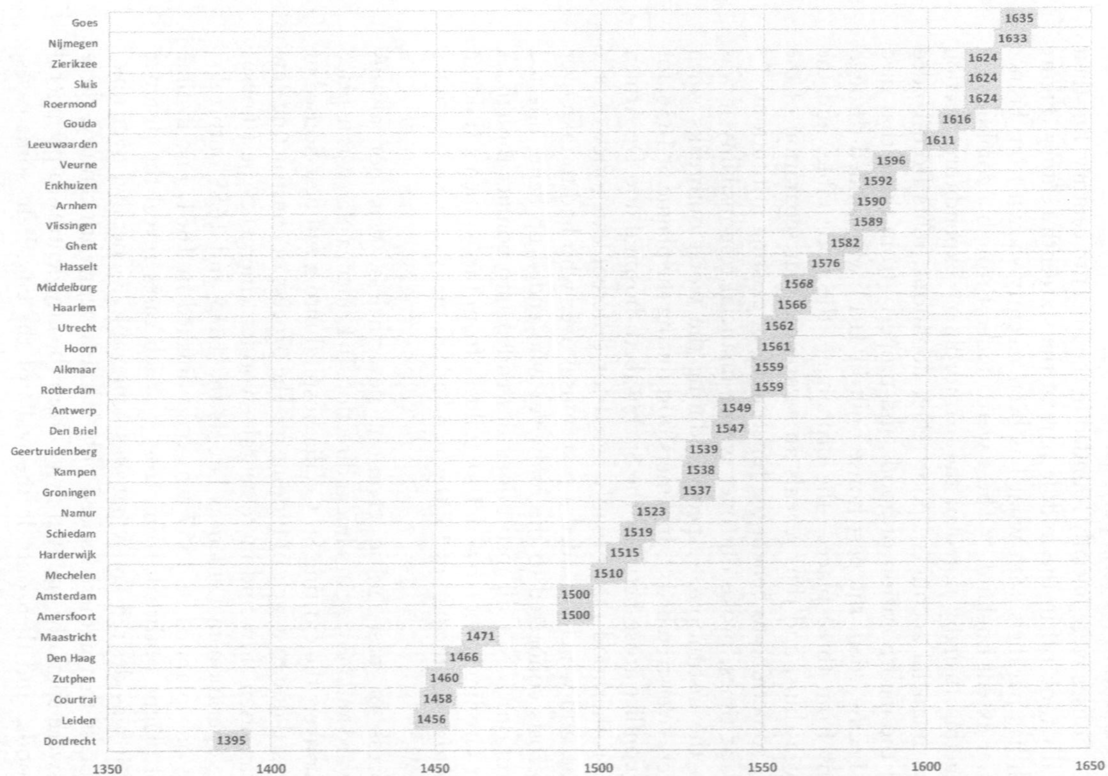

Figure 2.4 Foundation of pest houses in the Low Countries

Sources: Consultable in contracted form in the *pesthuizen* section of Curtis, ed., Original Burials Data, with full citations in the Bibliography of this book. This is a mention of the earliest foundation of a separate building or place specifically for those deemed to be infected with plague, as opposed to ordinary institutions such as monasteries where rooms were reserved for this purpose. Sometimes the lines between these distinctions are blurry and hence should only be taken as indicators. Sometimes we do not have clear insights into how the building was used.

on pest houses in England has presented two polarities in assessment—either ramshackle and temporary structures or permanent buildings of some significance—institutional isolation in the Low Countries was decidedly diverse and involved flimsy huts, purpose-built stone structures, and acquired and remodelled existing property portfolio.[157]

For those that died, many people in the late Middle Ages, particularly of high social status, were being buried inside the buildings of churches.[158] Nevertheless, epidemic disease outbreaks that led to exceptional mortality also required burials to be performed at separate institutions. The excavation of the cemetery at the St. Maartens hospital in Bergen op Zoom revealed 800 skeletons buried around the same time in a mass event (suggested, at present, to have been during the *pestis secunda* of 1359/60), and thus based on rough population figures from the mid-fourteenth century could have represented a quarter to a third of the inhabitants.[159] Over time, more ordinary church cemeteries were also constructed away from the church itself, especially from the fifteenth century onwards, which could accommodate more corpses.[160] For example, the cemetery in Leiden connected to St. Pieters church was lengthened to create more room in 1339 and 1400 (both epidemic years), and a new cemetery was created in Haarlem to the north side of the St. Bavo church around 1480.[161] Nevertheless, although the major drive for this development was space—thus, still somewhat pressurised by high mortality events such as epidemics—it was not necessarily forbidden for someone who had died of a disease such as plague to be buried inside a church, unlike the clear ban announced by the public health authorities of Florence during the 1630 plague.[162] And supporting that view, burial registers from the sixteenth and seventeenth centuries that explicitly distinguish between those buried in the church and those buried in cemeteries, such as at Haarlem, show spikes of burials for both locations during epidemic outbreaks.[163] After epidemics in 1635 and 1656 in Rotterdam, the building of the Prinsenkerk was twice expanded to accommodate more church interior burials.[164] Burial within church buildings remained a common choice within Low Countries communities well into the nineteenth century—despite prohibition by the revolutionary regime in the 1790s—representing roughly 25, 40, and 20 per cent of all burials in Alkmaar, Zwolle, and Den Bosch respectively by 1800.[165]

Nevertheless, especially by the seventeenth century, and in line with the greater frequency of plague ordinances being invoked, we do see increased administrative concern for burial practice. During plagues, graves had to be dug deep and closed quickly, bodies had to be conveyed along the shortest route from place of death to place of rest, and often by designated carriers at designated times, the precise conditions of which varied from locality to locality.[166] Greater caution was taken with burial decisions. During the outbreak of 1625 in Leiden, the criminal records noted a case of an inspection of a corpse, after which it was agreed there was no visible sign of the plague, and so permission was finally given to bury the body.[167] Also in the seventeenth century, we start to see prohibition of those coming from outside a city and dying of plague from being buried in that same city's church cemeteries—as what happened at Weert and Utrecht in 1636.[168] Indeed, at Utrecht, burials inside the St. Nicolaas Church were entirely forbidden on 11 August 1636.[169] Yet, still, it is unclear what the precise lines were between practical matters such as lack of physical room for bodies and culture of death matters such as the miasma-induced fears surrounding vapours and corruptions connected to the corpse's presence within a community. Supporting the first view at least, is that by the middle of the seventeenth century, we see increased reference to the buildup of coffins above ground, likely connected to the difficulties of finding space, and the lack of plots available in cemeteries.[170] One likely reason was the negative associations given to mass burial pits and the associated fears of being placed in non-consecrated ground, and thus the desire to still pack as many corpses into crowded church cemeteries was strong.[171]

A new theory but persisting practices

Although contagionist ideas became more prominent over the course of the early modern period, both providential and miasmatical frameworks for understanding disease origins and transmission remained steadfastly present as the Low Countries made their (late in northwest European perspective) transition to modern industrialisation—even if medics started to more explicitly question some of the unexplained puzzles connected to miasma.[172] In the Brabant village of Eersel around 1800, the Reverend Stephanus Hanewinckel noted how Catholic inhabitants kneeled in prayer in front of a lime tree (*lindeboom*) and stuck pins in the bark to be cured of an outbreak of fevers—even if we should recognise that this minister, within his many travelogues, tended to accentuate a perceived backwardness within the Catholic communities that he encountered.[173] Still in the first half of the nineteenth century, we see continual references to the infectious potential of atmospherics and the environment. In the resolutions announced by the village administration of Veghel, Brabant, in August 1808, for example, an assessment by the village doctor (*medicyne dorpsdoctor*) suggested that there were no stench-producing spots (*stankverwekkende plaatsen*) in the locality from which any rising contamination might be feared.[174] This was not solely a rural, and hence potentially interpreted as "backward", phenomenon either, since similar patterns of behaviour persisted in cities too. During the cholera outbreaks of the 1830s, in all the major Holland cities, citizens were instructed to keep their windows open, and were frequently using vinegar and chlorine—instructions that were frequently seen centuries earlier during plague and dysentery outbreaks.[175] Similar points have been made about cholera responses in nineteenth-century Italy, with many of the arrangements having their roots in anti-plague measures.[176]

In the first cholera outbreak in the Low Countries, in 1832, diaries produced in different contexts—from Amsterdam to villages in rural Frisia—continued to hold central ideas of providential punishment and faith.[177] And although the findings of John Snow during the cholera outbreak of 1854 in Soho, London, are credited with starting the incremental and slow acceptance across many parts of western Europe of germ theory ideas of disease transmission and spread, the case of the Low Countries shows how pre-existing frameworks of miasma, providence, and contagion remained significant even well into the second half of the nineteenth century. Prayer remained very common and important. For example, we see in Antwerp in 1866 that inhabitants were still verbally repeating a short prayer to combat cholera, asking for God's mercy despite their sins, and processions continued.[178] Antiphons devised originally in the late fifteenth century to deliver communities from *peste* and "sudden death" continued to be used and reformatted into hymns of the eighteenth and nineteenth centuries, as shown from the written music collections of the beguinage at Turnhout (Figure 2.5).[179]

Some older literature tried to suggest that epidemics such as cholera, in tandem with greater appreciation of germ theory, "forced" sanitation and hygiene reforms.[180] Structural improvements through cholera outbreaks were also argued explicitly for different cities in the Netherlands.[181] Most scholarship tended to disagree, however, and more recent studies have moved away from that.[182] Indeed, like what has been already argued for the medieval Low Countries, and echoing what has been maintained for nineteenth-century

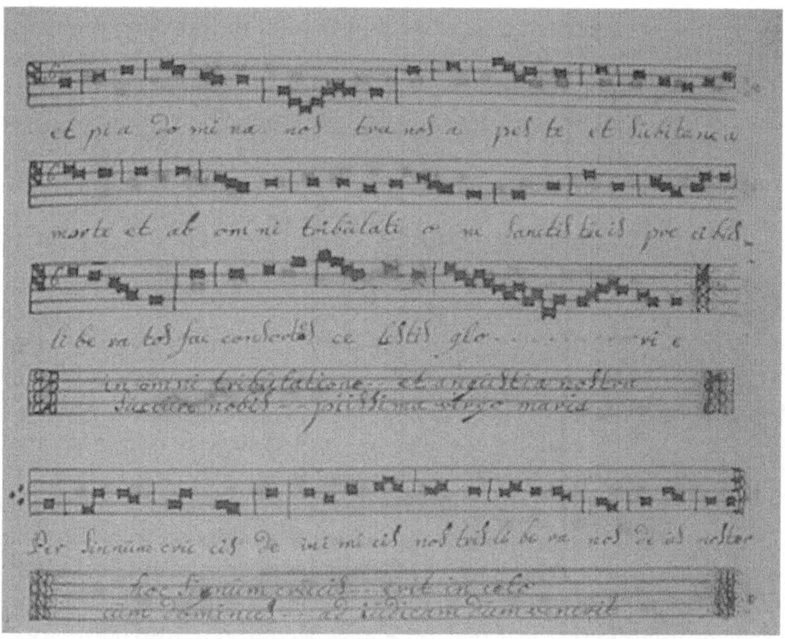

Figure 2.5 Late eighteenth-century hymn using the plague antiphon, Turnhout beguinage

Source: Vanden Bossche, Een pest-antifoon, 13.

England, Italy, and northern Germany, epidemic outbreaks of diseases such as cholera or tuberculosis did not take a leading role in creating strong and substantial structural reform for public health change in the industrialising Low Countries.[183] Although outbreaks could be used by political authorities to lend support to particular ideological convictions as suggested for Antwerp during the cholera of 1866, it has been noted in the city of Utrecht, for example, that while attention and resources were made available to help the plight of the poor during the severe cholera outbreak of 1866, the immediate interest quickly waned in the years thereafter, offering little structural improvements to those most likely to be afflicted.[184] In Haarlem, the distribution per capita of wells and cesspits—important public infrastructure necessary to avoid water-based disease outbreaks—even declined across the nineteenth century, and thus hardly an epidemic-induced "sanitary awakening".[185]

Conclusion

In Chapter 2, I have focused on the long-term dimensions of how communities in the Low Countries tended to interpret and understand epidemic disease. Overall, I show that there was some change over time—in particular, the idea that disease becomes a product of external dangers rather than internal moral corruptions starts to become much more prominent around the sixteenth century, although still with a complicated co-existence of the two ideas. Gradually, there were also developments in the types of social groups identified as connected with epidemic disease. In the sixteenth century, we see the first signs of the links being made between plague and poverty by contemporary observers and authorities, roughly corroborating the chronology posited for northern and central Italy, but in the seventeenth century, we see a much more coherent "outbreak narrative" develop, where women and physical outsiders are more explicitly condemned and restricted.[186]

Nevertheless, there were also strong continuities in understanding epidemic disease in the Low Countries—from the late Middle Ages onwards we can observe a complicated mix of providence, miasma theory, and contagion, where it was impossible to separate the three in causing moral corruptions. Some contagionist ideas are perhaps found earlier than we expect, even in the late-medieval period, while the influence of religion remained present well into the late nineteenth century, even as germ theory among medical elites takes hold. The interpretation of epidemic disease, and how to be rid of an affliction, did not merely travel in one linear direction and was not a timeless essence—the primacy of ideas oscillated over time and were accentuated under certain contextual pressures.[187] Perhaps most fundamentally, and in accordance with other preindustrial public health history produced recently, Chapter 2 supports the idea that epidemics were rarely instigators for massive changes or developments in public health practice, institutions, and infrastructure.[188] That is not to say that a "timeless Galenic vacuum" existed though.[189] Instead, adaptation occurred incrementally over time, building on developments occurring outside of epidemics, and supported by a collective memory within communities of epidemics which had already recurred—and it is the recurring nature of those anticipated hazards that is the subject of Chapter 3.

Notes

1 Green, A New Definition. But, of course, not limited to plague, and sometimes looking at the interaction between plague and other diseases: for example, Dittmar et al., Tuberculosis.

2 We should distinguish between two definitions in the literature. The more precise definition of plague is a specific disease caused by the bacterium *Yersinia pestis*, which is the definition of plague used in this book. Sometimes the generic term "plagues" is used in the literature to mean various epidemic afflictions of the past, although this is an unhelpful inexact practice.

3 Green, The Four Black Deaths; Spyrou et al., The Source. Also, for the First Plague Pandemic from the sixth century onward: Keller et al., Ancient *Yersinia pestis*.

4 Vermunt and van der Kallen, *Opgravingen*, 90–9. The *Yersinia pestis* evidence from the Bergen op Zoom site had been discussed in a major genetics literature, although with differing views on the dating of the evidence, which have not been fully resolved. Initially dated to the Black Death of 1349–51 on the vague unreferenced basis of "soil stratigraphy, artifacts, and coins": Haensch et al., Distinct Clones, 5. The first questioning of this dating of the sample from Bergen op Zoom, initially dated to the Black Death, was made by Monica Green, who suggested an alternative of *pestis secunda*. The whole contextualisation of this discussion since the original 2010 study in: Green, Out of the East, 303–4. Since then, acceptance of *pestis secunda* for the sample can be found in: Roosen and Curtis, The "Light Touch", 45; Barbieri et al., *Yersinia pestis*, 30; Namouchi et al., Integrative Approach, e11794; Parker et al., 14th Century, 2. More vaguely, the "late fourteenth century" in Spyrou et al., Phylogeography, 3. In my view, the dating cannot be classed as definitive yet as it does not come through contextual evidence of the mass burial site itself but simply that other 1B lineages of this *Yersinia pestis* DNA from St. Mary Graces in London and Bolgar (capital of the Volga Bulgaria) have been dated to *pestis secunda*: Curtis, Plague, 85. Potential supporting evidence from documents was lost in a fire at Bergen op Zoom in 1397: Van Ham, *Macht*, 249.

5 Keller et al., A Refined Phylochronology, 8. It has been suggested that *Yersinia pestis* DNA evidence has recently been uncovered from a skeleton in Mechelen, apparently datable to the Black Death, although at the time of writing this remains unpublished: Soens, The Black Death; Soens, pers. comms. [23/10/2024].

6 Beneker at al., Urbanization, 21–2 and supporting documents 1.

7 Curtis and Roosen, On the Importance. Though these quantitative limitations should not obscure the fact that this information is highly valuable: Sarris, New Approaches, 339.

8 On the issue of representativeness of these sites: Kacki, Digging, 264–5; Cessford et al., Beyond Plague Pits, 497, 514.

9 For the recent incorporation of epigraphical evidence: Slavin, Death.

10 Arrizabalaga, Problematizing; Alter and Carmichael, Classifying.

11 Cohn, *The Black Death Transformed*, 247.

12 Theilmann and Cate, A Problem.

13 Carmichael, Universal.
14 Carmichael, *Plague*, 21.
15 Benedictow, *The Complete History of the Black Death*, 450.
16 Green et al., Diagnosis, 314.
17 Jones, Apostumes.
18 The initial two-volume classic: Biraben, *Les hommes*. Subsequent digitisation of the appendix: Büntgen et al., Digitizing. For the scientific literature involved and a criticism: Roosen and Curtis, Dangers. Some scholars have interpreted our criticism as directed towards Biraben; for example: Benedictow, Biraben's Lists; Desierto and Koyama, The Political Economy, 500. This is incorrect. We hold the initial text of Biraben in quite reverential terms but criticise the appropriation and application of his appendix by others, often in the natural or social sciences, to create datasets unfit for purpose. In subsequent work, Benedictow has repeated the misinterpretation and then inaccurately referred to Roosen and Curtis as "Dutch historians": Benedictow, *The Complete History of the Black Death*, xxiv; Benedictow, *The Complete History of Plague in Norway*, 237. Other work continues to use unfit-for-purpose datasets of "plague references", and then even combines this with other unfit-for-purpose datasets of "war references": Kaniewski and Marriner, Conflicts. See the criticisms of the broader trend in Van Bavel et al., Climate. Some scholars are starting to think of productive ways to improve the datasets, although it is a slow process: Krauer and Schmid, Mapping.
19 It might have been a plague bubo but also conceivably a sign of anthrax, since we do not have information on the location of the body: Hamaker, ed., Historische aanteekeningen, 138.
20 Coomans, *Community*, 234.
21 See the *fivres contagieux* mentioned in 1438 in Liège: Hélin, Les recherches, 176.
22 Van Schaïk, *Belasting*, 305–6; Hélin, Les recherches, 176. For the severe prolonged drought in the Low Countries: Camenisch et al., Extreme Heat, 3.
23 Arickx, De armendis, 177.
24 In 1497/8, it was likely syphilis rather than smallpox, and we see similar references around the same time in Leiden, Rotterdam, Haarlem, Middelburg, and along the Maas in Limburg and Liège: Curtis, From One Mortality Regime to Another? 140; Fokker, *Onderzoek*, 14–17; Hélin, Les recherches, 177. Previously, in the literature it was suggested that syphilis begins to be recorded in Europe in the 1490s after being brought back from the Americas in the context of the Columbian Exchange: for a useful summary: Harper et al., The Origin. The surge in references in the Low Countries in the 1490s lends support to this view. However, palaeopathological evidence of syphilis in three skeletons has recently been produced from a hospital in Kampen from earlier in the fifteenth century, perhaps pointing to earlier exposure: Schats and Klomp, In Sickness, 113–14. It could also be the case that both scenarios are correct. Syphilis was not unknown in Europe, but the Columbian Exchange brought about the first virulent form of the disease leading to discernible epidemics in the late fifteenth and early sixteenth centuries. On this epidemic form, see Arrizabalaga et al., *The Great Pox*, 16, 266–9.
25 Huisman, *Stadsbelang*, 23. On the 1529 sweating sickness in the Low Countries: De Moor, Adriana Stoffelsdr.; Ladan, De Engelse zweetziekte; Van Schevensteen, Un traité anversois. The Haarlem city administration announced a procession on 1 October 1529 against the "new sickness" (*nieuwe siekte*), which shows how societies were clearly able to acknowledge afflictions they had never seen before, and could still make distinctions: Ladan, *Gezondheidszorg*, 56. Earlier scholarship on the subject had suggested that the sweating sickness, often referred to as

sudor Anglicus, was confined to regions of England, which is incorrect: Dyer, The English Sweating Sickness, 383.

26 Den Braber, ed., Overlijdensregister, [15/2/1715].

27 Example noted in Van Besouw and Curtis, Estimating, 16.

28 Creemers, ed., Kronijk, 192. This outbreak occurred in the aftermath of a well-known famine at the start of the Eighty Years' War: Kuttner, *Het hongerjaar*; Van Dixhoorn, The Grain Issue.

29 SB, Vestbrieven, no. 765, fo. 193–4 [26/3/1549]. Noting the differences, while simultaneously acknowledging the similarities in its contagious nature with other diseases. For the Den Bosch case: Coopmans, *De rechtstoestand*, 17, 197 (Coopmans uses an incorrect date on page 17).

30 GA, Kerkeboek 1621–1743, Weiwerd, 124, DTB Groningen, no. 512, fo. 116v [AO]. On the likelihood of this disease in this area: Knottnerus, Malaria.

31 De Keijzer, ed., Nieuwpoort, 8; Anon., ed., Lottum.

32 One of the standout examples of a burials series that includes plague markers next to the names of those buried fully and consistently over time is the *momboirkamer* of Utrecht from 1624 onwards. For example, during the significant plague outbreak of 1636, 3,512 burials out of a total 5,050 (69.6 per cent) have a plague marker, and removing those we see the remainder of the burials equates roughly to the normal mortality trend: Rommes, Op het spoor, 120; and for extra data: Curtis, ed., Original Burials Data.

33 A good example is the consolidated series from seventeenth-century Leiden where the initial plague outbreak in 1601–5 has seemingly full registration of explicit plague markers (more than 50 per cent of the burials in 1604, for example), but the same completeness is then not seen in the rest of the series. For the data, see Curtis, ed., Original Burials Data.

34 SAB, Parochieregisters, Poppel (Ravels), St. Valentijn, 1604–64, fo. 13v [AO]. Here we have a reference to someone as *nigronisa* (blackened) during an epidemic outbreak in the Campine village of Poppel in 1629, but this does not necessarily refer to a bubo, especially since 1629 is not a known plague outbreak.

35 Jacquet-Ladrier, Les épidémies, 134.

36 SR, Archieven van de Notarissen te Rotterdam en daarin opgegane gemeenten, 18, 498, no. 42, fo. 73 [14/7/1643].

37 Calculation based on rental values extracted from 1632 fiscal records in Leiden: Van Besouw et al., Epidemic Mortality.

38 Deneweth and Wallis, Households.

39 As seen in the small Brabant village of Princehage in 1582: Kappelhof, Verzorging; and in Tilburg in 1599: De Brouwer, "De aenclevende sieckte", 5–7.

40 Mentink, De rode loop, 138, 140.

41 On Douwe Ales: Jensma and van Lieburg, *Het "doktersboek"*, 15–16. On cattle plague and lay veterinary practitioners: Van Roosbroeck, Experts; Van Roosbroeck, Caring.

42 Coomans, *Community*, 216–17.

43 Mitchell, Historical Sources, 184. The (usually female) "searchers" used for codifying and announcing causes of death in London, for example, did not appear in the Low Countries: Munkhoff, Searchers. See Chapter 4 for more details. In late-medieval and early modern Milan, this codification process was performed by a combination of state-appointed (male) officials working in tandem with elite physicians: Carmichael, The Forensic Tradition. This might explain the higher level of detail found in the Books of the Dead for Milan.

44 The painted red plague cross, as seen in sixteenth- and seventeenth-century London, however, does not appear in Low Countries sources: Brookes, Plague Markings.

45 Anon., ed., Beek.
46 Arrizabalaga, Medical Causes; Gijswijt-Hofstra, Inleiding, 9.
47 This is the easiest way of understanding what Bruno Latour meant when he said that the Pharaoh Ramesses II did not die (thirteenth century BCE) of tuberculosis as tuberculosis had not yet been "invented".
48 Van den Boomen, The Imperfections.
49 The earliest mention of the *gave Gods* seems to have applied to a man from Gouda in a Delft chronicle from 1426: Oosterbaan, ed., Kroniek, 109. However, earlier general mentions of receiving *pestelencie* from God can be found such as the Carthusian chronicles of 1385 describing the death of famous deacon Geert Groote in Deventer: Brinkerink, ed., Biographieën, 423.
50 Tramper, De pest, 3.
51 Bergsma, ed., *De wereld*, 29.
52 Kerkhoff, *Per imperatief plakkaat*, 38–9, 253.
53 Van den Brand, ed., Maashees, 1.
54 Jensen, "Disaster Upon Disaster", 55–6.
55 Sundberg, Building the Social Cascade.
56 De Vos, ed., Remedie, 62.
57 Pettegree and Der Weduwen, News, 112.
58 Kohle, The Road, 73.
59 Maillard-Luypaert, La tradition.
60 Hulshof, ed., Gebed. The requests for salvation from the outbreak were directed towards St. Anthony, a known and venerated plague saint.
61 Pauly, Pestepidemien, 58.
62 RAZ, Inventaris van de collectie Johannes Gimberg (1850–1930), 0142, no. 68, fo. 1 [AO]; Coomans, Policing, 21.
63 Viaene, Judocus Clichtove.
64 Vanden Bossche, Een pest-antifoon, 12. A poem referring to the dead during the 1635 outbreak in Leiden was later found in a collection of devotional songs: Pollmann, Hunger Tales, 125.
65 Geldhof, De pestepidemie, 307; Heijmans, ed., Nadere toegang, 251 [5/10/1603]; Van der Wiel and Ekamper, Kromme sikkel, 86.
66 Coomans et al., Plague, 596.
67 RtL, Archief van de Onze-Lieve-Vrouwparochie van Hamme, 880/47, no. 34296 [AO].
68 Noordegraaf, Calvinism.
69 Huisman, De maatschappelijke reacties, 26; Boschma, "Een pest", 72. Although later in the eighteenth and nineteenth centuries, providence was used to both reject and support inoculation, depending on context: Van Lieburg, Revisiting, 219–20.
70 Faber, Cattle-Plague, 5; Duiveman, Praying, 546.
71 Some continuities in practice were even seen during the 1570s and 1580s in Antwerp, where the city authorities switched from Catholic to Protestant and back again in this short period: Coomans et al., Plague.
72 For Rotterdam: De Iongh, De ontwrichtende pest?; although rebutted: Noordegraaf and Valk, Rotterdam. For Doesburg in 1624, mostly retreating to the south around Angerlo: Vermeesch, *Oorlog*, 144.
73 At Gouderak in 1514 during the general inquiry into the conditions of the towns and villages in Holland and Friesland, a priest was unable to come and declare details for the report because of those "languishing in the parish, lying sick from the hot sickness" (*heeter siecte*): Fruin, ed., *Informacie*, 401. The Count of den Bergh could not travel from Bergh in 1567 to meet with the Duke of Gulik on account of the *pest*: EAL, Huis Bergh, 1227–1842, 0214, no. 358 [17/7/1567]

[AO]. Later in the same file a letter explains that the Count cannot access his feudal registers (*leenboek*) because of raging plague: EAL, Huis Bergh, 1227–1842, 0214, no. 3268 [17/7/1578]. At Gorinchem in 1533, the local administration warned a husband-and-wife couple that they "may not and dare not" travel from their home during time of the great sickness (*grote sieckten off crenckten*): Van Dooren, ed., Thuisisolatie.

74 EAL, Huis Bergh, 1227–1842, 0214, no. 7258 [30/8/1556] [AO].
75 Van Lieburg, Kinderziekten.
76 Frijhoff, Gods gave afgewezen.
77 Dekker, Coping.
78 Sundberg, *Natural Disasters*, 51–88, 212–50; Van Roosbroeck, Experts; Rommes, "Geen vrolijk geloei".
79 Dijstelberge and Noordegraaf, eds., *Plague*.
80 Sentiments seen in both his original *pest-boeck* of 1600 and his later *Preservatiif voor de Pest* of 1624: Van Asperen, Nothing Else than Decay, 15.
81 DAA, Huisarchief Batinge, 0617, Recepten tegen de pest, het koliek en het maagkoliek, no. 340 [AO].
82 See, for example, the case of the priest Houbraken at Veghel in 1652, with a remedy for *pest* and fevers (*koorts*): Van Asseldonk, Recepten. Similarly, a priest at Baardegem, near Aalst, began one of the series of the parish registers with a remedy for those in plague-infected houses (*de gheene, die in besmette huijsen van peste sijn*), but still only freed by the "grace of God": SAB, Parochieregisters, Baardegem (Aalst), St. Margaretha, 1639–1843, fo. 2r [AO].
83 See the recipes against *pest* of the Frisian farmer, Douwe Ales, who came up with a remedy for those who were going into houses (*Voor de pest als ghij in die huisen gaet*): Jensma and van Lieburg, *Het "doktersboek"*, 82, 162. It should be noted that Douwe Ales (1682–1714) lived after the final plague outbreak in the Low Countries, although he was obviously not aware of that.
84 A good insight into Galenism and the development of community prophylactics against disease: Geltner and Weeda, Underground, 126–8; and an important overview: Coomans, *Community*, 31–82.
85 On this complex relationship between the senses, human bodies, and the environment, see the latest on seventeenth-century London: Turner, Intersensory Experiences.
86 Naaktgeboren, Policing, 163.
87 De Ketham, Een tractaet. The importance of connections drawn between celestial configurations and the incidence of epidemics in the early modern period is recently asserted in Pfeffer, Astrology.
88 Casteels, *Looking for Justice*, 265.
89 Van Adrichem, Een pest-instructie, 49.
90 Noordegraaf, Zacharias Heyns' Pest-Spieghel.
91 Groenendijk et al., "Away with all my Pleasant Things in the World", 275.
92 Duiveman, *Nature Triumphed*, 84.
93 On the distinctive features of this outbreak: Van Maanen, De grote epidemie. For the crime: Van den Heuvel, ed., Crimineel klachtboek, 286 [24/2/1677].
94 Coomans, *Community*, 22–3.
95 Curtis, Preserving, 284; Van Zalinge-Spooren, "Die contagieuse sieckte", 57. In 1567, a Groningen magistrate paid 15 rijder (value equivalent to guilders) and 3 stuivers to labourers to clean waterways and burn and bury materials described as plague-infected: Huisman, *Stadsbelang*, 27.
96 Van Zalinge-Spooren, *Gemeint*, 217.
97 In response to a plague outbreak in Flanders in 1424, the aldermen of Arras forbade second-hand cloth dealers from purchasing from infected localities:

Bocquet, *Recherches*, 76. In Courtrai in 1474, the city aldermen asked the town fullers not to purchase a house and yard by the town hall, for fear of the plague: Curtis, Preserving, 291. Fears associated with cotton and wool extended well into the eighteenth century, since the products were thought to "retain infection" for a long time, being difficult to fumigate: Pannier, From Crisis Management towards a Mediterranean Model? 44.

98 Coomans, Food Offenders, 124; Coomans, *Community*, 233; Weeda, The Porous City, 100, 106.

99 Van den Driest, Hondenbaan, 38; Callewier, De hondenslager, 2–3. The financial rewards were not high—at the end of the fifteenth century only eight *mijten* (one sixth of a stuiver in value) were offered per dog killed, which for the 1400/1 total of 242 dogs corresponded to just over two guilders for the arduous task. In 1401, a similar fee of a quarter of a stuiver per dog killed was offered in Courtrai. Anxieties about dogs and cats and their connection to outbreaks were already seen in the late Middle Ages: Marsilje, Aangelijnd, 62–4; Béghin, Entre le coeur. And they continued through to the final plague outbreak of the 1660s, as seen in the observations of Oomius, *Des Heeren*, 61.

100 Callewier, De hondenslager, 8.

101 Coomans, *Community*, 228. On the concern over domestic pigs: Coomans, Varkens; Camphuijsen and Coomans, De middeleeuwse stad.

102 Riguelle, Que la peste soit de l'animal!

103 Riguelle, La police.

104 Riguelle, Que la peste soit de l'animal!, 109. A phenomenon noted more broadly outside the Low Countries: Audoin-Rouzeau, *Les chemins*. For the rat finds in excavations: Lauwerier, Ratten, 36–7.

105 Bogaers, Geleund, 361.

106 Frijhoff, Gods gave afgewezen, 154.

107 Hollewand, Funeral Consumption, 70.

108 Noordegraaf and Valk, *De gave Gods*, 120.

109 Term borrowed from the recent work on the noises and silences connected to Gilles li Muisis' narrative of plague in Tournai: Singer, Hearing.

110 Champion, *The Fullness of Time*, 38; Schmitz, Schiedam, 129.

111 Coomans, *Community*, 250.

112 Rombach, Zenuwzinkingkoorts, 17. For the summer temperatures in Europe, 1766–2000: Schurer et al., Disentangling.

113 Coomans, *Community*, 228. Blood was seen as a corruptive source linked to plague, and especially a perceived putrid intrinsic quality of the poor: Siena, Poor Bodies, 126.

114 Rabinow et al., Intestinal Parasite Infection; Rabinow et al., Continuity; De Cupere et al., A Multidisciplinary Analysis; Deforce et al., Analysis; Graff et al., A Comparative Study; Rocha et al., Paleoparasitological Remains.

115 Van Tielhof and van Dam, *Waterstaat*, 1857. On smell and the amelioration of water flow in Leiden: Buning, Stench.

116 Foncke, *Water's Worth*, 61.

117 Anon., ed., *Ordonnantie by de magistraet der stad Leeuwarden gemaeckt*, no. 20 [12/8/1636].

118 Koene, *De Caeskopers*, 65.

119 Prak and van Zanden, *Pioneers*, 25. Although there is no tangible evidence to corroborate that supposition: Vogelzang, Et in arcadia ego? 23.

120 Kaisin, ed., *Annales*, 310–11.

121 On the nuances of the interactions between the three: Coomans, *Community*, 225–6.

122 Kerkhoff, *Per imperatief plakkaat*, 48–51.

123 Noordegraaf and Valk, *De gave Gods*, 45. That the plague had already been seeded in 1663 is also noted in a document where it is mentioned that a ship returning from Cadiz, Spain, in 1663, had to remain in quarantine at the beginning of the year 1664 because of the *pest* in Holland. SA, Archief van de Notarissen ter Standplaats Amsterdam, 1578–1915, 5075, no. 3607, fo. 98v [19/9/1668] [AO].

124 On populationist and mercantilist ideas underpinning this development: Pannier, From Crisis Management towards a Mediterranean Model?

125 Ermus, *The Great Plague Scare*, 7, 55. A chronology questioned in Murphy, *Plague*.

126 For more coordinated strategies in Italy: Henderson, Coping. Italy only experienced one major seventeenth-century plague outbreak in the north and centre in 1630 and one in the Papal States and the Kingdom of Naples in 1656–8: Alfani, Plague; notwithstanding localised or regional flickers of plague such as in Palermo and surrounding areas of Sicily in 1624 or Puglia in 1690–2: Fusco, The Importance; Macrì, Quarantena.

127 Some scholars have linked the timing of integrated strategies and the disappearance of the plague in the Dutch Republic without any consideration of the broader chronology of plague disappearance in the neighbouring territories: Noordegraaf, Dearth, 59.

128 Curtis, Was Plague an Exclusively Urban Phenomenon? 145–6.

129 Furthermore, an integrated strategy might have been difficult to implement earlier in the seventeenth century given that the 1624/5 and 1635–7 epidemics did not come from outside via ships but were internal to the Low Countries and connected to ongoing military conflict: Van Besouw and Curtis, Estimating. It should be noted also that although Kerkhoff in *Per imperatief plakkaat* suggests that an integrated approach only emerged for the final outbreak of the 1660s, the Dutch Republic successfully confined the 1655/6 plague to a very territorially restricted area including mainly localities in Holland, Utrecht, and Frisia: Curtis, Was Plague an Exclusively Urban Phenomenon? 149.

130 GAA, Graven en hertogen van Gelre, graven van Zutphen, 0001, Rekeningen van de overste rentmeester Arnold van Ghoor, 1438–1450, no. 2997, fo. 168v [AO].

131 The kinds of institutional interaction discussed more broadly in Ogilvie, *Controlling Contagion*. Some scholars have suggested that economic health mattered more than public health, for example: Bourgois, Les Provinces Unies, 201. This is likely an exaggeration since both economic and public (collective) health were intrinsic components of the maintenance of the common good.

132 De Vries, *Barges*, 317.

133 Agresta, From Purification.

134 Coomans, *Community*, 219.

135 Coomans, Food Offenders, 139.

136 Gooskens, Pestepidemieën, 42.

137 Auwerda-Berghout, ed., Voorne, 75.

138 For example, at Den Bosch in 1616: Van Zuijlen, ed., *Inventaris*, II, 1228; and refusing beggars and vagabonds at Aalst in 1625: Boterbergh, Burgers, sections 3.6 and 3.7. In 1599, an official announcement by the Antwerp government said it was forbidden to take in anybody from the nearby town of St.-Niklaas on grounds of the *infectie vande peste* that had spread there: Anon., ed., *Gheboden ende uutgheroepen* [27/7/1599].

139 De Brouwer, "De aenclevende sieckte", 6. For the wages conversion: De Vries, An Inquiry, 82–3.

140 Janssens and Van den Branden, De pest, 72. This intervention was not successful as, in the years thereafter, Gierle suffered two of the worst epidemic outbreaks in quick succession—losing a third of their inhabitants in 1624/5 and again in 1636/7.
141 Nijssen, Zo ging dat, 52 [25/5/1624].
142 ZAM, Vrije van Sluis 1584–1796, 7, Stukken betreffende maatregelen tegen besmetting met pest, 1605, 1770–1771, no. 363, fo. 3r [AO].
143 Wiel and Ekamper, Kromme sikkel, 76. Coomans, *Community*, 241.
144 Van Malenstein, Het Sint-Petersgasthuis, 73.
145 't Hart et al., *Gepokt*, 51.
146 Rommes, Plague, 68; Noordegraaf and Valk, *De gave Gods*, 196. More than two-thirds were founded in sixteenth-century France from a sample of 46 pest houses: Murphy, Plague Hospitals and the Provision of Medical Care, 827–8; and on their broader characteristics in early modern France: Murphy, Plague Hospitals and Poor Relief. In England, pest house use takes off from the second half of the sixteenth century, although just over half of the sample of 66 pest houses were founded in the first half of the seventeenth century, and thus show a later chronology: Udale, *The Plague*, 118.
147 For example, at Rotterdam in 1648, a skipper decides to rewrite his testament, instead giving a third of the silver cups that he had kept in the pest house to the institution's personnel: SR, Archieven van de Notarissen te Rotterdam en daarin opgegane gemeenten, 18, no. 4, fo. 10–13 [28/10/1648].
148 Spaans, *Armenzorg*, 156–7.
149 These costs were substantial. A woman overseeing the Onze Lieve Vrouwe hospital at the town of Geraardsbergen, southern Flanders, paid a sum of 70 pounds for medicines because of the *contagieuse sieckte* in 1636, which was also noted in a letter to the governor of Ath: De Vos, *'Onser Liever Vrouwen' hospitaal*, 378.
150 AEA, Sint Elisabeth Gast- of Ziekenhuis te Amersfoort, 1500–1970, 0102, no. 445 [AO].
151 Manuscript found in http://www.cartago.nl/nl/oorkonde/kfh341.xml. Ludeke Jarges was a Groningen woman who died a century earlier in 1469 and left her considerable wealth to religious institutions in the city.
152 An original case for a separate pest house for the city was made even earlier by Jan van Hout, Leiden secretary, in a Poor Report from 1577: Van Asperen, Nothing Else Than Decay, 3.
153 Dröge, De bouwgeschiedenis, 75–82. This delayed construction process might account for the exceptionally severe epidemic outbreaks in Leiden in 1635 and 1655 when considered in a relative perspective: Van Besouw et al., Epidemic Mortality.
154 Wan, Paradox of Isolation. Although not always totally in accordance with this process and chronology. Thus, for example, at Harderwijk, a wooden shed was set up in 1515 on a piece of land outside the town, and divided into two parts, where those suffering from plague and other infectious diseases were treated. Then, later, during the plague outbreak of 1602, the pest house was moved inside the city in the brewery of a nunnery in the Oosterwijk: Penning, Het vroegere pesthuis, 3569. For the view that pest house construction outside the city was largely a seventeenth-century phenomenon: Coomans et al., Plague, 594; but perhaps a slight exaggeration if applied to the whole of the Low Countries.
155 For example, the wooden huts at Herbatte, used to house the plague-infected from Namur: Jacquet-Ladrier, Les épidémies, 132, 134. In villages, these were often set up on local commons, as seen at Hogemierde, Brabant, in 1560: Vera, *...dat men het goed van den ongeboornen niet mag verkoopen*, 81; and at Boxtel, also Brabant, in 1607: Coenen, *Baanderheren*, 117. People were sheltering in

huts on the heaths according to magistrates during a local flickering of disease in Hapert, Hoogeloon, and Casteren: Leuris, De pest, 177. Temporary huts tended to be a more prominent feature of epidemic disease response in smaller towns and villages of Brabant, perhaps linked to the greater number of common pastures and wastes there: Hoppenbrouwers, The Use.

156 De Brouwer, "De aenclevende sieckte", 6.

157 For England, for the two polarities, compare: Udale, *The Plague*, 114–43; Slack, *The Impact*, 277.

158 For example, in the city of Delft: Bonenkampová, Waren "rijke stinkerds" rijk?; and the rural village of Dudzele in coastal Flanders: Dombrecht, "Edel, arm en rijk, maakt de dood gelijk?" 283–6.

159 Vermunt and van der Kallen, *Opgravingen*, 90–9.

160 For a general chronology of these cemeteries increasing importance: Noordegraaf and Valk, *De gave Gods*, 196–200.

161 Van Oerle, *Leiden*, I, 99–104; Curtis, From One Mortality Regime to Another? 134–5.

162 Cipolla, *Cristofano*, 166–70. In sixteenth- and seventeenth-century London, the practice of burying those who had died of plague seemed to go on in and around churches, with the attitude of the urban administration quite ambiguous: Harding, Burial. Higher status burials inside churches were effective revenue streams for these institutions: Jenner, Death, 628.

163 Curtis, From One Mortality Regime to Another? 151.

164 Wiersum, Grafschriften, 7–10.

165 Van Oosten, The Cursed Side, 154. For prohibition: Jenner, Death, 616.

166 Burials having to take place at night or early morning in some localities such as 03:00 to 04:00 and 20:00 to 21:00 in Namur, where fewer people were out: Jacquet-Ladrier, Les épidémies, 126; while in others, burials of the infected were only possible in certain daylight hours, and thus infringements were observable: Curtis, Preserving, 285; Van Asseldonk, *Veghel*, 307. At the St. Pieters Church during epidemics in seventeenth-century Leiden, children were buried in the morning and adults in the afternoon: ELO, Stadsarchief van Leiden, (1253) 1574–1816 (1897), 0501A, no. 1319, fo. 167v–76v.

167 Van den Heuvel, ed., Crimineel klachtboek, 295 [19/5/1625].

168 Wassink, *Van stad en buitenie*, 259; Rommes, Plague, 57–8.

169 Van der Weyde, Over begraafplaatsen, 101.

170 As at the cemetery of the Utrecht Buurkerk in the plague of 1664 where 200 coffins were at one point waiting to be buried: Wiersma, Observaties, 2620; and the lack of space noted in the burial registers at the Naarden cemetery in 1656: Anon., ed., Naarden, 35; and in certain Rotterdam cemeteries during the 1624 outbreak: Moquette, Pestepidemieën, 17–18.

171 As argued for England: Harding, *The Dead*, 55, 67; Houlbrooke, *Death*, 334–5.

172 Why similar environments did not lead to the same disease outcomes, or why not everyone in a household got sick or died, for example: 't Hart, *Utrecht*, 24.

173 For the tree observation: Van Asseldonk, *Veghel*, 305. For the negative sentiment towards Catholics by Reverend Hanewinckel: Hamans, The Observations, 233. Hanewinckel also referred to the "dirty way of life" (*morsige levenswijze*) in the same communities that likely led to sickness, especially within the houses of farmers: Van Asseldonk, *Veghel*, 307.

174 Van Asseldonk, ed., Regesten, fo. 65v–6v [6/8/1808].

175 Mathijsen, *De gemaskerde eeuw*, 117. See, for example, the wine vinegar (*wijnazijn*) used as a recipe against *pest* in 1665 in the Drenthe village of Dwingeloo: DAA, Huisarchief Batinge, 0617, Recepten tegen de pest, het koliek en het maagkoliek, no. 340 [AO].

176 Valenti, From Plague.
177 Dommerholt, "O heere".
178 Anon., ed., Gebed; Bruyndonckx, *Een cultuurgeschiedenis*, 66–7.
179 Vanden Bossche, Een pest-antifoon.
180 Hamlin, "Cholera Forcing".
181 De Zwaan, *Zorg*, 132–8.
182 For the older disagreements: Visscher, De Rotterdamse zorg; 't Hart, *Utrecht*, 250–1.
183 For the medieval Low Countries: Coomans, *Community*, 25, 293; for nineteenth-century England, Italy, and northern Germany: Pelling, Epidemics; Valenti, From Plague; Evans, Epidemics, 143–4; Kappner, Did Cholera "Force" the Reform?
184 Two valuable recent MA theses on this subject: Bruyndonckx, *Een cultuurgeschiedenis*, 78–89; Tanis, *An Epidemic*, 59. The findings of Tanis' thesis were recently condensed into Tanis, "To Think Seriously".
185 Van Oosten, The "Great Sanitary Awakening", 111.
186 Only three out of 288 plague tracts linked plague and poverty in northern and central Italy in the period 1348–1500 and just four from 1500 up to the San Carlo Plagues of 1575: Cohn, *Cultures*, 208–11. A chronology supported by Henderson, Charity, 78; Pullan, Plague, 106–7. References to the poor in French plague treatises begin around the mid-sixteenth century: Jones, *From Diseased Bodies*, 315. For the outbreak narrative concept, previously applied to the twentieth century, but perhaps of deeper temporal significance: Wald, *Contagious*.
187 Van Lieburg, Revisiting.
188 Coomans, *Community*, 25; Geltner, *Roads*, 27–31.
189 As observed by Cohn, *Cultures*, 294.

3 The many faces of epidemic disease

Severity, spread, seasonality, and selectivity

The concerns of this chapter appear straightforward—how many and what kinds of people died during epidemics in the Low Countries between the fourteenth and the nineteenth centuries?[1] Simple questions on the surface, however, do not necessarily make for straightforward answers—mainly because for most of the period in question we lack the kinds of modern population censuses that allow us to pinpoint the number of people at risk in any one place over time. Instead, we often must make do with proxies for mortality impact, especially for the Middle Ages, and even for the early modern period with the emergence of series of standardisable burial registers across large areas (although not entirely standardised, as explained in this chapter), we must employ methodologies where relative change in the number of deaths compared to an estimated backward-looking norm is often our main indicator for severity of an outbreak. Meanwhile, deaths in institutions do sometimes provide us with better insights into more precise populations at risk, and how many of the sick and infected end up dying—and yet we then have a different problem in that we must question to what extent these institutional environments such as monasteries, nunneries, hospitals, orphanages, and pest houses, are representative of trends within wider society. Of course, scholars have been dealing with these issues presented within preindustrial historical demography for decades, and despite these challenges, have still developed insightful findings as the basis behind important narratives and debates in social and economic history. When considering the mortality impact of epidemics in Europe, most scholarly discussion has been on the classic historical dimensions of change over time and differences across geographical regions.

Scholarship over the past 20 years has tended to push up the mortality estimates from the impact of the Black Death of the mid-fourteenth century, with many accepting the ballpark figures of 30 to 50 per cent death rates in the places it affected.[2] Still, however, there are some nuances to this. Although some have still described the Black Death as a "universal killer" or an "indiscriminate catastrophic event", other scholars tend to suggest that even this severe outbreak had some level of selection in line with pre-existing health frailties which were dictated by differences across socio-economic statuses, demographics, and lifestyles within communities.[3] Moreover, while we have become a little less assertive in suggesting that certain parts of

DOI: 10.4324/9781003694908-3

Europe *completely* escaped the Black Death, more accepted is the notion that mortality rates might have varied across different regions and from locality to locality.[4] Some areas were badly hit by the Black Death, while other areas found that *pestis secunda* (or another outbreak) was more severe.[5] Of course, this makes sense given the multiplicity of social, economic, health, climate, environmental, and genetic factors at play and difficult to untangle. Even the basic chronology and direction of spread is now subject to debate.[6] Nevertheless, the empirical basis behind differences in Black Death mortality across localities is still weak, largely due to the small quantities of evidence and non-comparable source base across areas. Figures plucked out of the air by contemporary observers should be taken with healthy amounts of scepticism, although scholars still use them, sometimes to exploit supposed "variation" in mortality as an explanatory variable for other developments, and more systematic, quantitative mortality evidence for the Black Death, while highly valuable (and rare), has obvious limitations and idiosyncrasies, and is often restricted to certain restricted geographical areas.[7]

Another area in which there is discussion about epidemic mortality is in perceived changes over time after the Black Death. According to some scholars, recurring plagues start to decline in mortality effect, and this is associated with changes in the profile of the disease. Indeed, recurring plague epidemics, especially from the early fifteenth century, are said to have been more focused and selective by hitting a particular profile of places and people. These changes were manifested in a disease that became an affliction of the poor and one that became increasingly focused on urban environments.[8] This perhaps helped support a view that there were clear differences between high-mortality late-medieval demographic regimes which gave way to a lower pressure regime in the transition to the early modern period—an issue elaborated upon in greater length later in this chapter.

Of course, some issues remain with these kinds of views. To begin with, it is still not clear to what extent the link between plague and poverty was "real", societal (elite) perception not grounded in empirical reality, or a rhetorical and moralising narrative. The fact that contemporaries were drawing links is not enough, as this can merely say something about changing attitudes to the poor in general or simply noticing things through experience—i.e., links that were already there. We are not helped by the fact that our mortality information for late-medieval epidemics is improving but still limited, and then a fine-grained analysis of the socio-economic profile of epidemic victims over time is entirely missing.[9] At best, the link between epidemics such as plague and poverty tends to be based on geographical association within poor neighbourhoods.[10] The idea that diseases such as plague became urban afflictions seems to be entirely disproven now, given recent findings on the wide rural spread continuing into the sixteenth and seventeenth centuries in both southern and northern Europe—and was a persistent narrative likely only based on a limited selection of mortality figures for restricted parts of early modern England.[11] The notion of plagues slowly and incrementally becoming less virulent over time in a linear progression was questioned by the findings from outbreaks in 1630 and 1656–8 in northern Italy and the Kingdom of Naples respectively—where it has even been suggested that these might have been the most severe outbreaks in any part of Europe since the Black Death.[12] Still, however, the lack of mortality evidence across long temporal spans *from the exact same type of source material* has limited our capacity to say anything definitive about whether epidemic disease became more or less virulent between the Middle Ages and the early modern period.

As well as debates over the characteristics of epidemic disease, scholars have also debated the causes and the drivers of their emergence, spread, and features. For a long time, production, trade, commerce, and water courses were seen as important economic drivers of preindustrial plagues—although the links are not consistent.[13] In some cases, we might see breakdowns in agricultural production as the precursors to harvest failure and famine-induced epidemic diseases, and yet other diseases such as plague do not appear to be automatically associated with food crises.[14] If anything, it seems as though plague outbreaks might be more connected to the presence of grain rather than absence—attracting vectors such as rats, and hence regaining a prominent position in recent literature on the long-distance transmission of the Black Death.[15] Elsewhere, for the early modern period, it is often suggested that poverty is a great underlying driver of epidemic disease—unsurprising—but with little indication of exactly which facets of poverty are causally responsible, especially specifically for plague, where the mechanisms of transmission have been persistently debated without resolution.[16] For the nineteenth century, the link between poverty and epidemics is better established—not least because the information exists to better demonstrate socioeconomic selectivity of mortality effect—although even there the connection is not inevitable, and especially in those cases where rich and poor alike could not avoid sharing communal assets such as water.

Finally, it has recently become fashionable to suggest that many epidemic diseases such as plague were driven by the dynamics of changing climatic conditions—which may make sense given that within individual years, epidemic mortality tends to respond to the seasonal patterns of precipitation and temperature.[17] Advances in historical climatology will help, but only if methods and approaches in historical epidemiology keep up—difficult given that the pool of historical climate evidence is ever expanding while information on disease mortality is more restricted and is "harder won" from documentary archives.[18] Still, however, the movement of and interaction between people still seems the most convincing driver of epidemic disease spread. For example, in the broader global Black Death literature, a prominent place is now reserved for violent expansion and military exploits of the Mongol Empire—something that appears consistent despite strong disputes in other domains such as the timing, chronology, and origins of the Second Plague Pandemic.[19] For the early modern period, scholars have demonstrated clear spatial and temporal links between military occupation, the presence of soldiers, and epidemic mortality—even if the direction of disease spread still depended on interaction with other variables.[20] Even this, however, is not enough. Movement—whether through trade, climate-related disruption, warfare, religious pilgrimage, seasonal work, or transhumance and nomadism—is supported or restricted by an institutional framework of markets, states, collectives, family networks, and household structures which strongly differ over time and space.[21] Thus, we have initial insights into how these institutions work in practice and interact with one another—but whether we can quantify institutional effect on epidemic mortality remains to be seen.

Quantifying late-medieval epidemic mortality impact

Although we have rough indicators of "difficult years" in the Low Countries going back to the late Carolingian period, the evidence to quantify the impact of epidemic diseases prior to the Black Death is very small, and before the Great Famine of 1315–17 *almost* non-existent.[22] One of the exceptional sources of information we have comes from Arras, the most significant town in the southernmost County of Artois, through a necrology for a fraternity for entertainers (*jongleurs*) and loosely defined citizens (*bourgeoisie*), and although a printed edition has been made available and other scholars have mentioned mortality for specific years through the source, it is surprising that it has not to my knowledge been put into a long-run series yet—especially given that it provides indicators for deaths that are both early and unbroken across the period 1194–1357.[23]

The necrology recorded deaths of all members who are explicitly named and, as far as can be discerned indirectly, the members' household relatives who are not often explicitly named and sometimes indirectly estimated through the higher fixed fees.[24] From Figure 3.1, we can see that the main mortality spikes in this period were in 1206, 1257, 1272, 1316, and 1340. Interestingly, the Black Death of 1349–51 did not show up in this series—an issue addressed a little bit further on in the book. Perhaps even more interesting was that the most significant clear spike in deaths among members and their families was in 1272—noted loosely as a vague crisis year in other parts of western Europe, but obviously not as entrenched in medievalists' collective knowledge as the Great Famine of 1315–17, or even the 1257/8 famines occurring around the same time as, though not necessarily caused by, the eruption of the Samalas volcano in Indonesia.[25] A mortality deviation of almost 250 per cent corresponds to almost a three and a half times increase in deaths above the normal trend—hence, if we were to accept an ordinary annual death rate of perhaps three per cent in this sample, we would be looking at around ten per cent of the fraternity dying. This normal death rate is very loose, as we do not know whether deaths associated with institutions such as this fraternity reflected the general situation within Arras as a whole—indeed, if we assume that fraternity members were of a higher status than non-fraternity members, then the overall death rate for the town was

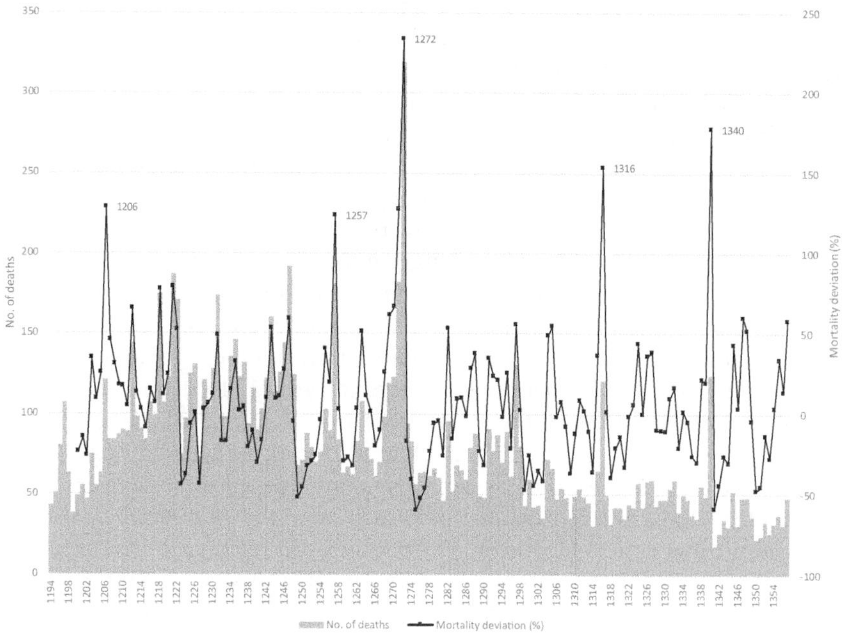

Figure 3.1 Deaths at the Arras fraternity for *jongleurs* and the *bourgeoisie*, 1194–1357

Source: Own database calculated from Berger, ed., *Le nécrologe*, II, 103–80. The mortality deviation is calculated relative to a backward-looking moving average of the previous five years (to minimise the impact of epidemic-induced change to population structure) but skipping a year and removing highest and lowest values to minimise the impact of exceptional or unusual mortality in calculating the average level.

likely higher. One thing that is notable from Figure 3.1 is that 1272 seemed to represent an important structural change for the fraternity membership in general—before 1272, the annual deaths of members and associates was over 100 while after 1272 this was closer to 50. Elsewhere in the southern Low Countries, 1272 has been identified as an epidemic year—in Mechelen, for example, it was the first identified year where a procession took place to deliver the community from sickness.[26]

Back-to-back harvest failures connected to the prolonged abnormal amounts of rain, wind, and low summer temperatures in the North Sea area and leading to famine conditions in the years 1315–17 likely led to the outbreaks of various diseases alongside starvation.[27] The impression created so far is that the southern parts of the Low Countries suffered greatly during this famine as one of the worst afflicted areas of western Europe.[28] We have less information for the north, although we do have chroniclers testifying to the extent of hunger and the simultaneous widespread deaths of cattle through pestilence in select parts of Holland and Brabant.[29] The effects of the famine in Zeeland remained in the collective consciousness, as the severity was mentioned by chroniclers centuries down the line.[30] Even within the southern Low Countries, however, the impact is suggested to also have differed across sub-regions—citing the importance of different arrangements of property rights and interactions between large landowners and smaller producers.[31] At Cambrai, at least, wealthier ecclesiastical institutions still maintained grain stocks during the period 1315–17, while the rural poor simply did not have enough to pay—a version of Amartya Sen's entitlements theory in practice, with the idea that food is there but some people cannot access it.[32]

Nevertheless, we have very few direct indicators of mortality impact for the Great Famine of 1315–17, while even broad indicators for demographic contraction are very low resolution and cannot really be separated from other simultaneous processes such as abandonment, desertion, and contracting rates of fertility.[33] As mentioned above, the year 1316 definitively stands out as a mortality spike in the Arras fraternity (Figure 3.1), although it is somewhat surprising, given the prevailing notion of its severe impact in the southern Low Countries, that the spike was only the third most severe in the period 1194–1357 and represented not much more than a doubling of deaths over the normal rate.[34] However, in line with the regional differences suggested above, indicators seem more severe for other places, even if the sample sizes are very small. At the coastal town of Calais in 1318, based on difficulties in composing its magistrate of 52 members, it has been suggested that mortality rates might have been around a quarter to a third, while further inland in Douai five out of 12 aldermen perished (41.7 per cent).[35] Again, these are estimates from more privileged segments of society. Further north, in Holland, all we have is a reference to the deaths of three abbots in a row in the monastery of Rijnsburg, 7 kilometres from Leiden, in 1316.[36]

Less widely known is that in the first half of the fourteenth century, between the Great Famine and the Black Death, there were also several other significant mortality crises. The problem, however, is that we have little indication of how to quantify their severity, and little definitive information on exactly what caused them. According to one work on the deaths of annuitants from Lille in the period 1328–69, two quite significant mortality spikes were discernible in 1333 and 1340, though the diseases involved are unclear—except they were largely products of harvest failures in the first case and a combination of famine and surges in fighting in the major theatres of war across Artois and Flanders in the second case.[37] Other findings from wills and necrology data suggest only modest mortality in 1332/3 for Douai, although 1340 seems to have been a significant event.[38] As seen from Figure 3.1, at Arras, 1340 represented the second most severe mortality spike across the period 1194–1257—exceeding the Great Famine. Estimates based on farmers returning their rents to the St. Julien hospital at Cambrai even suggest a mortality rate of one third—although again we should be cautious with the small sample and indirect nature of the evidence.[39]

As mentioned in the introduction, the former view that the Black Death did not occur in the Low Countries has long since been revised.[40] Nevertheless, we can make two qualifiers. First, the only convincing quantitative information we have on the mortality impact of the Black Death in the northern parts of the Low Countries comes from a necrology produced by the St. Lebuinus church of Deventer.[41] In this institution, 52 deaths were recorded in 1350 (48 of which came in June, July, and August), while in the entire 20 years prior to 1350 only 45 deaths had been recorded, and in the entire 20 years after 1350 only 54 deaths had been recorded. If an ordinary death rate in a confined religious institution was around two or three per cent then a 20-fold increase in annual deaths might reflect a death rate of 50 per cent.[42] The problem is that beyond descriptions of widespread death leading to problems such as abandoned and uncultivated land in rural areas close to Zwolle and Utrecht, our quantitative insights for the north remain limited.[43] Overall, we have more evidence of the Black Death impact in the northern Low Countries for areas around the central inland towns of Utrecht, Zwolle, and Deventer—the last two mentioned places both Hansa towns—which is interesting in that it might give further credence to a view recently proposed that the Black Death had multiple chains of transmission across Europe, including a route via northern Hanseatic trading towns separate to that via Sicily and the Mediterranean.[44]

Second, while the Black Death definitively occurred in the southern parts of the Low Countries, it remains unclear to what extent this was severe in a relative sense compared to other places where the Black Death struck.[45] Contemporary observers noted impacts such as fields going uncultivated for lack of workers, and city ordinances tried to encourage immediate burial of the dead in Tournai, for example—indicative of severity—but, of course, difficult to quantify and compare.[46] Indeed, while Black Death mortality has been revised upwards in more recent years, perhaps in the worst cases killing one in two people, research using other kinds of evidence and methods such as grain pollen analysis has also suggested that this 50 per cent death rate did not apply everywhere across Europe.[47] Some parts of the Low Countries might fit more with the second scenario. For example, in one paper it was stated of the Black Death in the Low Countries that the "losses were not as high as the 25 to 40 per cent [of the population] assumed for England and Italy".[48] Perhaps supporting that assessment, we might point to the relative absence of abandoned rural settlements seen in the (southern) Low Countries after the mid-point of the fourteenth century.[49] And as mentioned above, Figure 3.1 shows no kind of mortality crisis showing up in the necrology figures for the fraternity of Arras in the years 1349–51.[50] Combined evidence from wills and funeral palls in nearby Douai similarly pointed to modest or minimal effects of the Black Death.[51]

Nevertheless, some older, and some more recent work, cross-referencing fragmentary information and creating proxies for mortality from hospitals, orphanages, and poor tables for different cities such as Bruges, Ghent, and Lille tend to point to considerable Black Death mortality—also in the rural surroundings—but with the cautious and necessary qualification that any estimates are rough, based on small samples, and taken from difficult-to-interpret sources.[52] Recent work with mortmain records from the County of Hainaut, furthermore, has raised our impression of Black Death mortality to much higher than hitherto suggested, although still does not definitively provide a death rate comparable to other areas, and moreover, does not show the Black Death to be more severe than some of the later epidemics seen in the fourteenth and fifteenth centuries.[53] In the end, it is plausible that Black Death mortality in the more urbanised parts of the Low Countries might have been obscured to some extent by rapid demographic recovery through rural-to-urban migration, where barriers to migration such as coercive extra-economic obligations were not as prominent in many parts of the Low Countries compared to England or northern France, and accordingly, a more accurate picture of Black Death mortality might come from any estimates we can obtain from the countryside—if we can separate out deaths from outward migration.[54]

More concretely, we can say that, thanks to more serial forms of evidence that appear after the Black Death, the recurring epidemics seen in the second half of the fourteenth century and the fifteenth century were frequent and often severe across the Low Countries—and perhaps also contributing to a severe mortality regime of epidemic disease when considered in relative western European perspective.[55] Recent innovative evidence from the felling dates of construction timbers has shown that, from mid-to-later phases of the fourteenth century and first half of the fifteenth century, building projects, whether for domestic housing or public institutions, slowed and almost ceased in cities such as Bruges.[56] Indeed, repeat severe outbreaks make sense given that the Low Countries were an important theatre of medieval warfare, commercialisation and mobility were high, and cities and rural areas were closely integrated, although perhaps it is surprising in light of the demographic recovery of certain parts of the Low Countries—especially in phases of the fifteenth century.[57] The mortmain records suggested that the most severe outbreaks in Hainaut occurred during the *pestis secunda* of 1359–61, the plague of 1400/1, and 1439/40, which was likely a combination of plague and famine-related fevers.[58] In other places, such as Ghent or Leiden, emphasis has been on the third outbreak of 1368/9.[59] Compared to recent late-medieval mortality data from places such as Catalonia, the echo-epidemics of the late fourteenth and fifteenth centuries in the Low Countries were often much more severe.[60] More precision than that, however, cannot be achieved, as several methodological limitations remain with relevant sources such as the mortmain. Lack of information on the population at risk is a challenge that almost no medieval demographic source can overcome.[61] But more than that, it is certain that as a death duty payable to a territorial lord, the mortmain assessment applied to a very restricted sub-sample—perhaps only roughly 10 to 16 per cent of the population of the County of Hainaut.[62] Furthermore, as well as some fuzziness in timing of the assessment, as such a detested inheritance tax would have been widely resisted and hard to collect across dispersed towns and villages, it is unclear to what extent localities subject to the mortmain administration remained wholly consistent over time.[63]

One way to deal with the consistency problem to a certain extent is to use serial indicators or proxies for deaths from isolated institutions within individual localities. This information is not always presented in the same form, however, and medievalists must creatively search for this in difficult-to-interpret manuscripts.[64] Below I give a tangible insight into the distinct kinds of information that we have in the sources. For example, we have registers of coffins bought and graves dug by institutions such as the St. Catharina hospital in Leiden from 1392.[65] As seen from Figure 3.2, these figures are discerned from scouring the whole register for one number for each year and are located in amongst other irrelevant (for our purposes) information. Alternatively, we also have lists of deceased members of the Illustrious Brotherhood of Our Blessed Lady from 1381 at Den Bosch, a

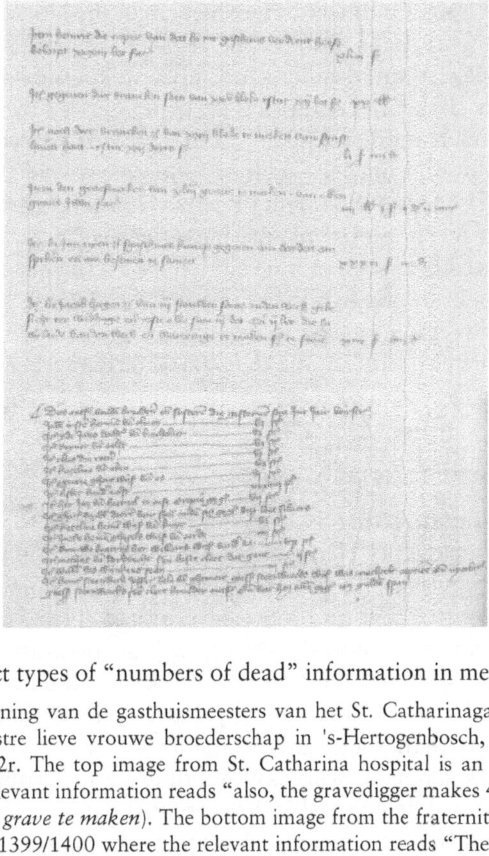

Figure 3.2 Distinct types of "numbers of dead" information in medieval sources

Sources: ELO, Rekening van de gasthuismeesters van het St. Catharinagasthuis, 334, no. 31, fo. 27r; BHIC, Illustre lieve vrouwe broederschap in 's-Hertogenbosch, (1291) 1318–2005, 1232, no. 117, fo. 2r. The top image from St. Catharina hospital is an entry from the year 1420/1 where the relevant information reads "also, the gravedigger makes 43 graves" (*Item den graefmaker van xliii grave te maken*). The bottom image from the fraternity at Den Bosch is an entry from the year 1399/1400 where the relevant information reads "These are the receipts of the brothers and sisters who died in the previous year" (*Dits ontfangst vanden bruederen en susteren die gestorven sijn int jair voirsch*).

religious fraternity founded in 1318.[66] Instead, this information is based on counting numbers of individual names per year.

While we can be more confident about temporal consistency, we lose something in representativeness—that is to say, confined ecclesiastical institutions might have displayed different mortality characteristics, both in normal and epidemic times, compared to society at large. That is why one of the most useful recent findings comes from my own large database of bells tolled and graves dug for burials of ordinary inhabitants at the St. Bavo church in the city of Haarlem, Holland.[67] Although only beginning in 1412 and containing gaps for some years, the source provides a large indicator of annual deaths (114 per year in an entire dataset of 10,360 deaths), covers deaths of men and women, and represented anything from a third to a half of all deaths occurring in the city in the period 1412–1547.[68] Corroborated by a useful death register connected to Haarlem's beguinage, the source strongly confirmed the exceptionally severe nature of the 1439/40 epidemic outbreak.[69] Furthermore, and supporting other work conducted on the life expectancies of nuns within St. Agnes nunnery at Gorinchem in the late Middle Ages,[70] the Haarlem *klok en graf* (bells and graves) register suggested that while 1439 represented the biggest and deadliest mortality spike, the final quarter of the fifteenth and early sixteenth centuries were characterised by smaller epidemic outbreaks, but much more frequently and repeatedly occurring, and connected to hardships and burdens such as food crises, warfare, and declining living standards.[71] More fundamentally, the Haarlem evidence shows that recent statements in big global plague narratives such as "Holland missed, or was little affected by, seven of nine epidemics [in the fifteenth century]" to be absolutely false.[72] In fact, while the impact of the Black Death in Holland is still unclear, the region seemed to experience the same kind of harsh late-medieval epidemic mortality regime that characterised other parts of the Low Countries.

Different preindustrial mortality regimes

One important question that is difficult to answer is to what extent the characteristics of epidemics changed over time in the Low Countries. In the wider literature, it was often assumed that medieval epidemics in western Europe were more frequent and more severe than those experienced in the early modern period—a contrast between a high pressure and a low pressure demographic system.[73] In an early work by Hatcher for England, it was stated that "by the 1530s contemporaries tell us that the times were less disease-ridden than they had been hitherto".[74] Even the *Cambridge Population Group* scholars, who saw nuptiality and fertility as the driving forces of preindustrial demographic development, still recognised a basic distinction between different mortality characteristics, stating for England that "the violent and frequent upsurges in the numbers of deaths recorded before 1565 look as if they might be the last throes of a late-medieval regime of widespread epidemic mortality".[75] This fits well with related narratives that epidemic diseases such as plague were changing over time—becoming more geographically restricted in spread,[76] or becoming more of a focused disease on the poor rather than a universal killer.[77] Not everyone has supported this clear movement from a sickly and crisis-ridden Middle Ages to a more salubrious early modern period, however. Some literature has instead shown strong temporal differences in epidemic mortality characteristics even within the confines of the late-medieval period,[78] and some have even suggested that life expectancies for certain sectors of the population in western Europe, driven by the weakening effects of recurring diseases, decreased rather than increased after 1500.[79] This last-mentioned interpretation would seem more appropriate for places such as Holland where it has been suggested that living standards for a large proportion of the population declined during the so-called "Dutch Golden Age".[80]

The issue of long-term dynamics and characteristics of preindustrial epidemics has been difficult to resolve because the source material needed for systematic analysis is often lacking. Very rarely have historical demographers been able to show a serial indicator for mortality across the medieval and early modern periods using the same type of source and still retain a large sample size.[81] Those that have tried to compare periods have tended to use very different types of material.[82] It is fortunate then that recent work with the accounts of the St. Bavo church at Haarlem has furthered our knowledge in this regard.[83] Indeed, the register of bells tolled and graves dug in the period 1412–1547 can be combined with a Haarlem burial record from 1598 onwards that is organised and structured in the same format and style—and importantly distinguishes between burials in the Grote Kerk (St. Bavo) and other institutions (such as the Nieuwe Kerk and St. Jans), and then burials in the church and the cemetery.

What Figure 3.3 shows below is that major plagues of the seventeenth century such as in 1624/5 and 1636, for example, do not appear to be as severe as the most significant epidemics seen in the same city of Haarlem in the fifteenth century—and nowhere near the worst outbreak of 1439. Comparable trends have been found in recent bioarchaeological approaches that can say something about respiratory health—respiratory disease prevalence in samples of both urban and rural communities in the northern Low Countries did not increase into the early modern period.[84] The finding from Haarlem would, on the surface at least, run contrary to more recently established revisionist views that medieval cities and towns in the Low Countries were more hygienic than previously supposed.[85] However, we should take on board two things. First, given that a larger St. Bavo cemetery was only constructed from c.1480 onwards in Haarlem, the absence of cemetery deaths in the records (not appearing until the 1660s) means that if it had been possible to include this information, we might have seen a less stark difference in the sizes of the spikes, if we make the reasonable supposition that the cemetery became more important for burials than the church over time. Second, it is by no means a

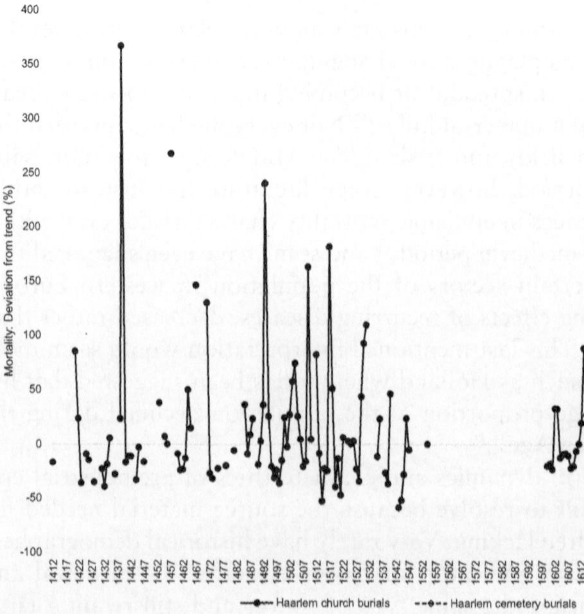

Figure 3.3 Mortality trends from Haarlem, 1412–1699

Source: Curtis, From One Mortality Regime to Another? 151. I express increase over the normal rate of burials as a percentage and calculated it in comparison to a backward-projecting average which uses the same method as Figure 3.1.

given that specifically epidemic mortality was causally connected to hygiene (hygiene might have been linked more closely to the endemic presence of disease) and could have been driven by other unrelated factors. Indeed, it is often presumed implicitly in the scholarship that a lack of hygiene was the most important direct stimulator behind epidemic activity.[86] As the upcoming discussion of the early modern burial registers in the Low Countries suggests, the interaction of warfare, environment, and climate were more important drivers.

Early modern burial registers

In the early modern period, we have sources that provide us with much more information about the demographic effects of epidemic outbreaks in the Low Countries compared to the Middle Ages. The parish registers provide lists of burials which serve as an index for mortality impact, and we also have lists of marriages and baptisms, which serve as indexes for indirect effects of epidemics on nuptiality and fertility. The burial registers, although highly valuable, are not a straightforward source, however. With such a diversity of administrations across the Low Countries, it is understandable that spatial and temporal coverage is neither complete nor consistent. Given that priests completed most registers and stored them in churches, and that the Low Countries were a major theatre of conflict directly involving different religious denominations, it is unsurprising that registers have been lost, damaged, or destroyed.

Some basic trends can be discerned. Over time we have more surviving burial registers. Thus, we have more for the eighteenth century than for the seventeenth century, and there are far fewer for the sixteenth century. Indeed, in most of the southern Low Countries burial registration was only formally required in 1614, although most institutions started later, and some on their own initiative started earlier.[87] Generally we have more burial registers from the southern Netherlands starting earlier (i.e., from the sixteenth century) compared to the north, and as mentioned in Chapter 2, Catholic scribes tended to record more details. Coinciding with density in patterns of settlement in the early modern Low Countries, we have many more burial registers for urbanised areas such as Holland and Flanders, and fewer for more rural and isolated regions such as Luxembourg or Drenthe. Spatial and temporal diversity in coverage was, furthermore, exacerbated by the fact that cities and towns tended to have their burials recorded across several different registers belonging to different parishes and churches, and these of course were not all founded at the same time given that neighbourhoods expanded and new ones were created. Finally, although many of these registers provide long runs of annual numbers of the dead, there are gaps or individual years where some of the months are missing, and the administration and recording process involved with registering burials might have been affected by hardship, too many deaths (for example, during an epidemic), or military activity.[88] We do have indications during epidemics in some records where certain churches were looking for priests on account of the previous ones dying, while in the burial records for the Guelders village of Horssen it was explicitly noted in the years 1673–7 that "nothing is recorded from the year of French invasion" (*In de Franse jaren is niet aengetekend*).[89] Similar administrative issues were seen for marriages and baptisms. So, for example, in Roubaix, today in France, baptisms were entirely postponed for the whole month of June in 1636 on account of the raging plague (*les cérémonies ordinaires des baptêmes n'ont pu estre remplies à cause de la peste*).[90]

Nevertheless, the burial registers record the burials of adult men and women well, even during epidemics, and tend to include the poorest segments of society. Although burials cost money, people could be buried in cheaper sites (outer lying cemeteries, for example) with fewer rituals, and the funeral costs of the destitute were often subsidised by the Poor Table.[91] Even poor recent migrants to a locality were recorded, sometimes anonymously but with their place of origin. Sometimes the documents provide other supplementary information such as occupation or status of the deceased, although not systematically, and usefully, for certain cities such as Leiden or Delft we have information on the exact street in which the deceased lived.

Although we cannot be sure that everyone who died in a locality is found in the burial registers, the proportion (of adults at least) is likely quite high given the precedence that communities across the Low Countries, just as elsewhere in preindustrial Europe, put on burial in consecrated ground—even if this precedence was higher for the Catholic Church than the Dutch Reformed.[92] Furthermore, we also have evidence of burials being mentioned in the registers even when they did not take place in a church or cemetery—at Wolvertem, north of Brussels, some are recorded as taking place in a garden, a pasture, and a small wood.[93]

Nevertheless, there are biases and blind spots that we should be aware of. Migrants who died in a particular city, for example, might have had their corpses transported to and buried in their locality of origin—although this was less likely during periods of epidemic-related restrictions. Burials, furthermore, were not on the very same day of death. Short gaps in time were obviously common, and usefully, sometimes both pieces of information, date of death and burial, are provided. During epidemics, of course, plague ordinances tended to urge rapid disposal of the corpse within one or two days. As well as the deceased going missing, we often have the opposite problem of new people or outsiders turning up in the burial registers of a locality. Although local communities were understandably reluctant to pay the costs of random soldier burials (i.e., the very people inflicting miseries upon them), they do turn up, sometimes in number, in the ordinary church burial registers. Given the connection between warfare and epidemics (as elaborated in this chapter below), this complicates our impression of the mortality effect of certain outbreaks. Nevertheless, still, more soldiers tended to be buried in cemeteries belonging to pest houses and hospitals.[94] Ordinary people were also buried in pest houses and hospitals, understandably increasing in number during epidemic outbreaks, and yet while we sometimes have the burial registers of these institutions, often we do not. Hence, mortality assessments in many localities via the burial registers during epidemics should be seen as absolute minimum estimates.

One point that needs to be emphasised is that children were not always systematically recorded in the burial registers—a fact sometimes explicitly confirmed in the registers themselves.[95] Although appearing in some, other localities did not record the burials of children at all, or perhaps even more problematically, recorded them but unsystematically.[96] Furthermore, even in those localities where children were recorded as buried, it is still often unclear to what extent that only included children that had been baptised. Hence, it is not clear whether those babies dying in childbirth or just after, or as still-born, were listed in the burial registers very often—although they explicitly are marked in some localities. In certain cities, however, we do tend to have more reliable and systematic listing of children, where we can separate out adult and child mortality during epidemics—as shown later in Chapter 3. One problem remains, nonetheless, in the interpretation of child status. Although ages of the deceased are found in select burial registers in the southern Low Countries, this is rare. Accordingly, we are unsure what references to *kind*, *enfant*, and *proles* constitute—and likely this differed over time and especially between localities. In some localities, child status might have been those under the age of 12, and in others under the age of 16 or 18 (often the ages at which individuals became personally responsible for various taxes), and in others it might simply have been a reference to unmarried adults still living in the household of their parents—something which likely had gendered implications as men married later than women, in general.[97]

Epidemic severity

When we look to individual direct documentary references to epidemic mortality in the sixteenth century, many estimates are quite modest. For example, according to Lutheran painter Godevaert van Haecht, 1,700 people (mainly children) died of *de peste* in Antwerp in September 1571—perhaps only two per cent of the population at the time—even if this was (a) likely on top of the ordinary death rate of three to four per cent, and (b) only a part of the year's deaths given that the epidemic did not cease until December.[98] Elsewhere, in one of the Bergh family letters—lords with large landed estates across Guelders—it was noted in 1578 that they could not access their *leenboek* (register of dues owed by feudal subjects) through raging plague in the summer, and by early winter, 150 people had died of plague in the village of Bergh, which was around ten per cent of the inhabitants.[99] Other cases seem more severe, however. Attached to one notarial protocol in the Brabant village of Boxtel in 1557, for example, a note is made on an outbreak of *peste*, the likes of which had never been experienced "in the collective memory". It also mentions, alongside the flight of the Lord of Boxtel and various traders, a death toll of 800 people—which from roughly 2,100 residents would be a death rate of 40 per cent.[100]

This case in itself, however, reveals some of the difficulties with reconstructing epidemic mortality in the Low Countries in the sixteenth century, as 1557 comes off the back of one of the most significant famines in 1555/6.[101] Indeed, epidemic mortality has been shown (especially in the Dutch Republic) to have been spatially and temporally decoupled from famine-related hardships in the seventeenth century, while in the late fifteenth and sixteenth centuries harvest failures, food crises, and epidemics tend to merge much more in both the north and south of the Low Countries.[102] Furthermore, sixteenth-century burial registers are sparse in the Low Countries, especially when compared to parts of England, France, and Italy, and most series are from cities and towns. Pure epidemic mortality becomes much easier to reconstruct in the seventeenth century, when we have better series of burial records and epidemic outbreaks that tend to occur very distinctly and separately from harvest failures or food crises.

I have collected seventeenth-century burials data from 568 localities (cities, towns, villages, and hamlets) in the Low Countries, corresponding to more than 2.5 million individual burials.[103] Only by collecting this information can we (a) escape conclusions drawn from myopic overfocus on particular regions or even individual cities, and (b) correct estimates that seem to come from nowhere.[104] In Figure 3.4, I show burials data crudely put together as deviations over average trends, not weighted by the population of each locality included (because we do not have accurate population estimates for all localities with burials data across all time periods).[105] Epidemics continued to recur quite frequently across the seventeenth century, including after the disappearance of plague after 1670. If we use an oft-cited deviation figure of 50 per cent as a rough indicator of a mortality spike year, and likely to be an epidemic, then we find that more than a quarter of the years in the period 1570–1699 fell into that category—providing more evidence for the anticipated nature of societies' experiences with recurring outbreaks.[106] In Figure 3.5, we see the same information but disaggregated by their status as urban or rural localities. Epidemic spikes in rural localities often were sharper than those from cities and towns—a point I establish more thoroughly via Table 3.1 and the following discussion below.

Compared to the consolidated averages of Figure 3.4, certain individual localities taken in isolation could be much more devastated by epidemic mortality. And, again, one thing that stands out from Table 3.1 is the rural profile of the worst epidemic outbreaks in the seventeenth-century Low Countries.

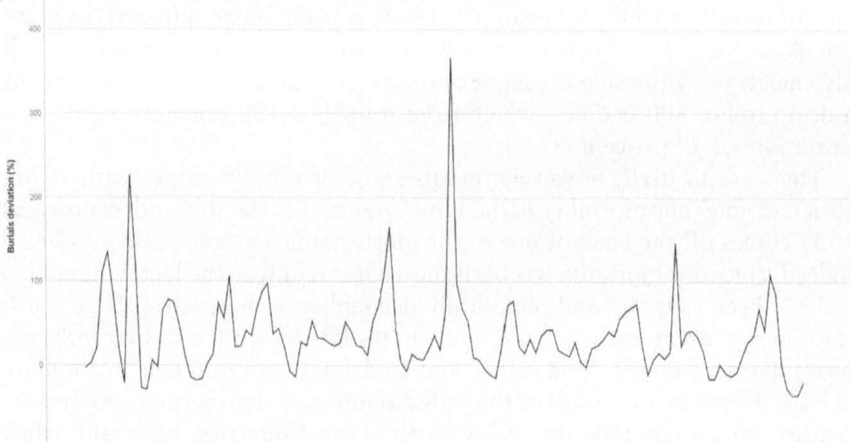

Figure 3.4 Average deviations in burials in the Low Countries, seventeenth century

Sources: Combination of burials data used in Curtis, Was Plague an Exclusively Urban Phenomenon?; Van Besouw and Curtis, Estimating. Full database now accessible at Curtis, ed., Original Burials Data. Only including localities that average six burials or more per year. I express increase over the normal rate of burials as a percentage and calculate it in comparison to a backward-projecting average which uses the same method as Figure 3.1.

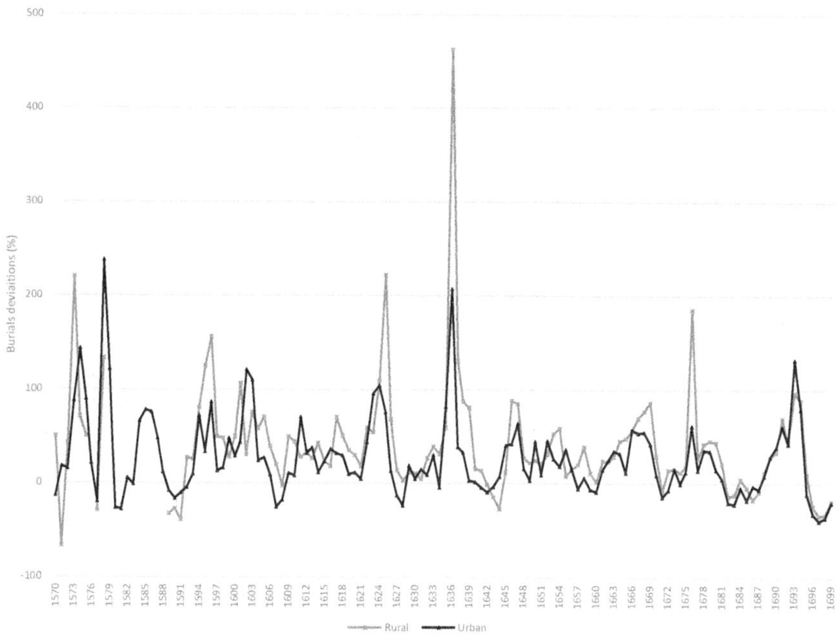

Figure 3.5 Average deviations in burials in the urban and rural Low Countries, seventeenth century

Sources: As in Figure 3.4. I decided urban and rural status of localities through population size, and this is consultable in Curtis, ed., Original Burials Data. I classify places with fewer than 2,000 inhabitants as rural, and 2,000 or more inhabitants as urban, even though understandably there is a wide diversity in classification of cities and towns. Almost all places with formal city rights (*stadsrechten*) inherited from the Middle Ages have more than 2,000 people. An excellent new source for population estimates of localities in the preindustrial Low Countries is Stapel et al., eds., (Re)counting.

Eight out of the ten most severe episodes came from villages, dropping only slightly to seven out of ten when isolating adult mortality. Previously, I have suggested that this might have been through exposure. Cities and towns in the urbanised cores of Holland and Flanders tended to experience higher regularity of epidemic outbreaks, but their regularity also meant that they often, but not always, faced more microbially resistant populations—with populations that were also more migratory.[107] Rural areas with more isolated villages tended to experience fewer but much more destructive outbreaks.[108] My findings are in line with recent palaeo-pathological evidence from the Low Countries, for example, which suggests that diseases connected to respiratory health were not, contrary to what might be expected, more prevalent in the early modern cities.[109] Furthermore, my estimates of rural mortality are likely an absolute minimum because sick and infected people from the countryside often ended up dying in urban institutions such

Table 3.1 Highest local deviations in trend of burials, seventeenth-century Low Countries

Year	*Place*	*Increase over the normal rate of burials (%)*	*Urban / rural*
1636	Ciergnon	7,100	Village
1636	Gierle	4,829	Village
1636	Doncols	2,960	Village
1634	Arcen	2,052	Village
1633	Maastricht (St. Nicolai)	1,860	City
1636	Huy (St. Pierre-en-Outremeuse)	1,833	City
1636	Torgny	1,740	Village
1693	Schriek	1,700	Village
1647	Schriek	1,650	Village
1636	Rochefort	1,548	Village
Only adults			
1636	Ciergnon	4,520	Village
1636	Gierle	2,840	Village
1625	Rijsbergen	1,630	Village
1636	Nijkerk (RK)	1,490	Small town
1636	Lille (BE)	1,390	Village
1666	Kropswolde	1,260	Village
1636	Fressin	1,240	Village
1636	Oudewater	1,210	Small town
1665	Louches	1,200	Village
1636	Huy (St. Pierre-en-Outremeuse)	1,150	City

Sources: Combination of burials data used in Curtis, Was Plague an Exclusively Urban Phenomenon?; Van Besouw and Curtis, Estimating. Full database now accessible at Curtis, ed., Original Burials Data. *RK* is the Catholic Church. BE refers to Belgium to distinguish the Brabant village of Lille from the French city of Lille. The top figures are based on aggregated data that includes both adults and children, hence should be interpreted with caution, although they are more comparable to other places such as northern and central Italy: see, Alfani, Plague. The bottom figures are disaggregated, removing all children from the data, hence are more accurate and precise, although less comparable to other studies.

as hospitals.[110] Interestingly, my findings on the rural severity of epidemics contrast with what has been found in England, where epidemics (in fact, specifically plague outbreaks) were more territorially restricted to cities and towns.[111] A point established more thoroughly in the next section of this chapter is that rural communities bore the harsher side of epidemic outbreaks because the countryside was generally far more exposed to the burdens of warfare in the Low Countries. The contrast with England supports that conclusion further given the low level of direct military presence there in the seventeenth century.

Nevertheless, the sharp nature of an individual year's spike in burials does not always say everything about the severity of an epidemic outbreak. Some outbreaks were damaging because of their persistence over multiple back-to-back years. Indeed, while it might be concluded that the outbreaks of

1624/5 and 1636 were the most severe in terms of deaths consolidated within one or two years, other outbreaks such as that of 1601–4 (sometimes even beginning in 1597/8) and 1666–70 were characterised by the longevity of raised burials over consecutive years. Sometimes this was connected to the presence of different diseases operating at roughly the same time, although not always—plague could linger in the same locality for numerous years.[112] In Tilburg, for example, the Dutch Reformed burial records show a *P* against 240 out of 852 names in 1666 (29.3 per cent), 46 out of 740 in 1667 (6.2 per cent), 253 out of 1036 in 1668 (24.4 per cent), 449 out of 1221 in 1669 (36.8 per cent), and 3 out of 668 in 1670 (0.01 per cent).[113] Put simply, then, severity assessments based on individual yearly spikes tend to understate the true impact in the Low Countries—as this was a place where epidemics did linger across years.

In fact, in line with the previous conclusions about the late-medieval regime of epidemic disease in the Low Countries, early modern epidemic activity in this part of northwest Europe should be seen as very severe—and this can be supported by comparing to other areas using the same kinds of measurements and methodologies. Indeed, back in 2013, it was stated that the plague outbreak of 1630 in northern Italy should be seen as one of the most severe for the whole of the preindustrial period in western Europe—not too far away from the mortality rates of the Black Death of the mid-fourteenth century.[114] In my view, however, the exceptional nature of these findings—in the process supporting a whole new "epidemiological hypothesis" for an early modern economic divergence between southern and northern Europe—appears exaggerated. Indeed, when compared to the most severe plague in the Low Countries, that of 1636, Table 3.2 shows a greater proportion of the localities in the Low Countries had severe outbreaks in 1636 compared

Table 3.2 Most severe plague epidemic compared: Northern/Central Italy (1630) and the Low Countries (1636)

	Northern/Central Italy (1630 plague)		*Low Countries (1636 plague)*	
Increase in burials	*No. localities*	*% of total*	*No. localities*	*% of total*
< 50%	27	25	31	18.1
50–299%	49	45.4	67	39.2
300–899%	22	20.4	55	32.2
900% +	10	9.3	18	10.6
Total	108	100.1	171	100.1

Sources: Localities for northern and central Italy are taken from the map produced in Alfani, Plague, 418; and localities for the Low Countries are consultable at Curtis, ed., Original Burials Data. Any mistakes in the interpretation of Alfani's work are entirely my own. An increase in burials of 300 per cent (a fourfold increase of the average) corresponds to a severe outbreak, and more than 900 per cent (a tenfold increase of the average) corresponds to an exceptionally devastating outbreak—potentially being a 30–40 per cent death rate. For the Low Countries, I only include localities with at least an average of six burials or more per year.

to northern and central Italy in 1630, and a greater proportion also had exceptionally severe outbreaks. The idea of a devastating Italian plague in 1630, significantly worse than other places in Europe, does not seem to hold. Indeed, this point is strengthened further when we consider that 1636 was not the only severe outbreak to afflict the seventeenth-century Low Countries, whereas in northern and central Italy, the 1630 plague was the only major one of the seventeenth century (although there were localised flickers of plague activity, and there were other non-plague epidemics such as typhus in 1651).[115] At best, what we could say is that the core area of the heartland of the Po Valley tended to have many localities with very high plague mortality in 1630, but then the very restricted territorial scope of this exceptional mortality then acts as an argument against the epidemiological hypothesis emphasising severity over a large area and powerful enough to shape macro-economic divergent trends.

Epidemic spread

In a recent article, we integrated two large datasets of adult burials and geo-located war events in the seventeenth-century Low Countries to show the relationship between military activity and civilian mortality with very high statistical precision.[116] We found that on average, localities within 30 kilometres of a war event saw their annual civilian mortality rates rise from roughly three or four per cent to roughly four and a half to six per cent of the population. War was omnipresent in the Low Countries in the seventeenth century, and thus this represented a significant burden of death for the area.

This spatial and temporal association between warfare and raised mortality was also seen during major epidemics—years where high numbers of localities across wide areas simultaneously saw spikes in burials in the Low Countries. Thus, out of the ten largest increases in epidemic-induced adult mortality for a particular locality in a particular year listed in Table 3.1 above, four were in places less than 30 kilometres from a war event and another four were in places 30–60 kilometres from a war event. Furthermore, strong statistically significant lagged mortality effects were seen in places 0–30 kilometres and 30–60 kilometres from war events—what we would describe as "lingering mortality", likely attributable to a spatial ripple effect of disease, occurring within the year after direct military presence of soldiers. Another key finding was that war-induced epidemic mortality was just as prominent in rural areas as it was in the cities and towns—not only contrary to the notion spread by some scholars that war-induced diseases particularly affected cities,[117] but also suggesting that claims for war-driven urbanisation through short-term flight from the countryside in search of safe havens have little support,[118] given the high rural excess mortality and limits placed on people's mobility from the countryside.[119] Of course, the mortality impact on the countryside should make sense given that notwithstanding individual city sieges, it was the rural communities that tended to be most exposed to the incessant burdens of roaming armies.[120] Related to this point, our study suggested that the gradual changes in the scale of warfare, involving larger and more manoeuvrable armies, could likely explain another significant finding—the wider territorial spread and durability (persistence over several years) of mortality effects after 1660, which is curious given the simultaneous disappearance of plague from the Low Countries.[121]

Although it has been suggested that previous scholarship might have been overly dismissive of armies' desire to be proactive with disease prevention, and their incorporation of medical expertise, the very fact that armies were frequently given numerous different instructions on how to maintain sanitary environments also points to the basic fact that military activity inherently brought with it serious public health issues.[122] Not only did soldiers expose civilians to unfamiliar pathogens, often by lodging directly with households, but they were vulnerable to sickness through prolonged exposure to inclement weather; ate fruits, fungi, and berries unsuitable for human consumption; brought and lived close together to other types of animals (sometimes also inadvertently seeding epizootics); received and passed on sexually transmitted diseases; created conditions conducive to the presence of vectors such as lice through unwashed cloth or mosquitoes through their constructed moats and trenches or enforced inundations;[123] had difficulties in effectively disposing of waste; experienced scarcities in access to drinking water; as well as making civilians themselves flee to temporary and less salubrious refuges out of fear, and occasionally deliberately poisoning or soiling water sources of enemies.[124] That is a large number of potential seeding mechanisms for epidemic disease outbreaks.

However, while showing the relationship between warfare and spatial distribution of raised mortality in precise statistical terms, one thing that we did not yet do was visualise this association very clearly. Below, therefore, I present a series of maps for two periods (1632–8 and 1672–8) that can demonstrate this in a more accessible way than the original regression analyses (Figures 3.6 and 3.7). Doing so also allows me to elaborate on two further points in this book. In some epidemics, and especially the most severe episodes of the seventeenth century (such as that of 1635–7), epidemic disease might have been seeded by military activity, but sometimes spread to areas well outside the confines of the direct presence of fighting or soldiers. Furthermore, the combination of the weather conditions and physical environment could also still shape the direction of spread.

In the maps, local deviations over the trend of adult burials are presented as circles of varying size according to magnitudes of deviation (using the same methodology as employed in the "Severity" section above), while transparent diamonds indicate burial series for localities present in the data but lacking a deviation estimate for that particular year. Also mapped is the 30-kilometre catchment area of all war events in the same year and the preceding year—dark grey circles indicate contemporaneous events, lighter circles indicate

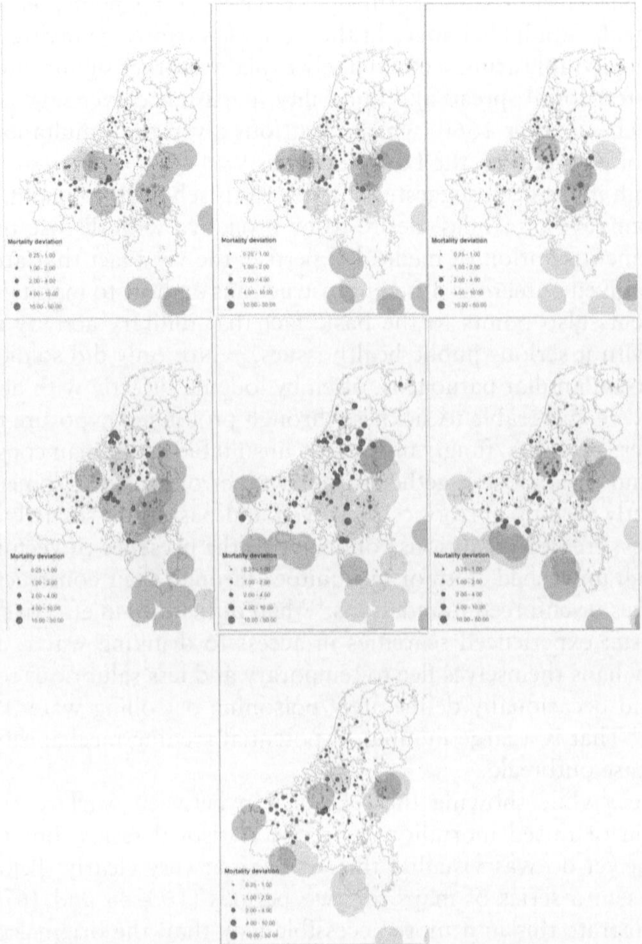

Figure 3.6 Spread of mortality and war activity across the Low Countries, 1632–8

Sources: Data used in Van Besouw and Curtis, Estimating. The combined work of Vincent Schippers and Bram van Besouw has created the maps. Top left is the year 1632; top middle 1633; top right 1634; second row left 1635; second row middle 1636; second row right 1637; bottom 1638.

the war events of the previous year, and their overlap produces the darkest shades.

In the context of the Thirty Years' War, military activity in the Low Countries in 1632–4 was concentrated on the northern strip of Flanders, and especially the Meuse Valley, following a sudden Dutch advance in 1633.[125] France entered the Thirty Years' War in 1635, embarking upon a notoriously vicious joint Franco-Dutch invasion of Spanish Brabant, which was rendered ineffective by disease among soldiers.[126] Clearly, raised mortality in

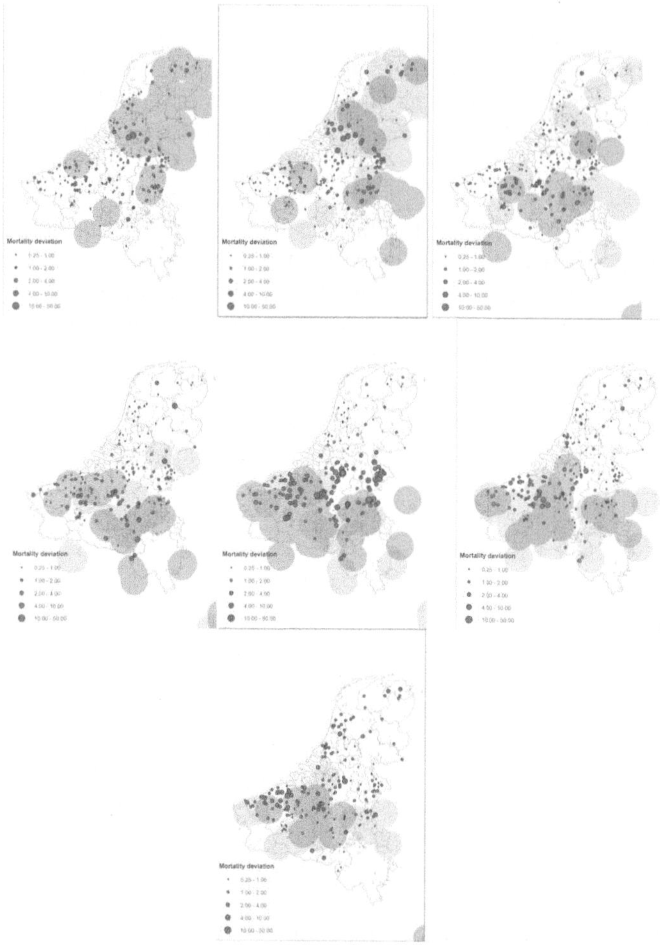

Figure 3.7 Spread of mortality and war activity across the Low Countries, 1672–8

Sources: Data used in Van Besouw and Curtis, Estimating. Maps created through the combined work of Vincent Schippers and Bram van Besouw. Top left is the year 1672; top middle 1673; top right 1674; second row left 1675; second row middle 1676; second row right 1677; bottom 1678.

these years was seen in close association with military activity—contemporaneous effects and occurring a year after war events—with raised mortality in Limburg in 1633 and 1634, epitomised by a severe plague in besieged Maastricht, and in Spanish Brabant in 1635, epitomised by a severe plague in besieged Louvain.[127] However, not all epidemic outbreaks were linked to military activity. Leiden was far removed from any military presence in 1635, and yet saw more than a third of its population succumb to disease—instead connected to a localised perfect storm of contextual economic and environmental factors including mass immigration of workers for the textile industry, pollution from said textile industry, sub-standard housing in hastily built city extensions needed to house textile workers, and increasingly dysfunctional sewers leading to waste being directly discharged into stagnant canals.[128] Similarly, as soon as fighting mostly turned southwards to areas of Artois and Picardy, notwithstanding a continued military presence in Cleves, a general widespread plague exploded in all directions of the Low Countries in 1636—afflicting the far north of Frisia, where a traveller was describing "pestilence at every door", to the far south of Hainaut, where the remaining few residents of the village of Torgny built a new chapel to mark the traumatic depopulation.[129] Spiked mortality in 1636 was even seen on small islands well separated from the mainland such as at Oost-Vlieland.[130] Thus, even if localised diseases could be seeded by military activity creating regionally constrained epidemics, it is clear that the most severe and pervasive epidemics (such as in 1636) had other means to spread beyond these constraints—divorcing themselves from the close military link. Interestingly, when the general plague died down, regional epidemic mortality once again continued to track with fighting—as the worst excesses of the Thirty Years' War turned to the far southern regions of Hainaut and Artois (see, for example, the famous ransacking of the Abbaye Notre-Dame d'Orval), towns such as Valenciennes and Mons experienced their worst mortality spikes,[131] while mortality remained high in 1638 in rural west Brabant in the aftermath of the siege of Breda in 1637.[132]

One of the most significant episodes of warfare that featured in the Low Countries was associated with the "disaster year" (*rampjaar*) of 1672, where the central, eastern, and northern parts of the Dutch Republic were overrun by French armies and their allies from Münster and Cologne.[133] Despite the intensity and scale of the occupation, however, mortality increases were relatively modest and regionally specific. If anything, it was the year thereafter, in 1673, that brought the more significant mortality effects—in line with our formal statistical analysis that highlighted the importance of lagged deaths from military activity.[134] The worst impact was seen in the western part of the Dutch River area linking southeast Holland, the western Betuwe, and western Utrecht, where most of the Dutch attempts to recuperate previous year's military losses occurred, and civilian flight is explicitly noted in the burial records for many places in this area as many towns and villages became exposed at the end of 1672 to French troops as a result of the freezing over of watercourses, making them passable.[135] Thus, for example, one woman from Amsterdam wrote in her diary that her deceased son's "pox and a burning rash" (*kinderpockgen and grootten brant*) was linked to their flight from the town of Woerden during the French occupation.[136] Epidemic mortality also followed closely with military activity further south in Limburg, and in the far north of Groningen and Drenthe with the incursions of the Bishop of Münster troops.[137] In 1674 and 1675, when military action began to converge on the southern Netherlands instead, the mortality increases were generally limited in severity, with higher ones concentrated around localised hotspots.

In contrast to the years 1672–5, the major dysentery outbreak of 1676, emerging in August and peaking in September and October, spread widely into areas far from actual military presence—as previously seen with the 1636 plague.[138] Indeed, this severe epidemic was omnipresent in parts of the southern Netherlands, especially Brabant and Limburg.[139] At the Campine village of Poppel, for example, there is an *uitvaarten* section of the burial records, where simply too many deaths had occurred for funerals to take place.[140] Yet it was also most pronounced in the southern parts of the Dutch Republic, especially Brabant and Upper Guelders, which were virtually the only parts of the Low Countries that had seen little direct military activity in the years up to and including 1676.[141] Another noteworthy feature of this dysentery epidemic was that it did not cross north of the central Meuse and Waal rivers, and exhibited a strong rural character south of them. This points to the interaction of environmental conditions guiding the geographical course of raised mortality with its initial origins in military activity. For this area, extremely hot weather in the summer and a wet autumn were recorded in 1675, which also resulted in grain price spikes, and led by 1676 to the formation of stagnant surface water pools in certain areas.[142] Indeed, in the city at the very heart of this area, Den Bosch, explicit reference was made in the financial accounts to the high waters making most paths and fields untraversable.[143]

Most places saw the height of mortality in September and October, but by November the epidemiç was also very swiftly over or nearly extinguished in the places it affected. While dysentery tended to cause as sharp spikes in deaths as that of plague, it did not linger (in the same localities, at least) for as long. The focus of raised mortality shifted from Brabant, Guelders, and Limburg in a westward direction towards (particularly eastern) Flanders, where military activity was most intense in 1677, and by 1678 was seen most prominently in the western parts of Flanders. Hence, mortality returned, once again, to the more localised coupling with the spread of soldier movements as the burdens on civilians ramped up. In one case from the small east Flanders village of Oostwinkel, it was noted in the burial records that one woman was robbed and killed by French soldiers even after payment of her *sauveguard* (right to free passage).[144] Rents and tithes went widely uncollected in the years 1677/8 across many parts of southwest Brabant and Flanders, and at the small villages of Bogaarden and Sint-Laureins-Berchem, for example, it was said that only a few houses were spared from being burned down.[145] The precise causes of deaths in these years are difficult to discern, but from the burial records we see mentioned an assortment of fevers and stomach and intestinal-related afflictions.

What we can learn from these maps, then, are two things. First, although there was a strong spatial and temporal link between military activity and raised civilian mortality through disease, it was not necessarily inevitable that the more vicious or intense the fighting or occupation, the more significant the mortality effect. Second, although many diseases might have been seeded through the activities of soldiers, some of the most severe epidemics, such as 1636 and 1676, were severe precisely because they were able to spread to other areas far from localised military presences—and potentially due to geographical, topographical, and environmental factors. In the Low Countries, many disease outbreaks had military origins, but those defining epidemics that hit hard and spread wide tended to be characterised by their decoupling from these same military origins.

Epidemic seasonality

The importance of environmental and ecological factors in helping shape the emergence and spread of epidemic outbreaks in the early modern Low Countries is also demonstrated by the information we now have on seasonality of mortality spikes. Within the course of a year, factors such as temperature and precipitation clearly varied, thus creating diverse kinds of pressures for epidemics to emerge. And if short-term weather conditions were important, then logically, long-term climatic movements that created the greater likelihood of diverse kinds of weather conditions should also be considered as important.

Although several types of diseases caused epidemics, which occurred in both cities and in the countryside, recurring and consistent seasonal patterns can be seen from the evidence of burials. Indeed, the dominance of the seasonal patterns is surprising given the variety of conditions and afflictions. In Leiden (Figure 3.8), the three major epidemic outbreaks of the middle segment of the seventeenth century each show a recurring trend where mortality starts to increase in the summer, ramps up in the late summer, reaches a peak in the autumn, before falling in the winter. In the most severe outbreak of 1635, almost one per cent of the city is lost in a matter of two days, when, by October, 200 people die a day. The same could be said for rural areas too. For example, from a sample of 34 localities across Limburg during the dysentery outbreak of 1702/3, leading to an estimated death rate of around six per cent, with localised highs of over 12 per cent, we see in Figure 3.9 deaths ramp up in August and September, reach a plateau in October, and fall in November and December. Various outbreaks in cities, towns, and villages across the seventeenth-century Low Countries have already been shown to have had this same late summer–early autumn profile.[146] Some exceptions were those mortality spikes connected to harvest failures, where the absence of a collected harvest across the autumn created some lagged pressures on communities in the winter—pressures which manifested themselves in the highest rye prices in the early spring.[147]

More research needs to be done on the connection between climate, weather, and seasonality of epidemic mortality at the micro level, and some progress has been made in recent years—confirming a broader northern

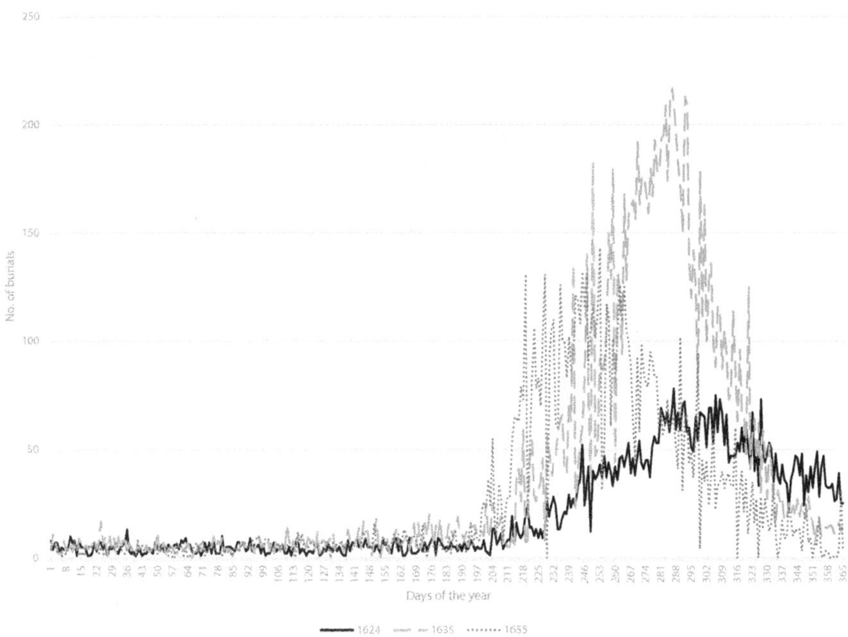

Figure 3.8 Seasonality of burials during three epidemic years in seventeenth-century Leiden

Source: Burials database used in Van Besouw et al., Epidemic Mortality.

European pattern of late summer and autumnal spikes.[148] Explanations, thus far, are speculative, but we could at least suggest that the reasons were diverse and likely dependent on the type of disease. Across the Low Countries, late summer and early autumn created the temperature and humidity supporting vectors such as mosquitoes that caused malaria and agues in the coastal and riverine areas. Particularly arid summers, which if followed by heavy rain, exacerbated the problems of drainage, and created stagnant pools of surface water, leading to dysentery, especially in the countryside in more inland parts. Plague outbreaks tended to have the same seasonal pattern—again temperature and precipitation were likely important in supporting an abundance of vectors such as fleas or hosts such as rats, even if we do not wholly understand the underlying mechanisms at present for this disease—or at least, only in theory rather than in historical context. We should not, however, discount the indirect effects of certain economic, social, and agricultural practices on seasonal epidemic spikes. First, given that the arable harvest tended to be collected from late summer onwards in the Low Countries, such large stores of grain invariably attracted rats—one of the most cited plague hosts.[149] Second, seasonal weather conditions also dictated military campaigns which tended to be restricted to the period between late spring

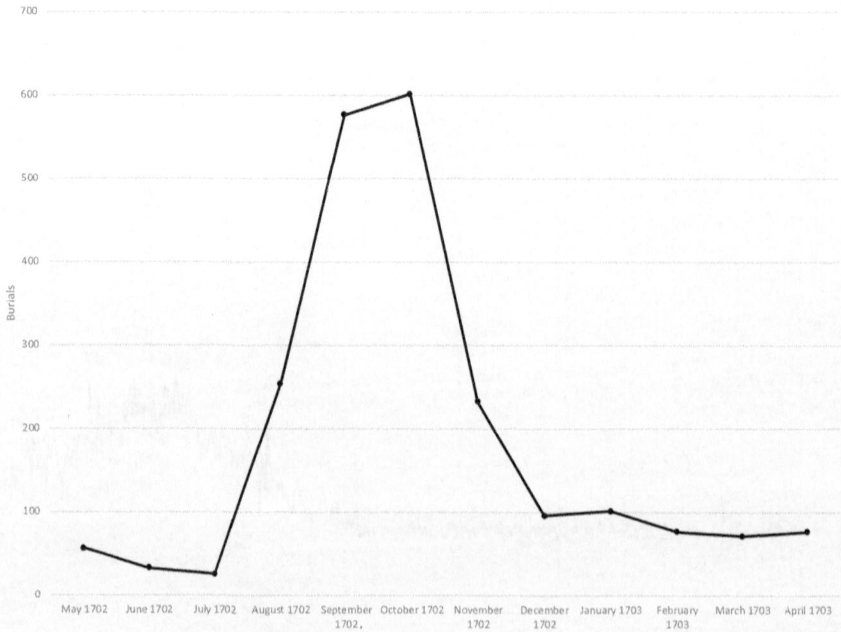

Figure 3.9 Seasonality of burials during a dysentery epidemic of 1702/3 in Limburg

Source: Calculated from data in Dings, Een dysenterie-epidemie, 5. The dataset comprises 34 localities with consistently present burials information. It includes mostly small villages of fewer than 2,000 inhabitants, and three small towns of roughly 5,500 inhabitants (Weert), 5,000 inhabitants (Venlo), and 4,300 inhabitants (Venray).

and autumn due to the adverse weather conditions for movement and support of troops in the winter.[150]

Epidemics and selectivity

One of the reasons why historical demography approaches to epidemic disease have remained focused on the nineteenth and twentieth centuries is that the sources available, such as censuses, allow for a much fuller reconstruction of the population at risk within a particular locality and a clearer differentiation of the statuses of the people involved. Accordingly, during and in the aftermath of COVID-19, we had a surge of interest from scholars arguing that nineteenth- and twentieth-century epidemic outbreaks within cities of the Low Countries tended to disproportionately afflict the poorer neighbourhoods—although the causal factors cited tend to differ from case to case. Smallpox in nineteenth-century Amsterdam, for example, "mirrored and exacerbated existing social inequalities", with the specific effects of wealth—which could also dictate access and desire to vaccinate—and housing quality cited as important factors.[151] Pre-existing health status discrepancies across the wealth spectrum were cited as important in socio-economic selectivity among adult male workers dying of influenza in the Netherlands in 1918–20.[152] Nineteenth-century cholera outbreaks, meanwhile, have shown to be related to socio-economic differences through the plausible spatial differences in provision of water disposal systems.[153]

Early modern burial records have fewer details to allow productive analysis of the impact of inequalities in wealth across communities, although there are some standout series, such as from seventeenth-century Delft and Leiden, that provide specific information on the streets of the deceased—information in the case of Leiden which is importantly highly complete and highly consistent over time.[154] While we have no direct information on the socio-economic status of those listed in these burial registers, this street-level index of mortality has been placed against a spatially detailed geo-located database of housing wealth distribution across Leiden neighbourhoods in the period 1632–68, covering three epidemic outbreaks in 1635, 1655, and 1664. Accordingly, it is possible to say something about the distribution of epidemic-induced mortality across streets—streets which are characterised by clear differences in wealth of the owners and profile of the occupants. As shown in Figure 3.10, in Leiden there was a clear inverse correlation between housing wealth and levels of epidemic mortality, and especially with the most

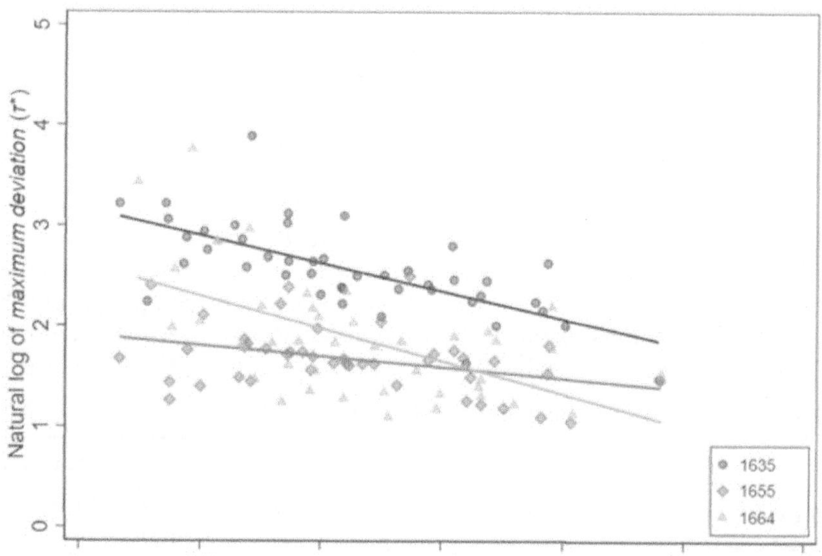

Figure 3.10 Epidemic mortality across Leiden streets of different average house values, seventeenth century

Source: Van Besouw et al., Epidemic Mortality.

severe outbreak of 1635. Whether the wealthy were better able to escape the city during these outbreaks is unclear—although it has been suggested for other cases in other periods such as fifteenth-century Louvain, where those with landed estates were able to retreat to surrounding villages in the hinterlands.[155] More importantly, in many poor areas of cities such as Leiden, low-value houses were technically owned by the rich as investors, but those occupying them were poor tenants, and thus the people that were dying during these outbreaks.[156]

I have also been involved in several studies that suggest that epidemic disease outbreaks tended to lead to proportionally more deaths in adult women compared to adult men, relative to normal or non-epidemic times.[157] Greater confidence in these results is attributed to the fact that these findings have now been established across three different areas of the Low Countries, at three different scales (individual city; regional; macro rural Low Countries), using three different types of sources (none of which clearly under-record women), and three different time periods (1349–1450; 1411–1547; 1600–99).[158] Indeed, in Tables 3.3, 3.4, and 3.5, epidemic disease is found to have presented a heavier burden on the life chances of adult women than men (relative to normal times) in the context of the fourteenth- and fifteenth-century mortmain registers of Hainaut, in the *klok en graf* registers of fifteenth- and sixteenth-century Haarlem, and in the context of a large dataset (the largest sex-disaggregated pool of preindustrial mortality evidence for anywhere in the world) of seventeenth-century rural localities in the church burial records across the whole of the Low Countries. Table 3.3 is important since it shows that the sex-selective impact of epidemic mortality holds even for the Black Death (since it does not deviate from the pattern of all the other recurring plagues)—providing further evidence to help revise the view that this outbreak was a universal killer.

Already, it is well known that during periods of food scarcity and famines, adult women should be able to survive malnutrition better than adult men, with the physiological reasoning being that women have greater amounts of body fat and thus greater reserves—and this is usually something supported by historical demographic data.[159] The same mechanism, however, should hold

Table 3.3 Adult sex ratios in mortality, Hainaut, 1349–1450

	Male	*Female*	*Unknown*	*Total*	*Sex ratio*
All years	11,292	10,559	396	22,247	1.07:1
Plague years	4,332	4,634	247	9,213	0.94:1
Non-plague years	6,960	5,925	149	13,034	1.18:1
Fisher's exact test	p value <0.0001				
Black Death, 1349–51	342	383	140	865	0.89:1
Other recurring plagues	3,990	4,251	107	8,348	0.94:1
Fisher's exact test	p value 0.5352				

Source: Curtis and Roosen, The Sex-Selective Impact, 253.

Table 3.4 Adult sex ratios in mortality, Haarlem, 1411–1547

	Male	*Female*	*Unknown*	*Total*	*Sex ratio*
1421	96	88	5	189	1.09:1
1439	135	158	0	293	0.85:1
1458	121	142	0	263	0.85:1
1467	79	74	0	153	1.07:1
1471	116	120	0	236	0.97:1
1493	95	133	1	229	0.71:1
1503	69	54	3	126	1.28:1
1504	73	63	1	137	1.16:1
1509	114	147	0	261	0.78:1
1512	88	64	0	152	1.38:1
1517	112	120	1	233	0.93:1
1518	56	56	0	112	1:1
1530	79	67	3	149	1.18:1
1531	73	89	0	162	0.82:1
All years	4,421	4,269	66	8,756	1.04:1
Epidemic years	1,306	1,375	14	2,695	0.95:1
Non-epidemic years	3,115	2,894	52	6,061	1.08:1
Fisher's exact test	p value <0.01				

Source: Curtis, From One Mortality Regime to Another? 144. The sex ratio in mortality during epidemics is even lower when isolating only major plagues. Outbreaks such of 1503/4, where more men died, were more moderate and attributable to syphilis.

Table 3.5 Adult sex ratios in mortality, rural Low Countries, 1600–99

	Male	*Female*	*Total*	*Sex ratio*
All years	134,205	128,780	262,985	1.04:1
Epidemic years	29,786	29,010	58,796	1.03:1
Non-epidemic years	104,419	99.770	204,189	1.05:1
Chi square	4.164 with 1 degree freedom, p value 0.0413			
Severe epidemics	9,296	9,458	18,754	0.98:1
Moderate & non-epidemics	124,909	119,322	244,231	1.05:1
Chi square	17.304 with 1 degree freedom, p value <0.0001			

Source: Curtis and Han, The Female Mortality Advantage, 61, 64. Only includes rural localities with at least ten data points and an average of six burials per year (a total of 293 settlements across the Low Countries). I distinguish severe epidemics from moderate ones as those outbreaks which increase burials by 300 per cent or more over the normal rate in a particular year, which is the definition used in Table 3.2.

for non-famine-related epidemics too, given that body fat provides higher leptin levels which are a key regulator of the immune system and help protect against various afflictions caused by bacteria, viruses, fungi, and parasites. Testosterone, in contrast, reduces immunocompetence.[160] Accordingly, my findings presented above confound theoretical expectations derived from the natural sciences (which emphasise biological explanations) and contradict historical demography findings which have been restricted to the nineteenth and twentieth centuries up to now.[161]

The question, then, is why? Understanding the drivers of the findings presented above—a sex-selective effect of epidemic mortality towards adult women—is challenging, and difficult to definitively answer with current levels of knowledge. However, the most plausible explanation connects to gendered patterns of expected behaviour guiding women's greater exposure to vectors or points of contagion compared to men. Although, of course, men treated and interacted with the sick, they also could find ways to more easily avoid this. Frequently, we find in Low Countries sources occasions where male priests refused to enter an infected household to read the last sacrament or hear out a deathbed testament—the task instead falling to maids or paid *schrobsters*.[162] Women, on the other hand, first tended to take on greater amounts of the care tasks, domestically, in other households, and in public or religious institutions, and second, likely found it difficult to escape or refuse these gendered norms.[163] These issues are discussed in greater detail in Chapter 6.

Put simply, social and cultural context mattered—and mattered more than posited predisposed biological resistance or vulnerabilities to disease between the sexes.[164] And I say this by referring to another case where, in contrast to the higher amounts of women dying during epidemics (relative to the norm), we consistently see more men dying during very severe epidemic outbreaks (relative to the norm).[165] Indeed, Figure 3.11 shows how in the city of Leiden in the seventeenth century, many of the epidemics saw vastly more men dying than women, and during the epidemic of 1655 this was highly exaggerated, where twice as many men died as women. On the surface, this seems odd. Indeed, the very fact that more men than women were dying as a rule (also in normal times: a male–female ratio of 1.16:1 as an average across the seventeenth century) suggests that more men were resident in Leiden—contradicting the generally accepted notion that by the early modern period more women lived in cities than men.[166] However, the point is that Leiden is a specific economic, social, and cultural context—one where the textile industry dominated, and where such a boom led to the mass immigration of women and men, but clearly, from the late sixteenth onwards, a skew towards single labouring men attracted by the work and wages.[167] These men worked in consolidated areas, and in large teams, and hence, we can understand why during epidemic disease outbreaks, the spike in burials in Leiden was much more pronounced among adult men—that is a wider gap than seen even in non-epidemic times.[168]

Another form of selectivity in epidemic mortality often discussed is connected to age. Understanding the age selectivity of epidemics is important because it could play a significant role in diverging rates of recovery. An epidemic that destroyed a community's adult population of reproductive age was likely more disastrous than an epidemic focusing on the elderly or minors—particularly given that working-age adults were more likely to be

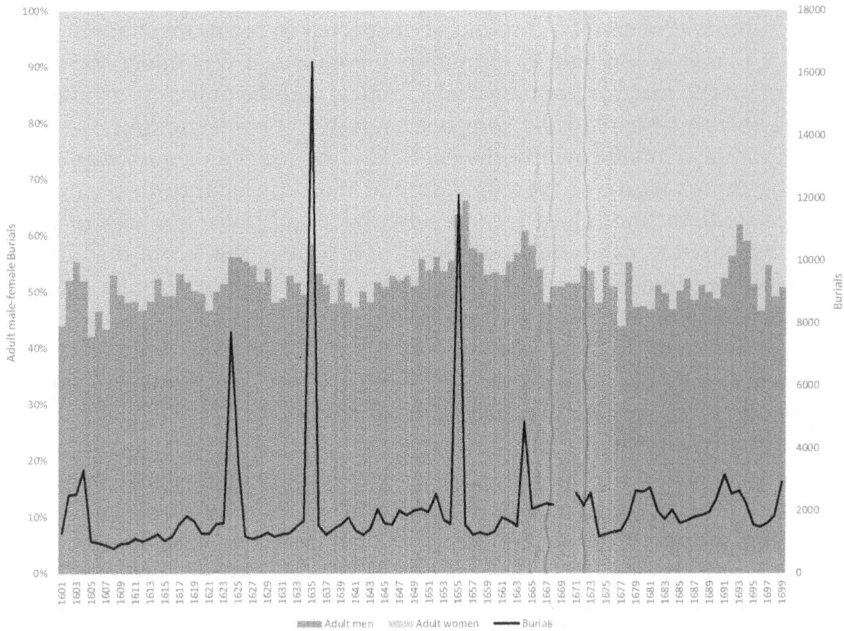

Figure 3.11 Adult male–female mortality in seventeenth-century Leiden
Source: Curtis, ed., Original Burials Data.

acting as care-givers—creating a set of secondary vulnerabilities.[169] Thus, for example, in the well-known diaries of Miquel Parets, a Barcelona tanner, during the plague of 1651, he made the point that children faced the prospect of being abandoned at foundling hospitals or became orphans, and hence "lost and wandering about the city begging".[170]

Some diseases such as smallpox were clearly afflictions that disproportionately affected infants and children, and with increased levels of immunity over time, this is something that simply became more entrenched in the eighteenth and nineteenth centuries.[171] For a long time, scholars have also tended to conclude that epidemics such as plague tended to selectively victimise children and sub-adults—a conclusion drawn from both the observations of contemporaries and demographic data.[172] Perhaps this is a reasonable assumption given that epidemics tend to end lives earlier than those following their normal course. Moreover, the notion that outbreaks such as *pestis secunda* or the third plague outbreak of 1368/9 hit children hard might be simply down to the fact that the age profile of communities was young given the mass mortality of the Black Death.[173] Indeed, more recent micro-demographic research, going into much more minute detail with reconstitution methods, has made the point that one of the flaws of all previous historical demographic research into plague and age-selectivity is that most have the basic limitation of not considering differences in the sizes of age cohorts. Put simply, it is entirely expected to see more children dying during a plague when half a community's population was under the age of 16, as often the case for preindustrial societies, and the only way around this is to be able to systematically compare against non-epidemic times.[174] Thus, at Nonantola, a small town in the Po Valley, during the plague of 1630, by knowing the structure of the population at risk, it was argued, contrary to received wisdom, that children and sub-adults had lower chances of death when compared to other older cohorts.[175] Of course, this is but one disease, plague. Other epidemics caused by other diseases likely had quite different pressures—victimising the very frail such as newly born infants or the elderly to a greater extent, for example.

Another way to deal with the flaws in not knowing the precise dimensions of the population at risk is to proceed as I have done with the sex-selectivity information above—rather than trying to calculate absolute numbers of people of different ages within a community dying during an epidemic, simply reconstructing relative change over time where adult–child profiles in mortality during epidemics are compared against normal times. As mentioned above, this relies on having a burial series, such as that of Leiden's, where over a long period of time, both adults and children are fully and systematically recorded—which is not always the case. As seen from Figure 3.12, seventeenth-century Leiden tended to conform to expectations

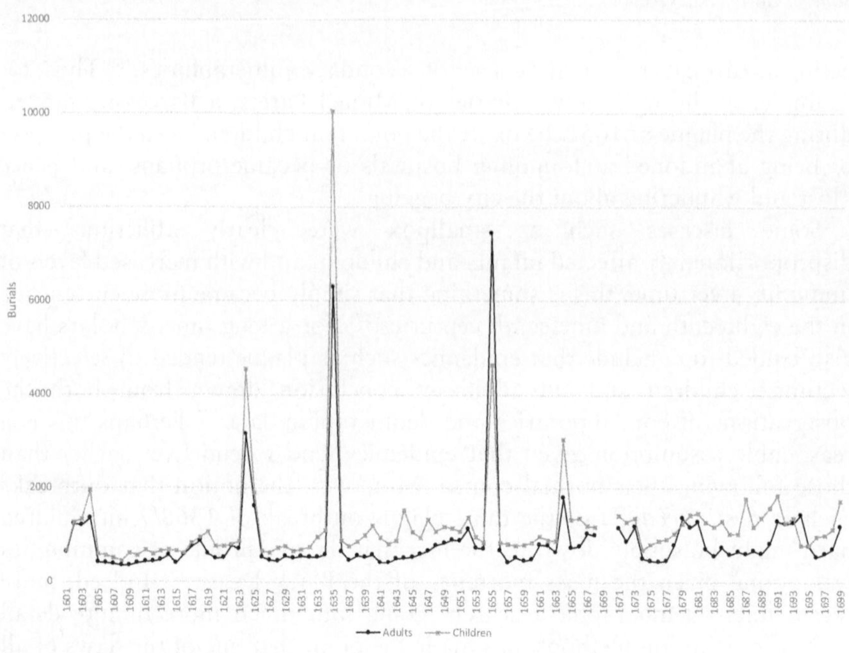

Figure 3.12 Adult–child disaggregated burials, Leiden, seventeenth century
Sources: Curtis, ed., Original Burials Data.

of more children dying per year than adults—a yearly burials average of 1,202 compared to 869—and a product of a young age structure, high birth rate, and high vulnerabilities for infants below one year old. These differences tended to be exaggerated during most outbreaks—especially when we look to the epidemics of 1635 and 1664, for example. Nevertheless, sometimes epidemics also inverted this usual pattern. If we look at the outbreak of 1655, almost twice as many adults died as children. This stands out when we consider that the 1635 epidemic was much more severe than all others, and yet based on just isolating adult mortality, the outbreak of 1655 had comparable impact—something of further significance when considering that, as mentioned above, 1655 also had a skewed sex ratio in mortality when almost twice as many men as women died. Certainly, differences between the epidemics in the adult–child mortality ratios suggest that very different diseases were at play in Leiden and remind us that we should not just dismiss all outbreaks as the same as plagues caused by *Yersinia pestis*.

Epidemics and recovery from sickness

Of course, it should be emphasised that not everyone who got sick or was infected during an epidemic automatically died. Disease morbidity rates (the proportion of people suffering from an affliction) were always higher than the disease mortality rates (the proportion of people dying from that affliction). How often did people survive diseases that led to epidemic outbreaks in the preindustrial Low Countries? We know, of course, from anecdotal cases that people recovered from terrible afflictions—even if survival led to knock-on health frailties. One notarial act from Rotterdam in 1665 noted that a woman aged 37 had suffered from dysentery (*roode loop*) and survived. However, she was left with many lingering complaints, and thus had gone to several medical practitioners to try and deal with this.[176] Another boy, Cesar, received eggs, bread, butter, and herbs from the Zwartzusters hospital of Breda in 1596 when suffering from dysentery, and apparently recovered, as he later left the institution.[177] Plague was also not an inevitable death sentence. Thus, Sister Elisabeth Strouwen came from Hasselt to Maastricht in 1633 to help care for those suffering from the *pestziekte* in the wake of the hardships born by the siege of the city by the Prince of Orange—she herself having recovered from the disease.[178] Recovery from plague was observed by ordinary people, and formed an important component of stories told—especially when coinciding with spiritual interpretations involving visions, shrines, pilgrimages, confessions, and miracles.[179] Streams of people afflicted with syphilis in the early sixteenth century found their way to the small Brabant village of Wezemaal in search of the protective and curative qualities provided by the devotion to the chapel of St. Job at the St. Martinus Church.[180]

Quantitative information from patients in institutions offers some of the best insights into recovery, even if we need to approach such evidence with caution—not least because, as mentioned above, we cannot be sure that trends from these institutions mirrored those out in wider society. Indeed, a recent study of morbidity and mortality during the plague of 1630 in and outside the pest house (*lazzaretto*) of Carmagnola, a small town just south of Turin, has concluded that although the poor were disproportionately sent to this institution (the rich could find ways to escape hospitalisation), in the end this worked in the favour of the poor who enjoyed better conditions than they did outside the *lazzaretto*, and accordingly had higher chances of survival.[181] That being so, we might conclude, if similar conditions were found in Low Countries institutions, that the case mortality rates in the pest houses and hospitals which I present below are lower bound estimates which might have been higher for those infected out in the community.[182]

At the Gouda pest house, we see from Table 3.6, that in the period 1617–35, just over 55 per cent of the patients that entered the institution died. This included three epidemic years of 1624/5 and 1635, with the other years providing indirect evidence for the lingering localised endemic form of plague. Although it is possible that some patients did not have plague, the criteria for entry into the pest house were strict, and much stricter than the above-mentioned Carmagnola. Indeed, upon the appointment of a new *pestmeester* in 1635, it was announced that no patient was to be taken in

Table 3.6 Deaths and survival in the Gouda pest house, 1617–35

Year	*Patients*	*Deaths*	*Survival*
1617	12	6	6
1618	2	2	0
1624	46	29	17
1625	285	147	138
1626	9	9	0
1627	2	2	0
1628	1	0	1
1629	11	8	3
1630	1	1	0
1634	3	3	0
1635	216	118	98
Total	588	325	263

Plague Year, 1635

Age Categories (Years)	*Patients*	*Deaths (%)*
0–10	48	21 (44)
11–20	46	26 (56)
21–30	33	14 (42)
31–40	18	10 (55)
41–50	17	8 (47)
51–60	10	5 (50)
Over 60	4	4 (100)

Source: Buwalda and Buwalda-Prey, Eenige gegevens, 5664–5.

unless they had visible signs of buboes or anthrax (*bubonen off antraxen*).[183] Interestingly, this ratio of roughly one in two people surviving was maintained across all age categories during the outbreak of 1635 (the only year with age-disaggregated information)—with the exception of the small sample of people over 60 who all died. Linked to the above, more younger people entered the pest house simply as a reflection of the age structure of society at the time—a classic preindustrial wide-bottomed population pyramid. It is unfortunate that information on the number of patients entered into the Gouda pest house disappears for the years 1636 and 1637, since 1636 was the worst plague year where almost 600 people died at the institution.[184] If we continue with the assessment that around one in two survived, then possibly 1,200 patients entered the institution in that year—roughly eight per cent of the resident population of Gouda.[185] Elsewhere, in nearby Rotterdam, the one in two survival rate is also suggested from the numbers of patients and deaths estimated from the pest house in the seventeenth century specifically during epidemic outbreaks (see Table 3.7).[186]

In other institutions, not necessarily specialised in those infected with plague, but as a hospital catering for a range of, often serious, injuries and illnesses, the proportion of patients surviving was understandably higher. We have good serial evidence from the *loodjesboeken* (lead token books) of the hospital at Middelburg in Zeeland, for example. At this hospital, poor residents of the city, migrants, and soldiers received entry into the over-burdened institution through acquiring a lead token. Based on Table 3.8, in the period 1584–99, roughly 10 to 15 per cent of the incoming patients died each year—which is perhaps not as high as one might expect given (a) ordinary death rates within the whole urban population were already likely three to four per cent, (b) this was a period of hardship driven by ongoing warfare (hence, in some years, there were many soldiers entering the institution), and (c) much of the older literature has tended to emphasise the lack of curative functions within early modern hospitals. Indeed, these kinds of figures from Middelburg lend support to more recent revisionist views that show specialised and professional care in these institutions, and far from their status as absolute death traps.[187] During the severe plague year of 1584, the proportion of those patients who did not survive went up to

Table 3.7 Deaths and survival in the Rotterdam pest house, seventeenth-century outbreaks

Epidemic years	*Patients*	*Deaths (%)*
1624–6	865	439 (51)
1634–5	578	281 (49)
1655–7	413	175 (42)
1663–6	599	291 (48)
Total	2,455	1,186 (48)

Source: Brunner, Pest-epidemieën, 623; Van Lieburg, Het dagboek, 244.

Table 3.8 Deaths and survival in the Middelburg hospital, 1584–99

Year	*Patients*				*Deaths (%)*
	Men (soldiers)	*Women*	*Children*	*Total*	
1584	856 (*21*)	555	100	1,511	474 (*31*)
1585	550 (*181*)	169	19	738	110 (*15*)
1586	547 (*183*)	164	5	716	128 (*18*)
1587	838 (*452*)	283	21	1,142	236 (*21*)
1588	432 (*230*)	158	6	596	114 (*19*)
1589	254 (*69*)	77	7	338	51 (*15*)
1590	254 (*85*)	101	5	360	55 (*15*)
1591	363 (*150*)	124	22	509	54 (*11*)
1592	392 (*168*)	122	21	535	60 (*11*)
1593	316 (*125*)	93	10	419	53 (*13*)
1594	218 (*82*)	69	3	290	41 (*14*)
1595	302 (*124*)	103	12	417	50 (*12*)
1596	836 (*686*)	154	26	1,016	178 (*18*)
1597	558 (*168*)	165	25	748	93 (*12*)
1598	489 (*159*)	160	25	674	74 (*11*)
1599	464 (*256*)	101	16	581	80 (*14*)
Total	7,639 (3,139)	2,598	323	10,590	1,851 (18)

Source: Calculated from Kool-Blokland, *De zorg gewogen*, 91.

31 per cent, hence raising the average for the period to 17.5 per cent. If we remove the normal number of patients and deaths from those figures (i.e., the yearly averages from 1585–99)—thus, 605 patients and 92 deaths—then we estimate that over 42 per cent of those patients likely in the hospital due to contracting plague survived. Again, we are in the ballpark figure of roughly one in two people infected with the disease surviving—which is well below the suggested case fatality rate of 80 per cent recently suggested for early modern plagues.[188]

Epidemics and demographic recovery

One of the recurring narratives in preindustrial Low Countries demographic history is the notion of rapid population recovery after severe epidemics. Rather than the notion of a light experience of epidemic mortality, the population growth in parts of Holland in the late fourteenth and fifteenth centuries likely points to mechanisms of recovery when experiencing a series of damaging outbreaks—the two main ones being (re)marriage and migration.[189] On that note, it should also be emphasised that post-epidemic demographic recovery was not inevitable, and often diverged across regions (sometimes regions close together) in the Low Countries—as suggested for late-medieval Hainaut—and thus likely involved endogenous mechanisms.[190] In previous work, I proposed a framework for understanding why (specifically rural) communities could work to better keep hold of and retain populations under pressure, emphasising diversification in economic activity.[191] However, in the absence of further high-resolution demographic data, the curious paradox of a severe epidemic regime co-existing with rapid population recovery is not yet possible to answer.

What data from the seventeenth century can do, by combining the burial, marriage, and baptism registers, is show the extent to which individual cities in the Low Countries could very quickly recover their populations from the most severe forms of epidemic disease. Figure 3.13 for Leiden shows how the outbreak in 1635 which killed at least a third of the inhabitants—one of the most destructive to occur in any place in the early modern Low Countries—saw a rapid demographic rebound. Only a few years later was the population not only at its previous level but moving beyond it—and entirely driven by inward migration.

It should be noted, however, that this inward migration worked in tandem with developments on the marriage market. In most places across the Low Countries, and especially in Holland cities, there were barely any barriers to remarriage for either men or women. Hence, many of these communities were able to experience to the fullest degree the highest proportion of spiked nuptiality possible after mass mortality events—and demonstrated quite consistently throughout the seventeenth century in Delft (Figure 3.14) after outbreaks in 1602, 1625, 1636, and 1679. Outbreaks that created observable

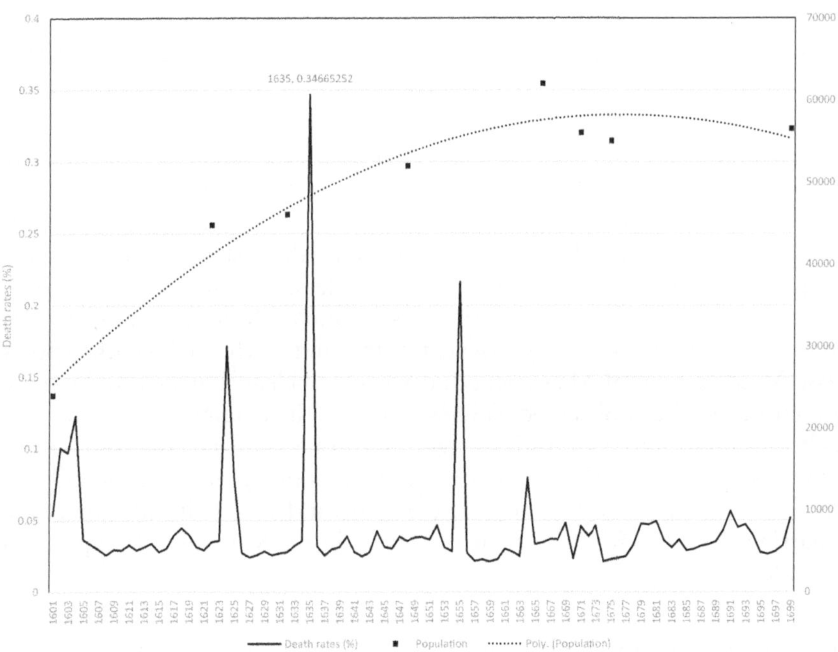

Figure 3.13 Estimated death rates and population figures, Leiden, seventeenth century

Sources: Curtis, ed., Original Burials Data.

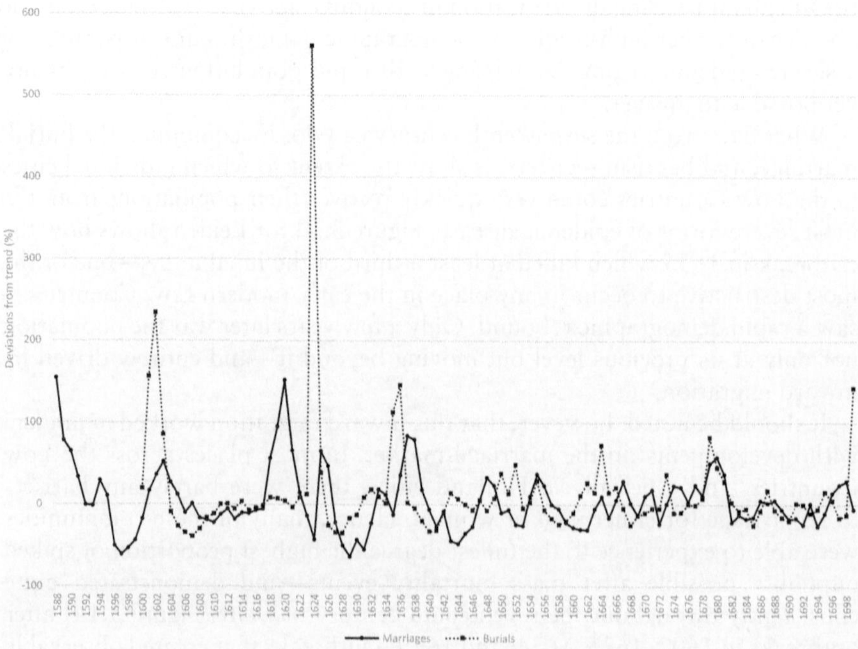

Figure 3.14 Epidemic-induced (re)marriage, Delft, 1588–1699

Sources: Curtis, ed., Original Burials Data. The epidemic year 1625 has a deviation in burials of 560 per cent (death rate of more than 25 per cent).

repercussions for survivors such as scarring from smallpox, might have dampened remarriage tendencies a little, although on this point, previous research from the Guelders town of Nijkerk has shown that surviving male cohorts had no observable differences in nuptiality, sterility, or fecundity compared to general populations.[192] Nevertheless, in conditions where epidemics occurred simultaneously to warfare and/or food crises, such as in rural communities of the late-seventeenth- and early eighteenth-century Basse Meuse region of Maastricht and Liège, the clear marriage spike trend has not always been observed as consistently.[193] It remains to be seen—and likely an important comparative project yet to be undertaken—whether the early modern Delft pattern is replicated when looking at epidemic-induced recovery in contexts where there were structural and cultural barriers to remarriage (particularly for women), as seen in the Kingdom of Naples, for example.[194]

Epidemics in the transition to modern industrialisation

Such is the prominent place of plague in the historiography that it has been suggested that the disappearance of plague after the 1660s in the Low

Countries raised life expectancies thereafter considerably—in Amsterdam, for example, perhaps by as much as four to six years (from birth).[195] More recent work on long-term mortality trends in Amsterdam has supported this view.[196] While plague was present up to the 1660s, mortality spikes were more frequent and sharper than those seen in the eighteenth century—where smallpox became the most significant form of epidemic threat in the city. Thus, death rates during epidemic outbreaks declined from 10 to 15 per cent before 1670 to 5 to 7 per cent in the eighteenth century.[197] By the time of the last outbreak of smallpox in Amsterdam in 1870–2, the disease added just an extra one per cent to the ordinary death rate in the city.[198] Similarly, while epidemics connected to winter airborne infections in Amsterdam remained present in the period 1856–91, excess winter mortality spikes existed even when removing deaths of this type—pointing to the impact of endemic and chronic afflictions shaped by environment instead.[199] However, we should also note that the recent mortality figures for Amsterdam across almost five centuries are not based on standardised source material—unlike my previously mentioned study for Haarlem between the fifteenth and seventeenth centuries—but instead bring together indicators from different kinds of documents. Furthermore, the population figures against which the mortality indicators are used to calculate death rates are not standardised across time either—with more frequent and more precise estimates as we move further into the nineteenth and twentieth centuries.[200] It is issues such as these which incentivise historical demography in the Low Countries to unfortunately remain firmly focused on the period after modern industrialisation.

Of course, Amsterdam is not necessarily representative of broader Low Countries trends. Indeed, mortality deviations in areas of the southern Low Countries were just as sharp, or in some localities even sharper, during dysentery outbreaks of 1676 or the epidemic fevers of 1693/4, as plagues from the sixteenth and first half of the seventeenth century.[201] Villages such as Schriek in 1693 and Izegem in 1694 saw more than tenfold mortality increases over trend for adults—equating to potential death rates of over 30 per cent.[202] Furthermore, epidemic disease outbreaks continued to occur across the eighteenth and nineteenth centuries—particularly in the countryside—although they became gradually less significant, not only through the eradication of plague, and the diminishing (but still present) impact of malaria, but the gradually diminished direct role that warfare came to play in rural inhabitants' lives after the Wars of Austrian Succession (1740–8).[203] Hence, a dysentery outbreak in 1748 linked to the movement of French troops had led to death rates of more than 35 per cent among poor agricultural labourers in the Brabant villages of Gilze and Rijen, located between Tilburg and Breda—but thereafter there was a clear link between reduced military activity and reduced excess mortality from epidemics in the second half of the eighteenth century.[204] When conflict returned with the French Revolutionary Wars at the end of the eighteenth century, epidemic mortality spikes similarly reappeared.[205] Sometimes these were contagions spread between military and ordinary populaces that did not raise mortality substantially—such as afflictions of the eyes like trachoma or ophthalmia—but still were both debilitating and characteristic of the poorer cities of Flanders up until the middle of the nineteenth century.[206]

One significant disease that remained a scourge of rural communities, rather under-emphasised in the previous literature, was dysentery—and especially present in the late summer and early autumn in the inland areas of Guelders, Brabant, Limburg, Hainaut, and Liège, highlighting the impact of climatic, geographical, and environmental factors that led to the formation of pools of stagnant water (as already mentioned for 1676).[207] Indeed, while it has been suggested that more effective administration and popular receptiveness to this administration might have accounted for the lower impacts of the dysentery outbreak of 1779–83 in the city of Brussels compared to the surrounding rural hinterlands, when we relativise with other dysentery outbreaks it seems more likely to simply have been differences in environmental drivers and presence of troops.[208] The rural environment throughout the eighteenth and nineteenth centuries also helped create epidemic activity in urban areas—as seen with the case of the so-called *Groninger Ziekte* of 1826 where around ten per cent of the inhabitants of Groningen died. Conventional historiography linked this outbreak to agues, some pointed to typhus, while a more recent statement suggests a multiplicity of malarial and enteric infections causing stomach and gut-related problems.[209] Nevertheless, whether we see the relevant vectors as either mosquitoes or bacteria in the drinking water—it is still clear that this is well associated with regional flooding events and seepage of manure into canals linking the city with the rural hinterlands.[210] Even as we reach the final decades of the nineteenth century, localised smallpox epidemics were taking place in thinly populated rural areas such as the Hoeksche Waard (a polder island southwest of Dordrecht)—the outbreak of 1883/4 in Oud-Beijerland, for example, leading to an excess mortality of four per cent, thus doubling the usual mortality rate, and was rooted in deficiencies in the effective administration of who had been immunised.[211]

Another development in the countryside was, after a temporary escape in the seventeenth century (at least in most parts of the Dutch Republic), the return of greater famine-related mortality—highlighting how famine reduction and mitigation was not a linear teleological progression.[212] In the Dutch Republic, this was seen more in the later phases of the eighteenth century,[213] although we should not discount major famines leading to epidemics of typhus and typhoid fever earlier in the eighteenth century in the southern parts of the Low Countries—for example, in 1739/40, with most mortality seen in 1741.[214] It is likely that the typhus outbreaks seen in rural communities around Utrecht in 1817/18 such as in Montfoort, Vreeland, Nederhorst den Berg, and Willeskop were connected to the impoverishment that had been induced by the famine conditions created during the Year Without a Summer in 1816.[215] More well known is that certain regions of inland Flanders were some of the worst afflicted by the mid-nineteenth-century failure of the potato harvest given the reliance on this subsistence crop,[216] which not only created the conditions for outbreaks of famine-related fevers, but also weakened populations exposed to other infectious diseases such as typhus in 1846, especially in west Flanders, and cholera in 1848/9 spreading from the port of Antwerp.[217]

Nevertheless, even if epidemics continued to afflict rural areas of the Low Countries in the nineteenth century, the major difference with the preindustrial era is that the toll of epidemic activity became worse in cities and towns compared to the countryside. An overview of cholera patients in 1832 in the province of Utrecht showed that 1,009 out of 1,147 recorded cholera sufferers were from the two cities of Utrecht and Amersfoort (88 per cent), of which 433 died (42.9 per cent)—leaving just 12 per cent of deaths in the countryside, although with a higher case fatality rate of 50.7 per cent.[218] Interestingly, there was no real linear progression in cholera afflictions becoming less virulent over time. Indeed, the cholera outbreak of 1866 in the same province of Utrecht led to the deaths of 64.2 per cent of those recorded as infected.[219] Overall, 46.5 per cent of cholera deaths in the period 1832–67 in the Netherlands were to be found in the densely urbanised province of South Holland despite containing only 18.4 per cent of the country's population.[220] Further south, in Namur and Luxembourg, death rates from cholera during the 1866 outbreak in the largest cities were more than four times what was calculated for the countryside—although the aggregate figures did obscure the finding that while certain villages were completely unafflicted, other villages had the highest death rates of anywhere in the two provinces.[221]

Accordingly, lasting regional differences in impacts could be stark. For example, in the western parts of the Netherlands in the nineteenth century, people tended to be significantly shorter than in the less urbanised northern areas—likely a function of children's (but not infants') exposure to scarring diseases including those affecting the digestive system such as dysentery and diarrhoea and those affecting the respiratory system such as tuberculosis.[222] While heights started to increase after the mid-nineteenth century, likely as a result of widespread improvements to the disease environment, where life expectancies of certain social groups increased substantially after 1850,[223] in areas where mortality from food and waterborne afflictions remained high, average heights were also slower to increase.[224] Further research into a sample of male prisoners in Bruges has suggested that exposure during puberty (but not birth) to high mortality and stress conditions such as in the 1840s, characterised by harvest failures and diseases, led to reductions in stature.[225]

By the later phases of the nineteenth century, pivotal sanitary improvements in cities such as Amsterdam began to emerge—even if large sections of the population still did not wholly benefit from them.[226] Overall, deaths through epidemic infections connected to dirty or polluted water tended to dampen down, and respiratory afflictions such as bronchitis and pneumonia became more prominent.[227] Cleaning up water sources and waste distribution, to a certain extent, was more straightforward than completely redesigning habitations for the poorest in society, which became the preoccupation of the twentieth-century modernist architectural movements. Nevertheless, one area of discussion that continues is on the drivers of the geographically differential trend towards higher life expectancies and reduced impact of epidemics as we approach the twentieth century. One factor that has been frequently cited as important is the impact of new medical insights supported by gradual movements away from miasma towards germ theory, although others have cited economic factors, and already mentioned above are the recent studies that have focused on socio-cultural aspects of regional demographic behaviour linked to religion.[228] Indeed, counter to the medical intervention arguments, others have suggested that medical practitioners themselves did not really share in any of the epidemic mortality improvements seen in the second half of the nineteenth century.[229] Thus, perhaps more than knowledge per se, more productive might be to look at how these new measures were implemented, and most importantly, the extent to which populations received them and took them up—a discussion on the relationship between elites and ordinary citizens advanced further in Chapter 4. Thus, for example, it has been suggested that in nineteenth-century Amsterdam, Jewish communities fared better with outbreaks of smallpox due to norms and values that heightened the willingness to accept vaccination.[230] Jewish physicians such as Ezechiel Joseph Goldmit, working in the early part of the nineteenth century, have been singled out for the efforts made to encourage vaccination take-up and compliance within Amsterdam neighbourhoods.[231] Meanwhile, this advantage in Jewish communities was not necessarily seen during cholera outbreaks, where disease was more contingent on shared poor quality water systems.

Conclusion

Bringing together a new wealth of quantitative information on epidemic mortality, we can draw some broad conclusions. The Black Death of 1349–51 had a severe impact in some parts of the Low Countries—although there is still very little definitive evidence for its presence in Holland, and furthermore, there is little definitive evidence to say that the outbreak was as severe or more severe than that shown for other parts of Eurasia where it hit. What we can be more definitive about is that the late-medieval epidemic regime of the Low Countries—the recurring outbreaks that came after the Black Death in the second half of the fourteenth and fifteenth centuries—was very harsh in both the north and south. The outbreak of 1439, one of the rare ones to coincide very closely with harvest failures, was the worst in its combined severity and territorial pervasiveness.

When we think of long-term dynamics, it is always difficult to compare across time with different types of source material—although standardisable evidence from Haarlem suggests that the late-medieval regime of epidemics might have been more severe than those coming later (this is just one city and trends might have been different in other contexts). More confidently, epidemic mortality in the sixteenth century, and especially in the first half, was less substantial compared to both the fifteenth and the seventeenth centuries—even if there were localised exceptions.[232] Likely this makes sense given that direct military activity with the presence of soldiers starts to ramp up from the final third of the sixteenth century onwards, and the importance of international trade and shipping links grows in the first half of the seventeenth century, especially for the Dutch Republic.[233] Furthermore, the reemergence of terribly severe epidemics that afflicted almost all places in the Low Countries around the same time, such as the plague of 1636, shows that there was no clear linear teleological path in the preindustrial period towards an escape from epidemic disease. Indeed, in this chapter I suggest that the severe and widespread plague of 1636 means that we should perhaps be more cautious with accepting the narrative of the plague of 1630 in northern Italy and the plague of 1656–8 in the Kingdom of Naples to be much worse than any other outbreak seen across early modern Europe.[234]

Another finding that persists regardless of period is the rural profile of epidemic disease in the Low Countries. Any argument for either the medieval or the early modern period that accentuates the urban character of epidemic outbreaks in the Low Countries should be definitively rejected. Plagues hit rural areas—and in the seventeenth century at least, tended to be more damaging for the lesser urbanised areas than the urban commercial cores. This makes sense if we accept an additional argument made in this book that privileges the seeding of epidemic disease through military activity—acts of war that tended to disproportionately burden rural communities—and likely explains why England's early modern plague regime was more urban. Importantly, the rural character of epidemic disease continued after the disappearance of plague after the 1660s in the Low Countries—and especially through the frequent appearance of dysentery outbreaks in the late seventeenth and eighteenth centuries. It was perhaps only around the middle third of the nineteenth century that epidemic diseases definitively could claim to have had a decidedly urban profile in the Low Countries, and hence in a later phase of modern industrialisation.

Finally, epidemics were selective, and this is something not easy to reconstruct for the preindustrial period—hence, we need to remain cautious, especially with explanatory mechanisms. Clearly, when we have good adult–child disaggregated burial data, we can see that many epidemics occurred where adult mortality did not track closely with child mortality, and vice-versa. This depended on the precise nature of the disease. Evidence from both the late-medieval and early modern periods in the Low Countries now suggests that, as a rule, adult women tended to be more severely afflicted by epidemics compared to men, relative to normal patterns of mortality—although there were always important exceptions driven by contextual social, economic, and cultural conditions, as the seventeenth-century Leiden case shows. Indeed, societal drivers were more important than inherent genetic or physiological vulnerabilities. A major piece of the puzzle that we miss is socio-economic selectivity of mortality—not least through lack of solid evidence of mortality disaggregated down the lines of wealth, but also because the precise mechanisms are always unclear. Scholars have shown for the nineteenth and twentieth centuries that epidemic mortality, perhaps unsurprisingly, tended to be in poorer neighbourhoods—something supported by our own work on seventeenth-century Leiden—but a close analysis of the dead distinguished by their different socio-economic experiences remains missing.

Notes

1 The demographic (mainly mortality) data behind Chapter 3 are openly accessible in a repository: Curtis, ed., Original Burials Data.
2 The higher-end estimate of 60 per cent is most often associated with Benedictow, *The Black Death, 1346–1353*, 380–4; and still adhered to in the updated: Benedictow, *The Complete History*, 650.
3 For the indiscriminate view: Margerison and Knüsel, Paleodemographic Comparison, 134; Naphy and Spicer, *Plague*, 171. For the selection view, mostly bioarchaeological approaches: DeWitte, Age Patterns; DeWitte and Hughes-Morey, Stature; DeWitte and Wood, Selectivity; although some with historical documents: Curtis and Roosen, The Sex-Selective Impact.
4 Regional differences in demographic impact emphasised with a plurality of methods. Using documentary sources: Roosen and Curtis, The "Light Touch"; Mengel, A Plague on Bohemia?; Guzowski, Did the Black Death Reach the Kingdom of Poland?; Bauch and Oertel, Late Medieval Plague Waves; using archaeological or epigraphical evidence: Lewis, Disaster Recovery; Slavin, Death; using palaeoecological data: Izdebski et al., Palaeoecological Data.
5 Not necessarily more severe, but *pestis secunda* is recently suggested to have had more substantial lasting demographic repercussions in England: Slavin, Plague Strikes Back.
6 Green, Out of the East.
7 We should be sceptical about the exactness of Black Death mortality estimates suggested in the likes of Christakos et al., *Interdisciplinary Public Health Reasoning*; which have then subsequently been used as independent variables in Voigtländer and Voth, The Three Horsemen; Jedwab et al., Negative Shocks; Finley and Koyama, Plague; Gingerich and Vogler, Pandemics; or alternatively these kinds of inexact estimates subsequently used as dependent variables in Wang and Rodríguez-Pose, Local Institutions; Gómez and Verdú, Network Theory. With critical remarks on the merits of this endeavour: Roosen, Severity.
8 Carmichael, *Plague*, 1; Cohn, *Cultures*, 209–10; Slack, *The Impact*, 195; Alfani, *Calamities*, 257; Alfani and Murphy, Plague, 326; Campbell, *The Great Transition*, 306–7.
9 Alfani and Murphy, Plague, 318.
10 Cummins et al., Living Standards; Cohn and Alfani, Households, 193–4; Monecke et al. Modelling. Less clear-cut in the case of plagues in Dijon in the first half of the fifteenth century: Galanaud et al., Historical Epidemics. Most studies tend to emphasise some facet of the urban environment linking plague and poverty, although socio-economic gradients in mortality have also been argued for rural villages, complicating the potential causal mechanism: Whittles and Didelot, Epidemiological Analysis.

11 Curtis, Was Plague an Exclusively Urban Phenomenon? We should also note the importance of severe mortality spikes in rural areas connected to epidemics of diseases that were not plague: Dobson, *Contours*. However, the original contention that specifically early modern plagues in England were mainly urban afflictions still holds in the latest research, although not becoming *more urban* over the course of the early modern period: Udale, *The Plague*, 59, 61, 70.

12 Alfani, Plague; Alfani and Murphy, Plague, 325–6. This contention I question with comparative information from the Low Countries later in this chapter.

13 Yue et al., Navigable Rivers; Yue et al., Trade Routes; Harrison, *Contagion*, 1–23; Namouchi et al., Integrative Approach; Siuda and Sunde, Disease; with a critique of some of this literature based on the plague databases being used: Roosen and Curtis, Dangers. For a summary of the commerce-epidemics literature: Curtis, Trade; Ogilvie, *Controlling Contagion*, 25–85; and likewise for water courses and transport: Udale, *The Plague*, 61–6.

14 Curtis, Plague, 91–5; Curtis and Dijkman, The Escape. Food crises can also occur after plagues, complicating their association: Espeel, Plague.

15 Barker, Laying the Corpses to Rest; Ditrich, The Transmission; Bauch and Büntgen, Climate-Driven Changes

16 Cummins et al., Living Standards; Cohn and Alfani, Households, 193–4. For recent literature speculating on plague transmission mechanisms: Dean et al., Human Ectoparasites; Barbieri et al., The Role.

17 Although admittedly with different emphases and interpretations of the role of local plague reservoirs across time and space: Green, Climate; Yue and Lee, Pre-Industrial Plague Transmission; Schmid et al., Climate-Driven Introduction; Campbell, *The Great Transition*, 294; Tian et al., Scale-Dependent; Slavin, The Birth. On seasonality and plague: Krauer et al., The Influence.

18 McMichael, Insights.

19 A basic notion agreed upon despite other more substantial disagreements: Green, The Four Black Deaths; Slavin, The Birth.

20 Outram, The Demographic Impact; Van Besouw and Curtis, Estimating.

21 Ogilvie, *Controlling Contagion*.

22 Chroniclers noting hard times (*twere zeit*) or dearth (*carestia*) in different points of the eleventh and twelfth centuries: Curtis et al., Low Countries, 119. An outbreak of ergotism caused by eating rye contaminated with fungus in parts of Flanders, Liège, Brabant, and Cambrai in 1089/90 is one of the earliest examples of persisting cultural commemoration of an epidemic across centuries: Stein, An Urban Network, 43; Coumans, Notes, 1129–30.

23 Mentioned in Roosen, *The Black Death*, 153; Roosen and Curtis, The "Light Touch", supporting documents, but without proper expansion on its value.

24 For how these are identified in the source, see the cautionary remarks in Berger, ed., *Le nécrologe*, II, 101–2.

25 Campbell, Global Climates; Sharp, *Famine*, 35–6. It should be noted that 1272 does not even appear on Campbell's list of spiked grain price years for England: Campbell, Global Climates, 90. As ever, indices for mortality are not present when considering these thirteenth-century crises, only remarks from contemporaries. On that note, observers note for both Scotland and Ireland that many people fell ill and the presence of pestilence in 1272: Campbell and Ludlow, Climate, 198–9.

26 Delafaille, *Hongersnooden*, 16–17. Priest Menko (1213–76) also mentions sudden death in the far north of Groningen at the Bloemhof abbey (*eodem anno coepit oriri hominum mortalitas et quidem etiam subito moriebantur*): Reilingh, *Geschiedkundig-geneeskundige beschouwing*, I, 11–12.

27 A visualisation of the low summer temperatures in the Low Countries (originally from Jan Buisman) in Soens, No Second Lord, 77. Literature from the nineteenth century originally saw the 1315–17 episode as a *peste* epidemic: Diegerick, La peste. Intriguingly, recent scholarship has once again started to suggest that mortality crises in the thirteenth century, and that of 1315–17, included plague: Green, Hidden Plagues. Green's assertion that *Yersinia pestis* was widely present in Europe before the Black Death is plausible in my view, but I also await more confirmatory and precisely datable DNA evidence if we are going to link it to specific episodes and thus am more cautious. The different Mediterranean cases that Green cites rely on "mean dates" from radiocarbon dating: Green and Oliveira da Silva, Shifting Paradigms.

28 Jordan, *The Great Famine*, 142–3.

29 Newfield, A Cattle Panzootic, 161–2.

30 Reygersbergh, *Dye cronijcke*, fo. 70v (folio number of digital scan).

31 Geens, The Great Famine; Speecke and Lambrecht, Social Inequalities.

32 Derville, L'hôpital. For the original theoretical framework: Sen, *Poverty*.

33 Curtis et al., Low Countries, 121.

34 This would correspond to the low death rates very loosely estimated in the older historiography for places such as Bruges (ten per cent) and Ypres (just over five per cent): Van Werveke, La famine; Van Werveke, Bronnenmateriaal. Recent literature suggests that revisions to these figures will be available soon: Speecke and Lambrecht, Social Inequalities, 225.

35 Derville, La population, 521; Dhérent, *Abondance*, I, 353; Dhérent, *Histoire sociale*, I, 98.

36 Ladan, *Gezondheidszorg*, 19. Although well known is the so-called Leiden breadstone, which revolves around a miracle occurring in 1315/16 where a woman asked another woman to share a piece of bread, and upon denying she had any, God turned it into stone—a story passed down through the centuries about the dangers of selfishness: Lenarduzzi and Pollmann, Bread, 63–6.

37 Aubry, Les mortalités lilloises, 334–5. There was also raised mortality a few years earlier in Lille in 1329 and corresponding with a spike in new registered citizens into the city: Derville, La population, 522.

38 For 1332/3 in Douai: Deregnaucourt, Le testament; see, also, Figure 3.1 for Arras.

39 Derville, La population, 523.

40 Two of the original views on how the Low Countries avoided the worst effects of the Black Death: Van Werveke, *De Zwarte Dood*; Van Werveke, Nogmaals; with the original critique: Rogghé, De Zwarte Dood.

41 Mentioned more than 40 years ago in Blockmans, The Social and Economic Effects, 843–4; and almost a century ago in Meinsma, *De Zwarte Dood*, 403–9.

42 Ordinary death rates as suggested for the St. Agnes convent in Gorinchem, Holland: Zuijderduijn, Living la vita apostolica, 20.

43 For recent references to these charters: Huiting, *Domeinen*, 163. The existence of one of the charters for Utrecht had already been mentioned, though not used, in De Boer, *Graaf*, 34.

44 Curtis, Plague, 79, 84. On the posited northern route: Green, Out of the East, 310–11. The Hanseatic League was a confederation of merchant guilds and cities and towns with markets from the thirteenth to the seventeenth century that stretched from the Baltics, across northern Germany, and to the North Sea area: see the maps, in Wubs-Mrozewicz, The Hanse, 27–9.

45 A non-exhaustive list of literature includes Blockmans, The Social and Economic Effects; Vermeersch, *1349*; Maréchal, De Zwarte Dood; Sivéry, La Hainaut; Billen and Boone, *Bans*; Vandeburie, De Zwarte Dood; Derville, La population;

Roosen and Curtis, The "Light Touch"; Delmaire, Contribution. The main mortality effects started to be observed in the early summer of 1349, despite some work referring to 1348, as seen in Despy, La "Grande Peste Noire".

46 Espeel, Plague, 355.

47 For the upward revisions: Benedictow, *The Black Death, 1346–1353*; Benedictow, *The Complete History*. For the diversity in mortality effect: Izdebski et al., Palaeoecological Data; with a conversation about the implications of the evidence as an index for specifically epidemic disease-induced mortality: Curtis, Reduction; Izdebski et al., Reply.

48 Blockmans et al., Tussen crisis en welvaart, 57. An estimated death rate of 16–25 per cent was later suggested for the Black Death in Flanders: Nicholas, *Medieval Flanders*, 266. Villages on the border of Luxembourg and the County of Bar are said to have lost one third of their populations: Noël, Première attaque, 745.

49 Sivéry, La Hainaut. Certainly, fewer noted than for parts of England, Germany, or Italy: Dyer and Jones, eds., *Deserted Villages*; Anon., ed., *Villages désertés.* Although desertions and contractions are more discernible for parts of coastal Flanders: Thoen and Soens, The Family, 197–8; Soens and Thoen, Vegetarians, 489; Thoen, De twee gezichten, 81–2; yet many of these were connected to water drainage and flood-related processes: Soens et al., Landscape, 147–8. Similarly, lack of clarity over precise causes and timing of late-medieval abandonments and contractions has been noted in the far north of the Low Countries in different rural regions of Groningen, although water features heavily in the explanation: Groenendijk and van Schaïk, Isolated, 319–20; Van Schaïk, De teloorgang, 11–14; Curtis, Danger, 113–14.

50 However, it was noted for Arras on 6 October 1349 that "the mortality was for the time being very great in the city" (*la mortalité était pour le temps moult grande en ladite ville*): Roosen, *The Black Death*, 153.

51 Deregnaucourt, *Autour*, I, 60; Dhérent, *Histoire sociale*, I, 114–17, Notwithstanding all the methodological limitations of using wills to calculate epidemic mortality: Roosen and Curtis, The "Light Touch", 36. Ongoing revised work on funeral palls broadly supports a low level of Black Death mortality at Douai: Stef Espeel, pers. comms. on research in progress [25/9/2024].

52 Vandeburie, De Zwarte Dood, 285; building on the earlier observations of Maréchal, De Zwarte Dood. See, also, Vermeersch, *1349*, 39–45; Derville, La population, 525; Derville contradicts previous evidence downplaying Black Death mortality in Lille: Aubry, Les mortalités lilloises, 342. An earlier work had noted the large numbers of registered immigrants into Lille in the years 1350–2, which was higher than the usual annual average: Desportes, Réceptions. For cautionary remarks about the sizes and representativeness of the samples in this type of work: Clauzel, Les maladies, 218–19, 224.

53 Previous scholars had already identified the Hainaut mortmain records as a valuable source, although understated Black Death mortality by not considering multiple deaths within a household and not incorporating one set of accounts for 1350/1 kept in Brussels, whereas most of the series is found in Lille: Blockmans, The Social and Economic Effects, 850, 856; Sivéry, La Hainaut. For the recent work on the mortmain: Roosen and Curtis, The "Light Touch".

54 For the lack of barriers to migration; Thoen *Landbouwekonomie*, I, 186–7.

55 Previous statements on the severity of "echo epidemics" in the southern Low Countries: Thoen and Devos, Pest, 20–1; Derville, *Les villes*, 145–7; Blockmans, The Social and Economic Effects; Thoen, Historical Demography, 577–80.

56 Haneca et al., The Ups and Downs, 9–10.

57 Although, as noted later in this chapter, urbanisation should not be seen as leading inevitably to higher epidemic mortality—and in fact, perhaps the reverse. See,

also, a theory on this issue posited in Benedictow, *The Complete History of the Black Death*, 877–85. For demographic recovery: Geens, *A Golden Age*, 39.

58 There was an awareness that the *pestis secunda* outbreak was generalisable to a wide area—for example, in a later Liège chronicle noted as "an epidemic which reigned in the world" (*ex epydimia qui tunc regnabat in mundo*): Hélin, Les recherches, 175. The noble, Jan van Blois, when visiting Geertruidenberg in 1360, decided not to stay in the main part of the city on account of the plague (*om der sterfte wille*): Janse, *Ridderschap*, 127. Of all the outbreaks, it also created the most severe pressures on food access in the southern Low Countries: Espeel, The Plague, 356. The year 1400 was already noted as a very severe plague in Sivéry, La peste noire; even when omitting a mortmain account from September 1400 onwards kept in Brussels: Roosen and Curtis, The "Light Touch", 41. Other literature has suggested that the 1439/40 epidemic was one of the worst in preindustrial Low Countries history: Curtis, From One Mortality Regime to Another? 137; Curtis, Plague, 91–2; Ladan, *Gezondheidszorg*, 60; Blockmans, The Social and Economic Effects, 861–2; Trio, De grote sterfte, 244–5; Neveux, La mortalité, 80–2; Barla, *Pour la necessitet*, 279–82. One testament from a woman from Schijndel, near Den Bosch, describes the 1439 outbreak as a *nieuwe pest*: BHIC, Mechelse aanwinsten van het bisdom Den Bosch, 1330–1719, 2006, Regesten, no. 82 [12/7/1439] [AO].

59 Described as utterly catastrophic for Ghent: Nicholas, *The Metamorphosis*, 290; a conclusion downplayed a little in Boone, *Gent*, 19–26. For Leiden in 1368/9: De Boer, *Graaf*, 73; and for the surrounding countryside: De Boer, *Graaf*, 98–105; and for the Land van Heusden in the south of Holland (now Brabant): Hoppenbrouwers, *Een middeleeuwse samenleving*, I, 60.

60 Many recurring severe outbreaks in the late-medieval Low Countries had death rates of 20–25 per cent: Curtis, Plague; Roosen and Curtis, The "Light Touch"; and this can be compared to death rates frequently under 10 per cent in late-medieval Catalonia: Benito Monclús et al., Assessing, 401.

61 Hatcher, Mortality, 38.

62 Roosen, Severity, 53. Roosen does not come to a firm conclusion on exactly which demographic groups are included in this sub-sample, although the diversity in values of the "best good" offered to the overlord does not necessarily suggest the poorest in society. Alternatively, for Namur, older scholarship tended to link mortmain payment to poorer groups: Génicot, Formorture, 508.

63 On popular resistance to this kind of tax on inheritance of "best good" in Flanders: De Waele, Subjects' Strategies, 314–15.

64 The difficulties of which are summarised in Curtis, Plague, 86; Smith, Measuring, 56–7.

65 De Boer, *Graaf*, 64, 80, 90; Ladan, *Gezondheidszorg*, 38, 234–5; Ligtenberg, *De armezorg*, 42.

66 BHIC, Illustre lieve vrouwe broederschap in 's-Hertogenbosch, (1291) 1318–2005, 1232, nos. 116–19 [AO]. Although the fraternity accounts go back to 1341, the information on deaths is not systematically displayed before 1381, and often intermixed with other categories of debt. Members accompanied by the terms *ex morte* or *obitam* have clearly died, but we also have members who are recorded as registering a testament, paying for candles or prayers, registered as unable to pay a debt, or simply just have their names recorded, and yet it is unclear whether these people have definitively died.

67 Bells were rung to let the community know that someone had died, to drive out the devil, and according to the miasmatical framework, improve the quality of the air through movement—hence, providing protection from epidemics and

storms. Different bells were rung according to wealth and status: Koslofsky, *The Reformation*, 96, 100; Champion, *The Fullness of Time*, 38.

68 Curtis, From One Mortality Regime to Another? The transcriptions and dimensions of the original data can be accessed at Curtis, Database.

69 NHAH, Kloosters te Haarlem, 2123, Fundatieboek. Register van de te houden memories, met aantekeningen over bezittingen, bestuur en geschiedenis van het Begijnhof, periode 1272–1630, no. 419, fo. 9–65v.

70 Zuijderduijn, Living la vita apostolica.

71 Conforming to the idea of distinct sub-periods of late-medieval mortality characteristics: Hatcher, The Great Slump, 239.

72 Belich, *The World the Plague Made*, 303.

73 Especially: Benedictow, New Perspectives; Benedictow, *The Black Death, 1346–1353*, 251–4. Also, Loschky and Childers, Early English Mortality, 91–5.

74 Hatcher, *Plague*, 64–6. A damping down of mortality by the end of the Middle Ages in England is also later supported in Nightingale, Some New Evidence; Oakes, Adolescent Mortality, 28–9.

75 Wrigley and Schofield, *The Population History*, 650.

76 Perhaps connected to the greater effectiveness in countering disease spread: Slack, *The Impact*, 83–110, 284–341. More recent work on England has suggested that epidemics did not become more restricted to cities and towns over the course of time: Udale, *The Plague*, 59, 61, 70.

77 Alfani and Murphy, Plague, 325–6; Carmichael, *Plague*, 63. Although in seventeenth-century Italy plague apparently reappeared with characteristics more in line with the concept of a universal killer, such was the extent of mortality in 1630 in parts of the Po Valley and in 1656–8 in parts of the Kingdom of Naples: Alfani, Plague.

78 Hatcher revising his earlier view from his 1977 pamphlet: Hatcher et al., Monastic Mortality; Hatcher, Mortality. Also, Harvey, *Living*, 112–45; Alfani, La popolazione, 37; Curtis, From One Mortality Regime to Another?

79 Cummins, Lifespans, 424, 426, 435. This data, however, is only for elites such as aristocrats, and is skewed towards England.

80 Van Bavel, *The Invisible Hand?* 204–7; Van Zanden, What Happened to the Standard of Living.

81 The problems of which are well discussed in Slack, *The Impact*, 59–63; Smith, Measuring, 56–7.

82 Kelly and Ó Gráda, Living Standards.

83 A more detailed discussion of the sources, the comparison of the two periods, the method of calculating deviation from trends, and the implications of the results is found in Curtis, From One Mortality Regime to Another? 149–53.

84 Casna et al., A Distant City.

85 Van Oosten, *De stad*, 211–12; Coomans, *Community*, 293–300; Lebon, *Een kijk*. With the original statement to the same effect for England: Rawcliffe, *Urban Bodies*, 3, 12–15.

86 This notion was already being questioned 50 years ago: Appleby, Famine, 510.

87 Lambrecht, Geboorte, 16; Devos and Van Rossem, Oud, 41–2. It should be noted too that baptisms and marriages were recorded more frequently and generally started earlier than burials—which makes sense given that baptisms and marriages represented information about the living and thus were more useful to church administrations and communities involved.

88 However, for the period 1620–99 at least, a Pooled OLS regression of burial register break points on spatial and temporal distribution of warfare showed no correlation: Van Besouw and Curtis, Estimating, 9.

89 Hence, in a letter by the commissioner of the Franciscan Church at Groningen in 1582, it was noted that almost all in the convent had died *aan de peste* and so needed a minister and priests: Formsma and Van Royen, eds., *Diarium*, 569 [25/10/1582]. The Horssen example retrievable in Curtis, ed., Original Burials Data.

90 Trénard, Roubaix, 184.

91 Teeuwen, *Financing Poor Relief*, 62.

92 One man at Doesburg died of the plague in 1567, and refused to receive the holy sacraments, but regardless was still buried in a consecrated cemetery: GAA, Brieven van en aan het Kwartier van Zutphen, 0124, no. 918, fo. 3285–6 [6/9/1567] [AO].

93 Spanhove, De pest, 338.

94 Hallema, Geschiedenis, 155; Ufkes, De verzorging. However, we also sometimes see soldiers turned away even from hospitals and pest houses during outbreaks, as during the plague of 1636 in Groningen: Hofman, *Sint Anthony Gasthuis*, 41–2.

95 During the plague at the far northeasterly Groningen village of Midwolda in 1604, the entry simply notes that more children died but were not recorded (*noch vele kinderen gestorven en uitgetekent*): GA, Doop-, trouw- en begraafboeken enz. in de provincie Groningen, Kerkelijke gemeente Midwolda, Kerkeboek 1596–1811, 124, no. 294, fo. 429r.

96 By unsystematic, I refer to three categories: localities where children are consistently listed every year but under-recorded; localities where the listing of children is random (occurring in some years but not others); and localities where the series of burial registers starts by not including children but then later adds them, and vice-versa. A good extreme example of the second unsystematic classification is from the Upper Guelders village of Arcen where hardly any year of the seventeenth century includes child burials, but then for the extreme spiked mortality year of 1634, with an 11-fold increase in adult burials, children are suddenly added to the total. If we do not carefully disaggregate adult and child burials, this gives a false impression of a more than 20-fold increase in burials over the trend: see Curtis, ed., Original Burials Data.

97 For example, in the burial registers of 1686–92 at Veghel, the priest starts to make explicit distinctions between adults and children, and those marked as 12 years and older were in the adult section, possibly linked to the ritual of First Communion: Van Asseldonk, *Veghel*, 210.

98 Van Haecht, *Kroniek*, II, 152. Relativised as modest in Coomans et al., Plague, 585.

99 EAL, Huis Bergh, 1227–1842, 0214, no. 358, 3268, 7282 [17/7/1578 and 21/11/1578] [AO].

100 Coenen, *Baanderheren*, 116.

101 In the northern Low Countries: Friis, An Inquiry; and the south: Segers, *Armenzorg*. On the drought and harvest failures: Buisman, *Duizend jaar weer*, III, 550–1.

102 Curtis and Dijkman, The Escape. In that sense, we differ from previous suggestions that dearth and plague are "phenomena which often occur together": Noordegraaf, Dearth, 61, 65; Noordegraaf and Valk, *De gave Gods*, 78–82. They might occur together but not inevitably, as discussed further in Chapter 5.

103 By localities, this could mean different parishes within a single city.

104 See, for example, the suggestion that the plague of 1636 in Nijmegen killed half the population, when the earliest burial registers we have start in 1673: Frijhoff, Gods gave afgewezen, 149.

105 Where available, population estimates per locality included in the burials dataset at the marker years of 1600, 1650, and 1700 can be consulted at: Curtis, ed., Original Burials Data.
106 Usually, a 50 per cent increase would be enough to prevent the generation born in the year of the mortality spike from fully reproducing: Alfani, Plague, 417.
107 A recent comment on my own work has suggested that I have stated that "plague likely affected Amsterdam more heavily than other places in the Low Countries": Francke and Korevaar, Housing Market, 4. This is the opposite of what I have demonstrated.
108 Curtis, Was Plague an Exclusively Urban Phenomenon? 169. On that note, it has been suggested that "one possible effect of repeated and selective plague outbreaks may have been to enhance the proportion of the population possessing such a genetic predisposition to immunity": Campbell, *The Great Transition*, 317.
109 Casna et al., A Distant City; Casna et al., Urbanization.
110 Goubert, Historical Demography, 47.
111 Udale, *The Plague*, 59, 61, 70.
112 Between 1624 and 1670, 27 out of 47 of those years (58 per cent) had at least one burial marked as a plague death: Rommes, Pest, 254.
113 Curtis, ed., Original Burials Data.
114 Alfani, Plague.
115 Cipolla, *Fighting*, 33.
116 Van Besouw and Curtis, Estimating. To clarify, most spiked mortality during these war events was not due to soldiers killing civilians. Although this did happen, it did not happen enough to shape the results, where violence was local and transitory: Gutmann, *War*, 163. We should not assume that this seventeenth-century situation necessarily applied to other periods, as the early years of the Dutch Revolt in the second half of the sixteenth century presented some brutal cases: Van Nierop, *Het verraad*; Adriaenssen, *Staatsvormend geweld*. In our material, the biggest danger to affecting the results was soldiers—external to the community in question—being buried in a local church cemetery. However, most communities understandably were reluctant to allow for burials of soldiers to take place in this way (see, Guttman, *War*, 163); many soldiers were buried in pest houses or hospital cemeteries; and we manually excluded all identifiable soldiers from the mortality data.
117 Voigtländer and Voth, The Three Horsemen.
118 Rosenthal and Wong, *Before*, 115–19; Dincecco and Onorato, Military Conflict; Dincecco and Onorato, *From Warfare*, 6–7, 37–8, 62–3.
119 Often forced to stay put by military commanders: Gutmann, Why They Stayed; Satterfield, *Princes*, 42–88; Goorts, *War*, 285.
120 Gutmann, *War*, 41–6; Mertens, Oorlog, 129–32.
121 Corroborating a suggested connection: Govaerts, *Armies*, 196. On these changes in army scale: Lynn, *Giant*, 112; Van Nimwegen, *The Dutch Army*, 13, 470, 515; Parker, *The Army*, 15–18.
122 For recent suggestions that militaries were also promoters of public health interventions: Govaerts, *Armies*, 183; Geltner, In the Camp.
123 Of related interest is the recent finding based on genetic analyses of 40 excavated individuals from St. Rombout cemetery in Mechelen, situated right next to the earliest military hospital in early modern Europe (used in the period 1567–1715), of eight cases of Plasmodium parasites that cause malaria. Furthermore, these samples exhibited non-local ancestry, suggesting troops from the Mediterranean: Michel et al., Ancient Plasmodium, 129–30. For the earlier excavations at the

St. Rombouts site, which included 3,617 graves and 4,158 depositions: Van de Vijver, Past Life.

124 Govaerts, *Armies*, 185, 193–4, 196–9, 208–9, 211, 215. Meanwhile, other frequently posited mechanisms such as the destruction of crops, while sometimes occurring, might not have been so usual as generally assumed, given the need for troops (especially in the seventeenth-century Low Countries context) to be maintained via the ordinary productive processes of rural communities.

125 Israel, *Conflict*, 42–3.

126 Van Nimwegen, *The Dutch Army*, 247–50.

127 The burial records for the St. Nicolai parish in Maastricht in 1633 show that 429 out of 588 deceased (73.1 per cent) had *pest* next to their names, with an almost 20-fold increase in burials corresponding to an excessively high death rate of 80 per cent (fifth on the list presented in Table 3.1): see Curtis, ed., Original Burials Data. On the severity of plague in Maastricht in 1633: Klinkenberg, "Dye quade siecte". For epidemics and soldiers in Louvain in 1635: Van Nimwegen, *The Dutch Army*, 246–51, 287, 296.

128 Van Oosten, The Dutch Great Stink, 715–16; Van Tielhof and van Dam, *Waterstaat*, 187. Accordingly, the 1635 outbreak in Leiden is often referred to as plague in the literature, with explicit references to *pest* by contemporaries: see, for example, De Kwant, "Waer datmen gingh/stont/ofte sach/". Yet, the seeding conditions might point to a different kind of water-borne disease. To be sure, a plague outbreak should have nothing to do with polluted or stagnant canals per se, unless these conditions are attracting rats.

129 On the campaigns in northern France: Parrott, *Richelieu's Army*, 68, 118; Israel, *Conflict*, 76; and in Cleves: Israel, *The Dutch Republic and the Hispanic World*, 255; Parker, *The Thirty Years' War*, 128. For the Frisia pestilence: Wassenbergh, ed., Reisindrukken, 164. For the Torgny example: Mardaga, ed., *La Patrimoine monumental*, 294; and seventh on the most severely afflicted localities list in Table 3.1.

130 See, Curtis, ed., Original Burials Data.

131 In the parish of St. Nicolas, Valenciennes, for example, 619 out of 1138 deceased (54.3 per cent) were explicitly marked as deaths through *peste* in the burial records, with a more than sevenfold increase over the normal burials level equating to a death rate of around a fifth to a quarter of the population: see, Curtis, ed., Original Burials Data. On the ransacking of Orval and the destruction through this area: De Moreau de Gerbehaye, Une dépêche cryptée, 425–8; Martin, *La Guerre*, 135–6, 370.

132 Schulten, Het beleg.

133 Van Nimwegen, *The Dutch Army*, 222, 331, 343, 346, 392–3, 407–8, 417, 422, 436–53, 459, 469; Lynn, *The Wars*, 113–18.

134 Van Besouw and Curtis, Estimating.

135 Spiked deaths in relevant afflicted places such as the large village of Oudewater were predominantly in December 1672 and January 1673 according to the burial registers: see, Curtis, ed., Original Burials Data. For the frozen watercourses: Van Nimwegen, *The Dutch Army*, 458.

136 Van Wijngaarden and van der Hoeven, eds., De familienotities, 15.

137 Ufkes, De verzorging.

138 Curtis, Was Plague an Exclusively Urban Phenomenon? 150.

139 An extensive elucidation in Bruneel, *La mortalité*, I, 213–317; also, Meulemans, Dysenterie, 36–40.

140 See, Curtis, ed., Original Burials Data.

141 Kappelhof, Pest; Dings, Een dysenterie-epidemie. North Brabant was more modestly impacted by the *rampjaar* of 1672 and the ensuing years of the Franco-

Dutch War but not completely unaffected: see the recent contribution in Knegtel and Cuijpers, eds., *Rampjaar of jubeljaar?*

142 Curtis and Dijkman, The Escape, 235; Bruneel, *La mortalité*, I, 521–2.

143 Van Zuijlen, ed., *Inventaris*, II, 1535.

144 Van Besouw, *On the Economic Consequences of Warfare*, 42.

145 Daelemans, Tithe Revenues, 32.

146 Curtis, Was Plague an Exclusively Urban Phenomenon? 154–6; Francke and Korevaar, Housing Markets, 4.

147 Curtis, Was Plague an Exclusively Urban Phenomenon? 156; Dijkman, Managing Food Crises, 49, 55, 63; for the famines of 1556/7, 1698/9, and 1816/17.

148 Krauer et al., The Influence, 4. Also, see the recent work on epidemic seasonality from a bioarchaeological perspective: Zazvonilová et al., Using Cementochronology.

149 The importance of grain stores and rats has seen a recent revival in the plague literature: Barker, Laying the Corpses to Rest; and the earlier: McCormick, Rats.

150 Van Besouw and Curtis, Estimating, 7.

151 Muurling et al., The Last Nationwide Smallpox Epidemic.

152 Rijpma et al., Unequal Excess Mortality.

153 Murkens et al., Transitory Inequalities; Riswick et al., Exploring the Mortality Advantage; Van Dam, The Fight.

154 For the period 1632–68, for example, 83.9 per cent of those buried had a street next to their name in the "old core" of the city—comprising roughly half of Leiden in the centre and the south: Van Besouw et al., Epidemic Mortality.

155 Van Uytven, *Stadsfinanciën*, 474; Van Uytven, De bevolking, 124.

156 Van Besouw et al., Epidemic Mortality. More on the significance of this issue in Chapter 5.

157 Indeed, most of these methodologies are about relative differences in sex ratios in mortality between epidemic and non-epidemic times rather than absolute numbers of men and women dying during epidemics, given that this is the most productive way of dealing with the challenges of not knowing how many men and women are living in a locality over time (we do not even know the general population at risk, let alone sex-disaggregation of risk). To be sure, in the approach of most bioarchaeological studies, this issue is almost insurmountable given the nature, scope, and scale of the evidence, and made more complicated by the inability to accurately identify the sex of all skeletons: Holleville et al., Nouvelles données, 11; Kay et al., Burial Archaeology, 349–50.

158 There is a plethora of other studies from other parts of Eurasia that support my findings from the Low Countries, but others are also ambiguous or contradict them (i.e., more men dying during epidemics). This literature is too extensive to list here but can be consulted in my own articles cited below.

159 On the biological and physiological theory: Speakman, Sex- and Age-Related Mortality Profiles. For references to historical examples of women out-surviving men during famines: Macintyre, Famine; Ó Gráda, *Famine*, 99–101; Zarulli et al., Women.

160 Lord et al., Leptin; Bouman et al., Sex Hormones. Moreover, mortality evidence for non-famine-related epidemics has shown the same trend of a female mortality advantage: Zarulli et al., Women.

161 The lack of historical depth to the sex-disaggregated findings was noted in Healey, Famine. Pioneering work has taken place in bioarchaeology, although with methods that are difficult to directly compare to demographic analyses: Yaussy et al., Frailty; DeWitte and Yaussy, Sex Differences.

162 Some examples: Martyn and Stevens, Testamenten, 35; BHIC, Schepenenprotocol Sint-Michielsgestel, 5121, no. 43, fo. 215r [17/5/1561] [AO].

163 See, also, Alfani et al., Pandemics, 35.

164 As stated in one of the original summaries on the issue back in 2002: Macintyre, Famine.

165 Matching up with recent work on sex differentials in epidemic mortality in early modern London: Didelot and Evans, London. Although the outbreak of 1665/6 saw a greater mortality impact on women—again, showing the complexities of context, exposure, and disease characteristics: Barnes, The Gendered Dimensions.

166 Burial records for other Holland cities suggest more women did live in these urban environments than men as a rule, but Leiden was an exception to this rule for the seventeenth century: see, Curtis, ed., Original Burials Data. Of course, this does not discount the notion that more women lived in Leiden in the sixteenth century, before the immigration boom: Daelemans, Leiden 1581. Another explanation for the high male–female ratio in mortality could simply be structurally lower life expectancies of men compared to women across the long term in Leiden.

167 Indeed, it has been argued that there was a demarcation in roles in the textile trade between men and women, but when wages began to boom in the seventeenth century, men dominated many of the best paying roles: Van Nederveen Meerkerk, Market Wage. It has also been suggested that between the end of the sixteenth and the first half of the eighteenth century, female labour participation increased a lot: Van Nederveen Meerkerk, Creatief, 26. But, of course, more women being recorded with formal occupations is not the same as saying that there were more women than men present in the city.

168 In a previous article, I mentioned that some of the discrepancy might have been caused by the fact that (a) during epidemics more people died in the hospitals and pest houses, (b) more women were to be found in these institutions, and (c) we do not have all the institutional deaths listed in the burial records: Curtis and Han, The Female Mortality Advantage, 59–60. Nevertheless, our subsequent work on the proportions of deaths in the hospitals and pest houses of Leiden suggests that this would not have been enough to account for the wide discrepancies in the adult sex ratios in mortality during epidemics—two per cent of all epidemic-year deaths (reaching around 3.3 per cent of burials during the two worst weeks of the most severe outbreak in 1635), of which, of course, not all were women: Van Besouw et al., Epidemic Mortality.

169 Benedictow, *The Black Death and Later Plague Epidemics*, 152.

170 Amelang, ed., *A Journal*, 40, 50, 58, 61–2, 68.

171 Rutten, In de schaduw, 182.

172 Alexander, *Bubonic Plague*, 258–9; Bradley, The Most Famous of All English Plagues; Zapnik, *Pest*, 241; Höhl, *Die Pest*, 299; Jirková, Plague, 231; Frandsen, The Last Plague, 358, 370; Whittles and Didelot, Epidemiological Analysis, 6; Schofield, The Last Visitation, 612–14.

173 For Leiden and the surrounding rural hinterlands in 1369, a cleric noted that this third plague outbreak particularly victimised pregnant women and children: Curtis, Plague, 89. We should also consider that this statement might be for rhetorical effect.

174 For the age profile of preindustrial communities: Curtis and van Besouw, Lifecycle, 1095.

175 Alfani and Bonetti, A Survival Analysis; also, for Carmagnola: Alfani et al., Pandemics, 36–7. Bioarchaeological findings for other places tend to support this view too, though with small sample sizes: DeWitte, Age Patterns; Castex, Identification; Séguy et al., Modélisation.

176 SR, Archieven van de Notarissen te Rotterdam en daarin opgegane gemeenten, 18, no. 452, fo. 390r [3/1/1665].
177 Kappelhof, ed., Kroniek, 56.
178 Timmers, Elisabeth Strouven.
179 Coomans, *Community*, 234.
180 Minnen, *"Den heyligen Sant al in Brabant"*, 63–9.
181 Alfani et al., Pandemics, 38–9. The favourable conditions cited for the poor were basic access to food and water, which was not guaranteed in the community when living in poverty. In Utrecht, the city government threatened to take away the distribution of relief for those poor infected during the plague of 1664 if they did not register at a pest house: 't Hart et al., *Gepokt*, 52.
182 Perhaps dissimilar conditions given that the case mortality rate in Carmagnola *lazzaretto* was 28 per cent, which is far below the rates seen in most Low Countries institutions: Alfani et al., Pandemics, 23.
183 Buwalda and Buwalda-Prey, Eenige gegevens, 5665. It stands out that they make explicit distinction between the black pustules—one as a bubo and one as an anthrax. Still, it was not always possible to be definitive in these distinctions. For example, one man declared that he treated another man's wound on his back that "resembled *pest*" (*op de pest geleek*): RAZU, Stadsgerecht Rhenen, 066, Rekesten, ingekomen bij het gerecht en de magistraat, no. 619 [22/4/1651] [AO]. This was not, however, a known plague year.
184 Buwalda and Buwalda-Prey, Eenige gegevens, 5668–9.
185 Roughly a population of 15,000 on the eve of the outbreak: Habermehl, Leven, 307.
186 Corroborated in Mentink and van der Woude, *De demografische ontwikkeling*, 55.
187 For this revisionist view: Cohn, *Cultures*; Henderson, *The Renaissance Hospital*; Rawcliffe, *Medicine*. And in line with the recent work on the *lazzaretto* too: Alfani et al., Pandemics.
188 Ogilvie, *Controlling Contagion*, 12.
189 These points are already emphasised in Curtis, Plague, 81–2, 98. The notion of migration obscuring epidemic impact has recently been empirically demonstrated for an area of Savoy before and after the Black Death: Epurescu-Pascovici, Facing.
190 Roosen, The Black Death.
191 Curtis, The Impact.
192 Rutten, Smallpox.
193 Gutmann, *War*, 188–90.
194 Curtis, An Agro-Town Bias?
195 Alter, Plague, 40–1.
196 Francke and Korevaar, Housing Markets, 3.
197 Stalpers et al., De sterfte.
198 Muurling et al., The Last Nationwide Smallpox Epidemic, 195.
199 Buzaski and Riswick, The Rhythm of Death.
200 Nusteling, La population.
201 Curtis, Was Plague Exclusively an Urban Phenomenon? 146.
202 Van Besouw and Curtis, Estimating, 16.
203 Malaria declined after 1750, although not in every region to the same extent: Brouwer, Malaria. We still do not have a complete explanation for this. In Denmark, agrarian improvements leading to drier surface areas have recently been posited: Ingholt et al., The Disappearance. This might hold for parts of the northern Netherlands such as coastal Groningen, which saw from the late eight-

eenth century onwards a shift towards very large grain farms: Curtis, *Coping*, 181–222; Knottnerus, Yeomen.

204 Schellekens, Mortality, 399, 402.

205 Devos and Rossem, Oud, 45.

206 Vandendriessche, Ophtalmia.

207 As shown through several localised studies with significant outbreaks in 1702, 1736, 1779–83, and 1794: Baumann, De dysenterie; Baumann, Bijdrage; Bruneel, L'épidémie; Bruneel and Coutiez, La dysenterie; Cnops, Het Sint-Elisabethklooster; Diederen, Schinnen; Dings, Een dysenterie epidemie; Van den Eerenbeemt, De "rode dood"; Indekeu, Van de "rode dood" verlos ons Heer!; Mentink, De rode loop; Meulemans, Dysenterie; Van de Westeringh, De rode loop in het schoutambt Heteren; Van de Westeringh, De rode loop in Andelst; Kayser, Le phénomène épidémique.

208 Meert, Bruxelles.

209 For agues: Baron, *'Het belang en de welvaart van alle ingezetenen'*, 1; for tyhpus: Kooystra, Een ramp; for different malarial and enteric infections: Ingholt, The Last Hunger Years? 492.

210 Van Tielhof, Droogte; Van Bavel et al., Economic Inequality, 12.

211 Beyerman, De (tweede) pokkenepidemie, 3, 6–8.

212 Curtis and Dijkman, The Escape.

213 Curtis et al., Low Countries, 128. This original claim for the return of famine-related mortality in the late eighteenth century in the Dutch Republic was made in Faber, *Dure tijden*. This was dismissed in some case studies such as for Leiden: Pot, *Arm Leiden*, 143.

214 Vanhaute and Lambrecht, Famine.

215 Rombach, Zenuwzinkingkoorts, 15, 25.

216 Beeckaert and Vanhaute, Whose Famine?; Vanhaute et al., The Subsistence Crisis, 37. Also, in certain regions of the Netherlands where the potato was dominant amongst agricultural labourers farming subsistence micro-plots such as the Oldambt of east Groningen: Paping and Tassenaar, The Consequences; Bergman, The Potato Blight, 404. The narrative of the potato harvest failure in the Netherlands is less established than for Flanders: Jensen, Remembered.

217 Devos, *Allemaal beestjes*, 113.

218 't Hart et al., *Gepokt*, 26.

219 't Hart et al., *Gepokt*, 27.

220 't Hart, *Utrecht*, 303. Calculation of South Holland population based on most up-to-date estimates provided for the year 1849 in Stapel et al., (Re)counting, file no. census_NED1849a.

221 Bourguignon et al., Le choléra, 12–14.

222 Quanjer, Height. On potential confounding factors such as nutrition and socio-economic profile: Van Poppel et al., Differential Infant and Child Mortality.

223 Van Poppel et al., Life Expectancy, 279; Van Poppel et al., The Life Expectancy, 630, 632–3.

224 For late-nineteenth-century disease and high mortality in southern parts of the Netherlands: Van den Boomen, *Born Close to Death*, 152–5; corroborating this focus on regional susceptibility but offering an alternative view on the impact of religious denomination: Walhout, *An Infants' Graveyard?* 162–3; for higher mortality of infants linked to less frequent breastfeeding, particularly among Catholic households: Walhout, *An Infants' Graveyard?* 117–43.

225 Depauw and Oxley, Toddlers.

226 Muurling and Ekamper, A World of (In)difference? 299.

227 Engelen and Schoonheim, Mortality, 90.

228 The classic modernist statement emphasising medical "progress": Hofstee, *Korte demografische geschiedenis*, 65–85.
229 Van Poppel et al., The Life Expectancy, 634;Van Poppel et al., Medische opleiding, 6.
230 Riswick et al., Exploring, 730. In The Hague in the second half of the nineteenth and first decade of the twentieth century, incidence of infectious diseases among Jewish households was less pronounced than that among Protestants and Catholics: Van Poppel et al., Religious Differentials.
231 Zaidman-Mauer, The Key Role.
232 Corroborating a claim made in Noordegraaf and Valk, *De gave Gods*, 46–7. For these authors, plague prior to 1550 had become localised and endemic and would have been on the verge of dying out had it not been for a virulent new form appearing after 1550 which was based around heightened intensity of long-distance trade networks and migration.
233 Rommes, Pest, 252.
234 For the comparison: Alfani, Plague.

4 The bonds of community during epidemics

Reception and resistance

It is now almost a cliché to link epidemics and the breakdown of social order. When we look to twentieth- and twenty-first-century cinema and television, for example, the prevailing outbreak narrative being told is a society turned upside down, with panicked faces, looting, avariciousness or selfishness, targeted violence against the vulnerable, and where a storyline plays out of recurring stock characters including heroes and villains, martyrs and scapegoats, and spreaders and helpless victims.[1] A plethora of scholarly literature and popular commentary produced over the years has asserted the likely impact of epidemic disease to incite disorder—with a specific emphasis on the attribution of blame to easily victimised groups. Indeed, although the West in the 1970s was optimistically considering a future without epidemic disease, driven by the eradication of smallpox via inoculation, HIV and AIDS in the 1980s created new waves of societal anxiety, ushering in a perceived age of emerging infectious diseases, and where widespread concern was drawn towards perceived "subcultures" of sex workers, gay men, drug users, and other categories comprising an economic underclass.[2] The resurgence of the "old pests" such as cholera in Peru in 1991 and then plague in Surat, India, in 1994, with the eruption of tensions down religious lines between Hindus and Muslims regarding the supposed poisoning of water systems, only reconfirmed the "timeless" disrupting and dislocating effect of epidemic outbreaks.[3] SARS, and more recently COVID-19, have intensified both popular and scholarly focus on the links between epidemic disease and heightened prejudice and discrimination.[4]

Historians tended to subscribe to this view too. In the 1990s, building on the pioneering older work on the climate of fear within preindustrial societies,[5] the previous decade's cultural turn led a new generation of scholars to focus on related topics such as the persecution and execution of witches in different parts of early modern Europe, which in turn helped stimulate interest in historicised patterns of blame attached to supposed plague poisoners or syphilis spreaders.[6] Historians became influenced by the growing profile of Michel Foucault and his associated concept of "biopower", where it was increasingly argued that many epidemics in the past were used as a tool by powerful social groups, perhaps elites or authorities, to repress and persecute weaker or less powerful members of society that were easy to target.[7] The

DOI: 10.4324/9781003694908-4

Black Death had for a long time already been a go-to example, where scholars pointed to increased lawlessness, breakdowns in administration, spikes in violence, antisemitism, and the abandonment of family members—all parts of the classic Boccaccian narrative of the time.[8] And this was supported by a broader range of examples, not only across early modern Europe, but in nineteenth-century colonial contexts—where epidemics of plague became vehicles behind the physical subjugation of populations, referred to as the "colonised body".[9]

Nevertheless, on reflection, there were several issues with these narratives too. Cultural historians, at least in these early phases of the field's growing popularity, were inclined to focus on the special, the standout, the curious, or the extraordinary. Issues of sample size and representativity—the supposed domain of economic and social historians—were not top of the agenda, and even actively dismissed.[10] Thus, we saw evidence of very extreme and important events—the burning of Jews and the public shaming and execution of suspected poisoners or spreaders, for example—but there was little reflection on to what extent this was a common or unusual epidemic response. Furthermore, as was frequently the case with research into historical epidemics, much of the narrative was based on findings derived from the Black Death. But the question since then is to what extent can we extrapolate findings from this outbreak, unrepresentative in its spread and territorial pervasiveness, to the broader history of epidemic disease over the past one or even two millennia? And so, it came to be that the pioneering line of research pursued by Samuel Cohn challenged the inevitability of the epidemic-disorder nexus previously entrenched within the literature. For Cohn, the Black Death did provoke *some* extreme dislocating features, not least in the targeted persecution of Jews—aspects that were very clear across parts of the Low Countries too, especially in the south (see Figure 4.1) and east.[11] Yet, these reactions were one of many complex responses to the Black Death, where individuals could defy our expectations in more modest ways, not necessarily seeing themselves as abject sufferers of God's wrath and even showing hopefulness and optimism.[12] Furthermore, when looking at the broader picture of plague and other epidemic disease outbreaks across a longer time span outside the Black Death, substantial upticks in extreme dislocating behaviour were not necessarily the norm.[13] Instead, often we saw unity, cohesion, and compassion, and on those occasions where disorder was in view, it was not necessarily the classic conception of the powerful targeting the weak and vulnerable, but the disadvantaged rising up against a perceived elite. The cholera riots of the nineteenth century are obvious testament to that, as well as the violent resistance of poor rural communities in western Africa against outsider influence during Ebola outbreaks of the past decade and more.[14]

The bond of cohesion within society was also one of the most significant issues discussed in *De gave Gods*. In this prominent book dealing with plague in Holland (and to a lesser extent surrounding areas of the northern Low Countries) after 1450, it is argued that these outbreaks had a clearly

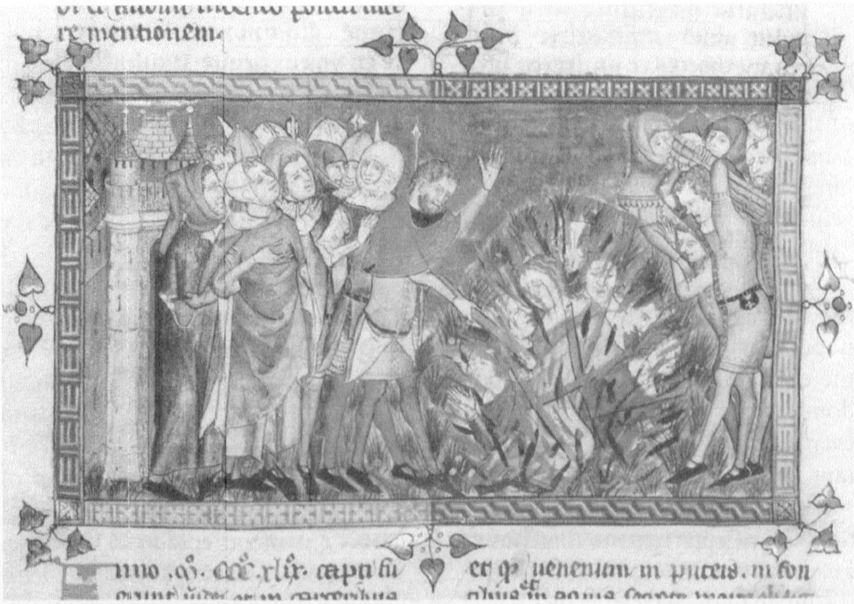

Figure 4.1 Depiction of the execution of Jews during the Black Death by Tournai chronicler Gilles Li Muisit, c.1350

Source: https://nl.wikipedia.org/wiki/Jodenvervolgingen_na_de_Zwarte_Dood.

disruptive impact on institutions, behaviour, and values that characterised everyday life—in the end, leaving no part of society untouched and loosening and fracturing existing societal bonds.[15] This argument was based upon a vast array of examples from different places and periods and included evidence from above such as aggressive regulation of mobility and implementation of isolation policies, and the denial of re-entry to towns for certain groups such as Jews and sex workers, but also disruptive acts perpetrated by medics, clerics, traders, and the general populace, which included refusal to treat (or engage with) the plague afflicted, usurpation of goods from infected houses for personal gain, disputes over inheritances, fights over access to unprepared coffins, flight from cities and the abandonment of vulnerable family members, and eruptions of violence towards targeted groups including plague workers such as gravediggers, cleaners, and pest house officials.

It was said that these dislocating aspects of plague in Holland and surroundings suggested in *De gave Gods* were even more disruptive in the early modern period due to the emergence of a Calvinist doctrine which encouraged communities to be passive and accept their fate when experiencing epidemics. Human acts of mitigation such as medical treatment, isolation, or migration were seen as redundant, where clerics instead privileged the religious weapons of prayer, piety, penitence, and repentance when confronted with disease.[16] The very fact that ordinary people were often ignoring these doctrines pointed to societies on the verge of chaos—abandoning the intrinsic social logic that was at the heart of how these communities were supposed to function.[17]

In the end, however, the sharp separation between religious ideology and conviction and societal practice was probably not so sharp. Already in Chapter 2 we emphasised the seamless interaction of preindustrial Low Countries societies' interpretation of disease—accepting the connection between providence, the regulation of morality and corruptions informed by miasmatical ideas, and concerns for physical spaces and environments creating contagions. Religious and institutional frameworks for societal responses to disease were not mutually exclusive but mutually reinforcing.[18] Indeed, individual case studies taken in combination since the original publication of *De gave Gods* tend to provide a more moderate view on the interaction between plague and society, at least in the early modern period, where the frequent reappearing nature of epidemic diseases, sometimes hitting the same communities again and again, working in combination with lingering localised endemic versions of the same diseases (within streets or neighbourhoods), meant that rather than total disorder or disruption, most outbreaks were incorporated into the general everyday rhythms of ordinary life.[19] The inherently moralising aspects of the providential interpretation inevitably meant that societies, communities, households, and individuals responded and adapted their behaviours, although these should not necessarily be defined as dislocating or inherently fracturing.

In this chapter, it is accepted that there are likely examples at both ends of the scale when considering the effects of epidemics on the bonds of society and communities in the Low Countries over the long term. Some epidemics might have created a disruptive effect in some domains of usual behaviour, while some epidemics might have stimulated minor adaptations incorporated into normal patterns of everyday life. However, what we define as the norm and deviations from the norm in daily practices might also be hard to pin down and separate from one another. Here, it is suggested that there might be more explicit interactions between disruption and normality than previously considered, blurring any sharp distinctions made between the two. Indeed, although one of the legacies of Foucauldian thinking is the idea that epidemics were used as an opportunity for repression or social control by elites and authorities, cracking down on vagrants, beggars, and sex workers, we currently have much less direct empirical information on communities' reception of and reactions to these responses.[20]

Building on one of my earlier contributions, this chapter further develops an argument that many of the epidemics seen in the preindustrial Low Countries were used as an opportunity to resist elite discourses and application of power.[21] However, this differed from nineteenth- and twentieth-century class-based urban proletarian uprisings seen across other parts of Europe during the cholera outbreaks in two ways.[22] First, this resistance was often on a much smaller scale, and although there was sometimes violent pushback, it was sometimes just characterised by passive foot-dragging. Second, this disruption—what we might define as a deviation from the normal patterns of behaviour—was not used to achieve social change or revolutionary objectives, but in fact paradoxically to preserve and re-entrench the status quo of tightly held ordinary customs and practices. Epidemics brought with them conservative ideals rather than radical ones and often represented a bargaining process established between political or economic elites and commoner majorities. Rather than disappearing when plague disappeared from the Low Countries after 1670, it was still something that characterised responses to epidemic disease outbreaks well into the nineteenth century after industrialisation.

Plague ordinances

As elsewhere across Eurasia, the repeat occurrence of epidemic outbreaks in the Low Countries drove territorial and urban governments, and sometimes even authorities at the village level, to impose regulations in response to the threat, or perceived threat, of disease—even if some of these regulations were mere reiterations and reemphasis on behavioural norms seen ordinarily outside of epidemic times. Although we have evidence of severe plagues in the second half of the fourteenth century, plague ordinances in the Low Countries only tended to appear from the fifteenth century onwards, where the earliest evidence comes from the southern parts of the Burgundian Netherlands such as the towns of Tournai, Valenciennes, and Saint-Omer.[23] Hence, for example, while it is well known that flagellants (penitents whipping themselves) were likely present in different parts of the Low Countries in the aftermath of the Black Death, although only from retrospective mentions through chroniclers, it was not until the plague of 1400, at least in the northern Low Countries, where we see for the first time normative administrative sources such as ordinances appearing on the subject—in this case, restricting the movements of flagellants in the Neder-Betuwe, part of the central Guelders river area.[24]

Like much of our documentary evidence connected to epidemic disease, ordinances and resolutions increase in number in the sixteenth and seventeenth centuries.[25] As administrations became acquainted with the same features of these outbreaks, earlier ordinances were often simply re-invoked, sometimes with small updates or further stipulations. Usually, there was just one ordinance announced during an epidemic, although exceptional cases could see as many as eight or nine ordinances announced in the same epidemic year, as seen in Antwerp in 1571 and 1601.[26] Although ordinances are often associated with plague, they were also sometimes announced in response to other diseases. Thus, in November 1669 in the Limburg town of Weert, regulations for dysentery were put in place such as the need for families to publicly announce when one of their relations had died, under threat of a 40-guilders fine.[27] Seven years later during the severe dysentery outbreak of 1676, the magistrates of Gestel, Brabant, similarly announced an ordinance to prevent *rooden loop* and *root melisoen* (terms used to refer to the bloody diarrhea produced during dysentery) from spreading any further in the village.[28] These same ordinances were being written and invoked well into the late eighteenth century.[29]

Many of the ordinances were so formulaic that they were often re-invoked by the same administrations. Sometimes this was close together in time—rules issued in the plague of 1473 were repeated in 1476 in Louvain—but sometimes the temporal gap extended for decades, as they were then reapplied in 1510.[30] The plague ordinance announced by the urban administration of Bruges in 1632 was effectively a reproduction and reprint from an earlier warning and instruction that appeared during the outbreak of 1604 in the city.[31] The ordinance presented at Roermond in 1615 was a repetition of a previous document from 1598.[32] Furthermore, different administrations copied from one another. For example, some of the regulations put down about vacating and renting out properties in which someone had died of plague in Haarlem in the ordinance of 1655 were almost word-for-word copied from a prior 1655 plague ordinance announced in Leiden.[33] Even across religious denominations, there was reproduction. In Antwerp, the regulations produced by the Calvinist administration in 1578 were copied almost verbatim from the regulations produced during the plague of 1571 under the Catholic authorities.[34]

The repetition and copying of these documents are understandable given the recurring nature of epidemic outbreaks in the medieval and early modern Low Countries, meaning that people often remembered and adapted behaviour to previous episodes.[35] In the diaries of the French school teacher David Beck, for example, writing in 1624 about the epidemic situation in Delft, he refers to a little instructive book against the plague (*boeckgen tegen de pest*) which had been produced during a previous outbreak in 1604.[36] Severe outbreaks of epidemic disease served as important points of collective remembrance that were instructive for how communities needed to deal with frequent anticipated outbreaks in the future.[37] Accordingly, some stood out for their perceived exceptional features. For example, a certification from 1613 mentions that in the early summer of 1604 there raged a *pest* in the isolated village of Winkel, part of West-Friesland, stronger than ever in time immemorial (*mensenheugenis*).[38] The *burgemeesters* of Leiden complained in 1683, thinking back to the memory of 1669, that almost all the city administrators had died from a sickness that had never been seen before (*waar men niet eerder van had gehoord*).[39] Some memories were marked by material culture. In the small town of Muiden, east of Amsterdam, the St. Nicolaas Church has a decorative board that commemorates the plague of 1602 said to have taken the lives of 650 inhabitants out of 900.[40] Much earlier, in 1526, the death of 31 children from the sweating sickness was marked by a reference to this fact on a small memorial table on a pillar in the left aisle opposite the third chapel in the St. Nicolaas Church in Ghent.[41] Some of these were intended as instructive lessons to hold resonance within communities over considerable periods of time, or instead were linked to morally suspect practices of the past. For example, in 1666, a Catholic wrote a mocking ditty —the *True year of sorrow of the image-breakers, of the Feast of All Cats Mewing*—which saw the ongoing plague as a logical product of a century of heretical misdeeds starting with the Iconoclasm a century earlier in 1566.[42]

As indicated in Chapter 2, the concerns of the governmental ordinances were drawn from the interacting frameworks for understanding and interpreting (and moralising) disease—providence, miasma, and contagion. Thus, each ordinance was mostly concerned with the same things—the isolation of the sick to protect the common good; the maintenance of private and public spaces to avoid corruptions connected to the senses of smell and sight; the regulation of trading and commercial environments, and specific types of people associated with these environments; and the maintenance of social order.[43] Of course, the exact nature of these components differed slightly in their accentuation over time, and demarcations about who these rules were aimed at sharpened over time. Indeed, and as already mentioned, it was not until the sixteenth century that we saw explicit connections in the ordinances between outbreaks of plague and the condition and behaviours of the poor.[44] At the Groot Gasthuis of Den Bosch in 1540, the urban administration instructed the institution to take in their own sick (*egheen siecken ontfangen*) but if the *pestilenciehuys* was clean (*suyver ende reyn*), those from outside the city with the *pestilentie* were not to be admitted.[45] As mentioned in Chapter 2, by the seventeenth century, communities started to become even more preoccupied with the external enemy rather than the threat within, and it is in that respect we can understand increased references to beggars and vagrants in the ordinances over time. During the epidemic outbreak of 1625 in Aalst, for example, the city guards were fined 12 guilders for letting in vagabonds and beggars. The act of begging itself was not punishable since Aalst inhabitants were encouraged to give alms to beggars of the city—it was the combination of begging and "from outside" that caused the most consternation.[46]

Enforcement of ordinances

Instructions were frequently announced to the residents of cities, towns, and villages on how to behave and what practices to follow during (the potential threat of) an epidemic outbreak, but clearly these were meaningless without enforcement and compliance. In theory, punishments were offered as a way of making citizens stick to the rules, and usually they came in the form of monetary fines, which were often substantial. For example, the penalty for continuing to trade as someone infected with plague in Groningen in 1598 was ten guilders. This was a substantial amount if we consider that in the late sixteenth century, an ordinary male agricultural labourer working on a yearly contract and attached to a specific household (*knecht*) in the northern areas of Frisia might only have received around 15 guilders—that sum not including the provision of board and food which had substantial value.[47] Other fines were even more exorbitant. In Utrecht in 1655, the hanging of cloth outside houses identified as infected with plague was prohibited at pains of 100 guilders, and the same amount was charged to those consuming alcohol at funerals of those who had died from plague in Delft in 1664. The seemingly innocuous practice of presenting elaborate funeral décor outside the houses of people who had died from plague in Rotterdam in 1664 was fined 200 guilders.[48]

Overall, the sums charged were so high that it is doubtful that these measures were robustly enforced, and most of the population were never able to pay anyway. A sum of 200 guilders was equivalent to about 15 years of rent of a labourer's residence in a seventeenth-century town such as Leiden, and many more years of rent in places outside the economic core of Holland.[49] Although fines did appear as income in urban financial accounts, my own survey of the budgets of 16 cities and towns across the Dutch Republic revealed that exceptionally high amercements did not ever feature.[50] During an epidemic outbreak of 1509, Leiden courts complained about the low levels of compliance with any of the regulations laid down in the plague ordinances.[51] In sixteenth-century Antwerp, it was mentioned in the ordinances that many had to be reissued because of the overall apathy or stubborn resistance.[52] At Amersfoort in 1599, the local justices of the peace complained that infringements against the ordinances such as going out to market without the white rod or throwing straw from an infected house into the canals were still not being paid.[53] It appeared that administrations anticipated poor compliance too. During the severe dysentery outbreak that hit rural Brabant particularly hard in 1676, an ordinance from the village of Gestel suggested that the act of throwing dirty sheets and other filth (*vuylicheden*) in the streets, watercourses, or on neighbours' property was to be punished at a rate of three guilders first time around, but a repeat offence was six guilders.[54] During the plague of 1636 in Namur, it was observed by the magistrate that the citizens were ill-disposed to observe the edicts promulgated (*mal affectionnés à l'observation des édits promulgués*) regarding the proper keeping of animals.[55]

Another way to maintain compliance was to focus on segments of society and accentuate feelings of personal responsibility. Sometimes responsibility for meeting the demands of the ordinances was placed at the feet of parents or employers, who were fined for the actions of their children or servants if found traversing streets when sick—as seen in the above-mentioned case of Gestel.[56] In one finding from the Utrecht *buurspraakboeken* in 1493, literally "book of the neighbours' meetings" and concerned instructions to residents on different aspects of communal wellbeing, parents were told to make sure that children from houses infected with *die pestilentie* did not come onto the street to meet other children and were forbidden from attending school.[57] In Leiden in 1467, parents were not allowed out to work while children were at home infected with plague.[58] Personal responsibility, of course, was sometimes helped along with individual incentives to intervene. Parts of the fines were sometimes promised to those reporting contraventions of collectively accepted good practice by neighbours—although surely being an opportunity for self-interested exploitation.[59]

In the late Middle Ages, many initiatives connected to healthcare were voluntary or less institutionally formalised, and thus these were less visible in the sources.[60] Sanitation tasks in the southern Low Countries were initially taken on by ribalds—able-bodied paupers, usually migrants, employed temporarily—and were viewed by authorities and citizens with a fragile mix of disdain and indispensability.[61] By the late fifteenth century, however, this started to change as these same tasks became more institutionalised—with epidemic-related work falling under the remit of *gasthuis* masters, *schrobsters*, *cellebroeders*, and the like. Accordingly, workers became incentivised to do their jobs with increasing vigilance under the pains of punishment. In Mons in 1529, the urban administration explicitly warned local police to imprison any person infected with plague who did not obey the ordinances.[62] The hopman and police master were reminded and urged by the urban government of Groningen in 1604 that the previous year's plague ordinance had to be enforced.[63] Later, in the same city for the administrative year 1666/7, the deacon accounts mentioned record income from fines after the epidemic outbreak of 1665/6—3,423 guilders, of which nearly 83 per cent came from being too late in carrying off dead bodies.[64] Already mentioned above were the fines meted out to city guards. Pest house officials also had to make sure nobody escaped from these environments and that nobody came in to visit the sick, as noted in the plague instructions to the personnel working in the Middelburg hospital in 1604 and the Amersfoort pest house in 1605.[65] In seventeenth-century Tilburg, failure to do so was even punishable by death by shooting.[66]

Nevertheless, administrations could not be too harsh on their enforcers. After all, they needed people to carry out these jobs. In Namur in 1598, magistrates simply paid the police extra to not only remain in place but enforce the rules.[67] Pest house masters were paid well but also difficult to find. In one case from the Campine village of Lille in 1607, a pest house master was newly installed and had to be placed temporarily in a villager's house—even having to lend him some sheets to sleep in.[68] In Liège, during an outbreak in 1634, the local council took pains to protect a renowned expert at fighting *les pestiférés*, lodging him near to the Jesuits.[69] At Herk-de-Stad, near Hasselt in Limburg, it took some time before the magistrate was able to agree terms with a pest house master from another nearby village of Heusden to come work for two months in 1624—receiving 100 guilders, lodgings, and expenses for fire, food, and drink, and the rights to free movement.[70] Pest house masters that were not paid fully or promptly were unafraid of bringing this to the magistrates, as seen in a complaint from the village of Meldert (near Tienen) during the plague of 1636.[71] Thus, the role of pest house master, while dangerous, could turn out to be lucrative—especially when salaries were topped up by personal payments and inheritances. At the village of Wouw, near Breda, in 1625, the heirs of Cornelis van Roije were instructed to pay 84 guilders to the local pest house master as a fee for his services rendered.[72]

Indeed, not all relationships between administrations and enforcers were coercive, and often much of the information provided to urban governments depended on knowledge, investigations, and surveillance conducted at the neighbourhood level.[73] In cities and towns, many of the rules and regulations connected to epidemics were implemented on the ground by so-called *buurtheren*, who were appointed individuals from different neighbourhoods who investigated issues regarding safety, security, and the maintenance of a harmonious environment, and reported infringements to the *burgemeesters*. Thus, in Leiden during the plague of 1664, some of these tasks included making sure the floors of houses in which someone had died of plague remained closed for 14 days, that renting of these houses and rooms did not take place until eight weeks after the previous death, and that inheritance decisions relating to the property did not occur until two months had passed.[74] Similarly, the *buurtheren* had to make sure the pest houses did not get overburdened, and had to regulate visits of family members by issuing official letters of permission.[75] Apparently, this was one area in which the city administration did come into conflict with those working at the street level, as the *buurtheren* were urged to be more sparing in issuing these documents.[76]

Criminalising behaviour during epidemics

Another way to gain insight into the issues of punishment and compliance is to look at serial sources that deal with the regulation of behaviour within communities—comparing epidemic and non-epidemic periods.[77] An important source for the medieval period is the *correctieboeken* (book of corrections), which have recently been thoroughly exploited for Leiden—especially for the fifteenth century.[78] Numerous noteworthy disease-related offences have surfaced including the failure to make visible the white stick (as an infected marker) in public (1483/4), keeping the plague dead in houses for too long (1519), throwing items from houses with infections into the city canals (1526), and consistent failures to demarcate people or property that has been in contact with the sick—seen again and again in 1467, 1509, 1515, 1518, and other years.[79] Curiously, however, these kinds of disease offences seem to disappear from the Leiden *correctieboeken* after 1539, despite the series of sources extending on well into the seventeenth century.[80] Around the same time in Leiden, in 1533, a new series of criminal records is available (*criminele vonnisboeken*), but while diseases are sometimes mentioned in this source (someone dying of *pest*, for example), they never serve as the context behind a punishable offence. In fact, by the eighteenth century they seem to be an instrument used to commute sentences to a much lighter punishment.

Frequently, we see stays in prison or correction houses (*tuchthuizen*) being shortened and the indicted being set free on account of an infectious disease (*besmettelijke ziekte*)—instead banned from Leiden and the surrounding areas for several years.[81] This situation clearly corresponds with the argument developed in Chapter 2 that over time in the early modern period, epidemics increasingly came to be seen as products connected to dangers from outside, or rather, immoral and corrupted behaviour perpetrated by outsiders.

Failure to declare infected status publicly by presenting the white stick was registered as a crime in the *sentencie bouck* of Nieuwpoort (coastal Flanders) in 1609, where the man was punished by having his bound hands and feet struck with a sharp rod and banned for six years.[82] Just like Leiden, however, where we have longer series of records, such as from sixteenth- and seventeenth-century Utrecht, we see an absence of direct disease-related offences, while in Den Bosch, plague was only criminalised on three occasions and all through failures of demarcating sources of potential infection to neighbours.[83] In the criminal records for Gouda extending from 1447 to 1810, disease was also hardly ever a context for formalised prosecution of criminalised activity, although on one occasion in 1523 a couple are found guilty of coming from Schoonhoven to Gouda, infected with the *pestilencie*, and yet do not declare this before coming into public spaces.[84] More tangentially, on another occasion, in 1482, a man is found guilty of publicly denouncing another person with something described as *St. Jans ziekte*—often referred to as a kind of dancing mania, while centuries later, we find several punishments for the sale of meat from a sick animal during a cattle plague in 1746/7.[85] However, rather than as a vehicle for criminalising behaviour, epidemic disease was sometimes instrumentalised by authorities to encourage compassionate and generous giving—in 1454, 1467, and 1519, for example, the punishment for an offence extended to providing donations of resources to institutions dealing with the sick and infected during outbreaks.[86]

Thus, while diseases served as a context behind criminalisation of behaviour, quantitatively speaking, such cases were not numerous—or at least not often registered formally. This can be seen in the specific case of witchcraft prosecutions and their associations with plague, which have been examined in certain regions of early modern Europe.[87] Some of the well-known cases of witch trials in the Low Countries did include cases where those accused eventually admitted to causing outbreaks of disease in people and animals—such as the Roermond trials of 1613.[88] In one extensive trial of Mechteld ten Ham, a widow of a city messenger, at 's-Heerenberg (eastern Guelders) in 1605, this woman stood accused of doing sorcery (*doet getoevert*) on children who were infected *van der pesten* in 1602.[89] Yet, when we look to the three series of criminal records mentioned above at Utrecht, Den Bosch, and Leiden, we see no links to disease and witchcraft anywhere, and despite the many offences of witchcraft and heresy listed for sixteenth-century Utrecht.[90] In Flanders, a valuable database of 226 convicted witches in the period 1589–1684 only managed to produce four cases connected to plague, and this was generally the result of publicly cursing someone with *peste*—though all in actual plague years, it should be noted.[91] Other scholars have downplayed the link between witchcraft or sorcery accusations and plague outbreaks in Holland and surrounding areas.[92]

Criminal records can also be a useful index of epidemics' capacity to provide the background behind general increases in misbehaviour and dislocation—even when not explicitly mentioning disease. The interpretation of the findings, however, has some complications. Scholars of preindustrial crimes have long questioned to what extent criminal records can serve as an index of criminality—i.e., literal increases or decreases in anti-social behaviour in the positivistic sense—or instead reflect how authorities perceived societal behaviour and how certain acts might be classified as "an offence" which at other times were not considered offensive or criminal.[93] Many conflicts tended to be resolved informally within neighbourhoods rather than formally brought to the courts, and we know that the balance between private reconciliation and bureaucratic administration in issues of anti-social behaviour changed over time.[94]

These issues are difficult to resolve though it has at least been suggested that certain kinds of social infringements started to occur in greater numbers around known epidemic outbreaks and food crises in fifteenth-century Ghent, Ypres, and Leiden.[95] When we look to general offences—i.e., not necessarily explicitly mentioning disease as part of the offence—in the sixteenth- and seventeenth-century criminal records from Leiden, Den Bosch, and Utrecht, however, we do not observe a close temporal association between raised criminal activity (or activities "made criminal" by authorities) and known years of epidemic disease outbreaks (Table 4.1). This seems surprising given the social control aspects of disease management said to characterise plague administration, but accordingly likely lends support to the view I expressed above that repression and coercion were things more apparent in theory than in practice. Similarly, when isolating classic "social control during epidemics" kinds of offences such as those relating to vagrancy or begging, there was no spike in activity. If anything, fewer vagrancy and begging offences tended to occur in these three cities, which perhaps points to short-term urban-rural exodus or some hindrances to policing this issue at the street level. When looking at the two consecutive years after epidemics, however, vagrancy and begging related offences did increase compared to non-epidemic periods in Leiden. This is perhaps understandable when we consider that Leiden experienced particularly severe outbreaks in a comparative perspective, especially the ones connected to the siege of 1573/4, and 1624/5, 1635, and 1655, and experienced rapid population replenishment each time via migrants from the southern Low Countries seeking respite from religious persecution and employment in the growing textile industries.[96]

Table 4.1 Criminal offences in epidemic and non-epidemic years in Leiden, Utrecht, and Den Bosch, 1530–1699

		All criminal offences		*Vagrancy/begging offences*	
		No.	*Annual Av.*	*No.*	*Annual Av.*
Den Bosch, 1548–1699	Epidemic years	106	8.2	14	1.1
	Non-epidemic years	1,256	9	156	1.1
	2 years post-epidemic	116	11.6	0	0
Leiden, 1533–1699	Epidemic years	426	26.6	29	1.8
	Non-epidemic years	3,944	26.3	489	3.3
	2 years post-epidemic	408	34	68	5.7
Utrecht, 1530–1699	Epidemic years	221	13	44	2.6
	Non-epidemic years	2,696	17.5	587	3.8
	2 years post-epidemic	223	15.9	51	3.6
Total	Epidemic years	753	16.4	87	1.9
	Non-epidemic years	7,896	17.8	1,232	2.8
	2 years post-epidemic	747	20.8	119	3.3

Source: Updated from Curtis, Preserving, 287; with epidemic years based on Curtis, Was Plague an Exclusively Urban Phenomenon?; Van Besouw and Curtis, Estimating.

Resisting epidemic measures

While previous literature tended to focus on the ways in which epidemics became used as a tool to implement repressive measures and social control, and to a lesser extent on the implementation of these policies, it is only more recently that interest has started to emerge on the societal reception of these policies.[97] In fact, I argue that plagues and other epidemic diseases in the late-medieval and early modern Low Countries often became a context behind the opposite kinds of tendencies, where ordinary people, sometimes on the lower rungs of a hierarchical society, vented their frustrations and fears. Although this could at times spill over into active conflict, sometimes even violence, directed at perceived elites, authorities, or agents of the administration, more usually people refused to cooperate with those seen to be creating impositions which conflicted with tightly held freedoms and customary rights or duties.

Indeed, this interpretation makes sense when we consider the number of cases where plague regulations interfered with the usual practice of events that brought people together which were both socially and commercially important—see, for example, the cancellation of the annual fair (*kermis*) in Nijmegen on account of the ongoing *contagieuse sieckte der pestilentie* announced to the brewer's guild in 1664.[98] Around the same time in the Brabant village of Veghel, the magistrates prevented children from singing to mark the New Year and stopped them from going from house to house and singing on Epiphany (*aende drijconenghe*), and in the same village during a dysentery outbreak in 1781, bird shooting at the *kermis* and celebrations in the inns were ceased so that the "thorn of God" was no longer directed to the community.[99] When it came to attendance of church, authorities often realised the distressing impact restrictions on the infected would have, pre-empting the resistance and uproar that might take place, and had already in the fifteenth century, in places such as Ghent, Deventer, Gouda, and Antwerp, started to devise alternative sites and times of worship for those that had been in contact with plague.[100] Afraid of false rumours and gossip, urban administrations made public announcements in newspapers, downplaying the presence of epidemic-induced sickness.[101]

One of the key areas in which epidemic-related resistance and conflict played out concerned the burial of the dead, and this is unsurprising given that it was also an area in which authorities tried to regulate most stringently. Evidence from the preindustrial Low Countries suggests that ordinary citizens often rejected attempted supervision and controls. Although people feared falling sick during disease outbreaks, this did not necessarily override greater fears about the encroachment upon the obligations (a customary neighbourly duty known as *burenplicht*) concerning the proper process of burying one's friend or neighbour.[102] This included tasks such as washing the corpse, closing up rooms of the house, placing the corpse into the prepared coffin and taking it to the burial site, attending the funeral, and attaching symbolic items to the body such as rosemary or flowers.[103] Some of these unpaid tasks remained part of burial practice until well into the early twentieth century, especially in the countryside, although they increasingly began to be replaced by paid labour.[104]

On occasion, there is some evidence that certain people were less enthusiastic about carrying out the neighbourly duties during epidemic outbreaks. During the plague outbreak of 1664 in the Mallemolen area of The Hague, for example, even financial rewards were not enough to entice neighbours to carry corpses to burial sites. Eventually one Anthonij van Dijck came forward, but only after composing an agreement that promised him a lucrative share of the inheritance if the remaining members of the household also died while he carried out these duties. Burial was still at the heart of this arrangement, even for Anthonij himself, as one of the conditions passed was that if he died, he would be allowed an honourable funeral paid for by the household, and a burial in the family's own allotted plots in nearby Scheveningen.[105] In another standout case during the early phases of an epidemic outbreak in Leiden in 1624 from the court proceedings (*gerechtsdagboeken*), the residents of the neighbourhood of Kranenburg (*de gemene buijerem vam Cranenbuch*) close to the St. Catharina *gasthuis* complained about their duty of having to bring corpses from that hospital to their final burial place.[106] Such resistance might have been a product of the exceptional number of deaths that were occurring at that institution during epidemics, and the fact that many of these deceased patients came from different parts of the city and thus were potentially outsiders to the surrounding neighbourhoods of the *gasthuis*.

More usually, however, it was the opposite situation. Ordinary people during epidemics were unhappy at being impeded from performing their customary obligations. Thus, neighbours often ignored the authorities' requests for officially installed personnel (*lijkdragers*) to be the only ones with permission to carry corpses of the plague-infected to burial sites, and often just continued to do so themselves. In Utrecht during the plague of 1602, the dead were only to be moved by the Alexian Brothers (*cellebroeders*),[107] and while threats of financial penalties were commonplace for ignoring this advice, ordinary people remained steadfast in carrying out these habitual neighbourhood duties.[108] Indeed, the lines between it being a required imposition and that of an honourable voluntary role are quite blurry. Some neighbourhoods such as the Vuilpoort area of Dordrecht were recognised by the local authorities for their part in burying the plague dead during the 1650s outbreak and collectively received a sum of 30 guilders for their service.[109]

A more famous example is known from the plague riots of Groningen during an outbreak beginning in 1623.[110] Already during the plague of 1603/4, the urban government of the city had reminded local officials to try to maintain popular compliance with the restrictions relating to isolation and hygiene imposed through the framework of the ordinances.[111] These restrictions were ramped up in the initial stages of the 1623 outbreak, with further resolutions that restricted drinking at funerals and only allowed the employed officials to come and carry the corpses of the plague dead—at a fee of ten stuivers per body.[112] Not only did this cut across neighbourhood ties and diminish customary privileges, but this was seen as profiteering—made worse by the fact that the poor struggled to pay these extra charges for the bodies, especially when more than one death had occurred in a short space of time.[113] Consequently, when the plague became more severe in the summer of 1623, ordinary people started to resist these officials, claiming, moreover, that these agents of the authorities had not shown reverence or respect for the dead.[114] In a tense standoff, the situation was escalated by the government sending in soldiers to physically enforce the rules, but these too were met with physical aggression leading to violence and were eventually pelted with stones.[115] Strangely, although no changes in the official rules occurred, the next severe plague to occur in 1636/7 in Groningen saw no real spikes in violence—at least not from what can be discerned in the written record—which perhaps lends support to the idea that street-level implementation often deviated from the principles and intentions bestowed from above. We can assume, however, that the desire to provide voluntary services to the plague dead within neighbourhoods persisted. In one medical treatise written during the plague of 1664, it was noted that there was a great social pressure within neighbourhoods to be present and provide aid when someone close by had got sick or died from the affliction—describing the reciprocal nature of this service and the threat of societal isolation.[116]

Given that urban governments in the Low Countries became much more concerned with regulating the behaviour of their citizens during epidemics in the early modern period, one might assume that resistance to these kinds of infringements upon social life increased over time. Perhaps this is correct, although acts of resistance were also already seen in the late Middle Ages. During the severe epidemic outbreak of 1467/8, for example, it has been shown that certain communities in coastal Flanders displayed heightened anxiety towards other kinds of disease officials—those entrusted with the task of caring for the infected in their houses, cleaning rooms, items, and surfaces, and sometimes helping with the preparation of the body for burial (known here as *reeuwers*).[117] Although we should be aware of the rhetorical effect seen in the views of fifteenth-century chroniclers such as Anthonis de Roovere or Nicolaes Despars, both pointed to numerous accusations levelled at these workers in the surrounding area.[118] In Ypres, it was said that a Willem Matthys poisoned two girls who had already recovered; in Wervik, the corpse of a child who had died from the plague was cooked and deposited into a well to contaminate the water sources; holy water was said to be poisoned in Bruges and Wervik; and suspicious poisons were said to have been collected from a known *reeuwer's* house in Oudenburg and Nieuwpoort—with the accused duly burned at the stake.[119]

Such cases reveal the complicated and blurred lines behind blame, punishment, and resistance during preindustrial epidemic outbreaks. The targeting of these individuals—just like with the corpse carriers mentioned above—was not entirely based on their perceived vulnerability, but because they were seen as official agents of an administration, and thus distrusted, despite the fact that these victims of abuse or violence might indeed be socially or economically vulnerable themselves. And although we might assume that those going into homes of the infected were doing so for the financial rewards and thus were likely coming from a poor or precarious position, indirect cross-referencing of juridical sources from 1468 has suggested several of these accused *reeuwers* actually came from relatively well-to-do groups, even if this was not always the case.[120] Indeed, the events in coastal Flanders have some conceptual and temporal parallels with a series of witch hunts that occurred in nearby Arras, Artois, in 1459/60, which did not wholly target the weak or the marginalised but were accusations levelled at wealthy merchants, magistrates, and even the chamberlain to Philip the Good, Duke of Burgundy—those that were not burned at the stake saw their properties confiscated.[121]

Of course, this same distrust of plague workers—cleaners, corpse carriers, gravediggers—did not ease over time. Thus, in the rural Meierij surrounding Den Bosch, Brabant, the magistrates' accounts show a number of cases where so-called cleaners (referred to as *schrobbers* and *schrobsters*) were arrested during the epidemic outbreaks of 1521–4, for example, for deliberately contaminating doors and their handles, and given an extreme punishment of being burned at the stake.[122] In 1557, upon mention of an outbreak of disease at Lith (*die pestelentie gaen off haestige sieckten*), a village on the Meuse in the central Dutch River area, the magistrates announced that foreign (*vreemden*) *schrobbers* were to be pushed out of the village, and anyone who encountered one of these *schrobbers* was allowed to hit them with weapons from the village.[123] In Delft in 1567, a plague ordinance reflected upon the upsurges in harassment of the masters of the hospital by people infected with the *Gave Godts*, and thus urged people to behave politely and to not treat the officials with "unmannered words, bad language, or rebellion".[124] During the plague of 1571 in Antwerp, citizens were warned about assaulting the *cellebroeders* tasked with carrying the dead bodies under instruction of the city authorities (as in Groningen in 1623, attacked with stones), and yet in the same year, these same authorities were also seeding their own conspiracies about the behaviour of the plague *schrobbers* and *schrobsters*.[125] About a century later in the outskirts of Brussels, the urban administration installed pest house masters in vacant houses along the Rue du Curé (Forest), but this was met with verbal intimidation and physical aggression from nearby residents.[126] An *aflezingboek*, a register recording all announcements, regulations, or judicial sentences that were read aloud to the public by magistrates, noted during the worst phases of the plague outbreak in Leiden in September 1624 that grave diggers were being harassed and especially mocked by local children.[127] And this harassment was not only restricted to the epidemic workers but also other people doing their ordinary work in the context of an outbreak—see the ridicule of Catholic priests offering the last sacraments to those on their deathbed during 1570s plagues in Antwerp.[128]

Not all forms of resistance were so dramatic or involved forms of physical violence or intimidation. In fact, much more common were the different ways in which ordinary people tried to passively resist new impositions, regulations, and changes brought on by the administration of epidemic disease—perhaps resorting to foot-dragging or reluctance to implement measures, and drawing parallels with a contestation of environmental administration seen in the countryside of late-medieval Piedmont, for example.[129] A good example of this is when people infected with a disease, people that had encountered the infected, or merely those suspected of being infected, were urged to leave their homes, and temporarily reside somewhere else. In most large-city contexts, this was within the confines of a pest house or hospital, but for smaller towns and rural areas this could be a series of hastily constructed isolated huts on the settlement periphery. The urgency of removing people perceived to be infected can be seen in a case from Tilburg in 1594, at the time no more than a village, where two people were forced to vacate their homes and move to isolated huts so quickly that they had no time to buy clothes and were made to pay 22 stuivers for replacements.[130] This was strongly resented. Indeed, in another case from the nearby Brabant village of Den Dungen, when a husband-and-wife couple died from the *pest* in 1631, the designated guardians of the surviving children were asked to bring them to an isolated hut on the moorland for their own protection. In such a traumatic episode, it is understandable that the children refused to go and managed to get their own way—when threatened with being put out onto the streets, a neighbour took them in as an "act of mercy".[131] Such fears were clearly great for children left to fend for themselves. In the Campine village of Lille in 1627, upon the death of their parents in these isolated huts, three children simply decided to flee rather than fall into the hands of the authorities.[132] Temporary huts seemed to be a frequent isolation method in rural Brabant—explicitly recorded much more often than other areas and sometimes erected on common land.[133] As is known about preindustrial commons in this area, uses and boundaries were often contested—and thus, it is no surprise to see a sixteenth-century case where two infected villagers were found disputing the exact location of their isolation huts.[134]

Other kinds of refusals were commonplace. A woman from Leiden during an outbreak of 1515 refused to carry the familiar white stick in public, after caring for those infected with plague in her home.[135] During an outbreak in Leeuwarden in 1538, one man refused to close off and vacate his house after his wife had been infected with plague—not paying the first fine, nor a second higher one.[136] Such hesitation to leave was understandable given the potential negative consequences. Indeed, another husband-and-wife couple in the Limburg town of Hasselt were asked by the local government to leave their house that was *pest geinfecteerd* in 1670, and yet upon her return, the wife, now a widow, found that she had numerous goods stolen valuing 423 guilders—the equivalent of more than a lifetime of rent for a house of an ordinary labourer living to their fifties in this area—the injustice of which led her second husband to petition for compensation.[137] This case echoes those where goods were stolen from houses of those that had actually died during an epidemic, as seen in Utrecht during the plague of 1636.[138] In places such as Vianden and Diekirch, guild masters resisted calls by the administration to isolate those infected during the same plague.[139] Some people also refused to work. Thus, during the plague outbreak in Groningen in 1575, a poor servant went to the local magistrate to complain that his master's house had become too dangerous to work in on account of infections.[140] Another form of resistance was made by those working on ships who refused to adhere to the maritime quarantine regulations upon arrival—especially after the increased vigilance seen in the eighteenth century towards vessels from North Africa and the Levant—and was seen in the refusal of a Venetian ship to leave the port of Ostend in 1781.[141]

Ordinary citizens often became frustrated at the carelessness of plague workers carrying out the tasks at the behest of urban authorities. Thus, at Breda in 1670, a man named Cornelis, living next to the St. Joos chapel, claimed six Flemish pounds in damages after grave diggers had misused his property—bringing bodies of those infected with plague through the garden to bury at the St. Joos cemetery.[142] People also used outbreaks of epidemics to criticise the work of governments more directly. In one letter written by Assuerus van Vierssen to his children about the "fiery" *Sieckte der Pestilentie* at the Frisian town of Leeuwarden in 1656, he used his fears to criticise the local administration for their cheating, corruption, and wickedness (*bedriegerije, coruptie en booshede*) which apparently went hand-in-hand with the usual actions of government.[143] During an outbreak in Kampen in 1519, Wolter Luytken was so enraged with the local government over the price of beer that he wished on them the *pest*.[144] Accordingly, urban authorities by the seventeenth century started to recognise the problems of enforcing rules and restricting citizens—especially in key areas of religious observance. Over time, we see key concessions in some of the ordinances. For example, at Venlo in 1615 many of the usual things are mentioned connected to isolation, hygiene, and funeral regulations, but on the specific subject of going to church, the infected were banned, but could visit the Onze Lieve Vrouw van Genooi chapel on Sundays and holy days up to 10:30 in the morning.[145]

The maintenance of ordinary social norms, however, was not solely a case of resisting authorities and agents of the elite. Local communities, and neighbourhoods within those communities, also used epidemic diseases to regulate ongoing breakdowns in appropriate behaviour among themselves. In one noteworthy case from Leiden during a plague year of 1603, for example, the court journals or minutes (*gerechtsdagboeken*) show how pre-existing residents of the Achtergracht in the Rapenburg area complained bitterly about the numerous recently arrived migrants from the southern parts of the Low Countries to work in the growing textile industry. These workers began to fill up the city canals with the polluting remains of their wool products, "so that over time the streets and wooden city wall fittings were no longer usable, and combined with the water in the canals created a terrible stink that it was barely possible to live there, and this was especially in this time of the hot sickness (*heete sieckte*) that creates daily victims".[146] These local residents then petitioned the urban administration to punish the polluters and erect a warning sign. Thus, what we see is not a crackdown from above on environmental infringements, but the regulation of what was seen to be the common good by ordinary citizens.

Ordinary people also challenged medical practitioners, especially when there was a perceived negative outcome. At Kampen in 1520, one man went to a doctor who promised to cure him of his *pokken* (in this case likely syphilis rather than smallpox) for a fee of four guilders. The man registered a formal notarised complaint that the symptoms came back, and then his wife contracted it, meaning that he could not sleep next to her.[147] Similarly a notarised complaint was produced by a Rotterdam miller in 1652, who noted that 24 years ago (hence in 1628) he went to a surgeon after being stabbed in the back, but heard while being treated that the surgeon had kept his sister in the same house who had the *spaanse pokken* (either smallpox or syphilis).[148]

Resistance to medical authority, however, stepped up a level when doctors were framed as outsiders. As mentioned in Chapter 2, access to a medical practitioner was not straightforward for all people in the medieval and early modern periods, particularly in rural areas, with instead much of the healthcare interventions provided by localised access to herbs, spices, and potions. Often these were remedies suggested by local trusted clerics that they had prepared themselves.[149] This situation persisted well into the late eighteenth century within some rural communities. Hence, during the severe epidemics of dysentery in 1778/9 and 1782/3, for example, rural residents of isolated villages in the Duchy of Luxembourg were said to reject outside intervention and advice.[150] Similarly, in the Guelders villages of Doornspijk and Oosterwolde around the same time, the spread of dysentery was attributed in moralising terms to the "unforgiveable squalor of the residents and the closing up of their houses", and yet not one recommendation by the doctor M.J. van Cooth had been followed when he returned a week later.[151] Other physicians that visited Voorst, near Zutphen, in 1783 suggested that prejudices of the inhabitants made them loath to accept any means and advice, and the physicians were met with such hostility that they were reluctant to make future return visits. Of course, an additional factor was poor rural people's concerns about the costs—in the case of smallpox, for example, some households rejected advised medicines in favour of buttermilk.[152] It is important to note, however, that not all community members, even in relatively enclosed villages, thought the same. Indeed, in the aftermath of the smallpox outbreak of 1883/4 in Oud-Beijerland, some residents requested (re-)vaccination from the local medic, and yet under the instruction not to reveal this to neighbours or employers.[153]

Just as was seen in earlier plague outbreaks in the sixteenth and seventeenth centuries, interference and changes to burial practices still were a point of contention in the late eighteenth century and beyond. While administrative ordinances and medical advice instructed that the corpses of dysentery victims had to be buried "in a far place on moors, deep underground", one man from Olburgen and two parents from Velp still wanted to bury the bodies of their family members in consecrated church grounds.[154] In the end, magistrates conceded to these requests, although also noted that this information was not to be made public among the other local communities—controlling the outbreak narrative. Simultaneous concerns were raised during the dysentery outbreak in the nearby town of Arnhem. The decision by the local government in 1782/3 to force the poor to bury their dead at a new cemetery outside the Velperpoort led to the gathering of an angry group of citizens outside the town hall and then the market.[155]

Kindness and compassion

As well as resistance to authorities and elites, people also showed kindness and compassion to one another during epidemic outbreaks in the preindustrial Low Countries. Of course, there were acts that we might describe as particularly discriminatory or hateful. During the 1655 plague outbreak in Alkmaar, for example, the urban administration made it forbidden to rent houses out to Jews from outside the city and shippers could not transport Jews or their goods to the city.[156] Other groups from outside remained free to come and go as they wanted in Alkmaar in 1655. Such concerns were seen in a contemporaneous document from 1656, where the administration of the small Achterhoek town of Groenlo was satisfied to declare that a Jewish man, Philips Magenets, upon visiting his father-in-law, was not infected with the *pest*.[157] Yet in line with what Cohn has suggested, by the early modern period, the most terrible forms of antisemitic violence during epidemic disease had dissipated—especially when contrasting with the awful pogroms seen during the Black Death.[158] And while we have the naming of diseases after particular people and ethnic groups—for example, in the criminal records from Leiden, we see reference to syphilis as the "French Disease" (*morbum gallicum*)—this hardly can be placed in the same category as burning certain targeted groups of people to death.[159]

In fact, to begin with, administrations themselves were also not always wholly repressive—perhaps not out of kindness or compassion per se, but simply because it did not always suit the goals of authorities to coerce and repress. At Namur during an epidemic in 1569, public aid was offered to those confined to their houses and who were conforming with the isolation protocols.[160] Taxes were sometimes reduced with the explicit rationale of helping deal with the demographic damage caused by epidemic disease mortality, even if we do not know whether petitions by local communities themselves were always honoured by state officials.[161] Although perhaps more often to be found in the accounts of churches and poor tables, we also find several city accounts (*stadsrekeningen*) where sums were given out to those family members either looking after someone afflicted or had lost someone to a disease—whether this was quantitatively significant is something discussed in Chapter 5. Similar payments were made when families were split up and healthy children could not follow their parents into the pest house or hospital, as seen in Den Bosch in 1625, and in Amsterdam during the plague of 1664, the city made payments for ringing the church bells for the propertyless (*onvermogende*) that were infected with the *contagieuse sieckte*.[162] In 1617, the Amersfoort city administration suggested that if the households could not find the ten stuivers necessary to pay the gravediggers to take away the corpse from the plague-infected house, the urban government would honour the payment.[163] Although from the sixteenth century onwards there was increased unease in the connection between a kind of perceived "culture of poverty" and the spread of epidemic disease, a paternalistic moral economy also created forms of civic pride in successfully lowering the burden for those badly affected.[164] This persisted through to some of the epidemics of modern industrialisation—both Rotterdam and Antwerp administrations proudly vaunted their generous efforts to help poor migrants during the late-nineteenth- and early twentieth-century cholera outbreaks.[165]

We do have examples of clear unkindness among communities. At the village of Rhenen, near Utrecht, it was noted in the criminal records that after God had ignited a sad pestilence over the house of Aert Rutgersz in 1668, a group of people that attended his funeral had dared to rejoice "godlessly" with the outpouring of "very vile words".[166] Yet more often, rather than victimisation, there were calls for solidarity. At Helmond during the plague of 1636, several compassionate gifts were made to poor plague sufferers, including a special collection organised by the inhabitants of the small town in June.[167] Similar voluntary collections were made in October 1634 for the infected poor (*pauvres infectés*) at Liège and at Luxembourg in May 1636—where bare necessities were left in a tree by a gravedigger.[168] Inhabitants of plague afflicted communities came together to mark exceptional levels of death in collective memory—already mentioned is the example of the decorative board for the plague at Muiden, and at the small hamlet of Torgny in (Belgian) Luxembourg, locals built a chapel to this same end marking the cessation of a plague outbreak in 1637.[169] Private individuals similarly had built a plague chapel on the road to Roth from Vianden in 1587.[170] Although the cliché view of epidemics tends to emphasise greed and even thievery from vacated houses, which of course did happen on occasion,[171] it is interesting that a plague cleaner (*schrobber*), Hanrick Huijberts, found some loose cash (*kontant geld*) in a house that he served in during the occupant's life and then after the occupant had died, but simply handed the sum of two and a half guilders over to the surviving children's guardians.[172] In one case from Leiden, a widower by the name of Frederik Jacobsz was attacked by a debtor, and witnesses in support of his good character came forward to say that some years earlier during the *pest* of 1655, Frederik had worked day and night to help both poor and rich neighbours.[173]

Such cases continued into a period well beyond the disappearance of plague from the Low Countries. At the village of Gestel during the 1676 dysentery, it was announced in the ordinances that the sick could not come into public or common spaces, but if there was exceptional need, they should ask for help from their neighbours.[174] Similarly, during the dysentery outbreaks in late-eighteenth-century rural Guelders, authorities were also conciliatory—allowing friends and neighbours to care for the sick if they came from the same village, but not if they were associates from outside the community in question—conforming to the "dangers from outside" interpretation developed in Chapter 2.[175] Compassion was less likely to be extended to physical outsiders—and yet even occasionally on these grounds we have evidence of women at Namur going out to beg for resources in aid of the infected "foreigners".[176]

There were times in which help was refused to certain groups—see, for example, the plague outbreak of 1579 at Namur where a doctor had refused to treat the poor, but tended to urban professionals—yet this can be placed against an example from the same city just 20 years later where a doctor was met with incredulity by the same group of urban elites for his continual commitment to treating the infected poor in their temporary isolation huts built on the periphery of the city in Herbatte.[177] At Herk-de-Stad, Limburg, during the outbreak of 1623, the newly acquired master of the pest house agreed terms with the local magistrates where he promised to treat all those afflicted with the *gave Godts* both rich and poor (*reijcke ende arme*).[178]

Similar situations could be seen with clerics. On occasion we see reluctance and refusals. At Soignies, a small town in Hainaut, the Franciscan convent of the Grey Sisters outright refused to treat the plague afflicted in 1556.[179] A group of nuns (known as the *susteren van Reyde*) came to the city of Groningen in 1533 looking for residency in one of the monasteries, but on account of their infected status (*in die pestilencie bevallen*) none would dare take them in—eventually receiving five Emder guilders from the Stadtholder in compensation.[180] At Delft, priest Jacob Gerritsz of the Oude Kerk refused plague sufferers the last sacraments—a decision that would have knock-on consequences as the pest house similarly refused to take in the stricken that had not received the last sacraments.[181] In Alkmaar in 1598, priest Venator refused to treat plague sufferers because in Nijmegen three priests had died from it, including his brother.[182] Similar scenes were found in rural areas. At Haren, a small village in Brabant, someone was noted as having been infected with *de gave Gods*, but when the priest was asked to give the last rites and witness the testament, he did not do so out of fear of infection.[183] One infected child in Tilburg was brought to the house of the poor table in February 1625, but it was stated in the accounts that nobody wanted to help her.[184]

Yet, such cases often exist side-by-side the many reports we have of treatment by religious personnel inside and outside of formal ecclesiastical institutions.[185] Again at Namur, during the epidemic of 1555, it was noted that two *cordeliers* (members of a Franciscan reformist movement) spontaneously started attending to the infected.[186] Sisters at the St. Elisabeth monastery in Bergen op Zoom agreed in 1525 to take care of those infected with *pest* or dysentery (*root melisoen*) at a pest house linked to a newly constructed hospital, and where the poor table covered half the daily treatment costs of those unable to pay (a fee of 4.5 stuivers per day).[187] In one case from Ghent in 1603, the efforts of a Capuchin brother who died in the service of plague sufferers was martyred (*charitatis martyrio*) for his works.[188] At Roermond in 1618, Jacobus Carisius, priest of Montfort, was recognised by the magistrates for his many services during the time of the *pest*.[189] An Alexian brother from Lier, Jan van den Bolck, is found in the probate records to have received numerous sums of money from different families that he helped during the epidemic outbreak of 1661/2 in Princenhage, close to Breda—including a large sum of almost 88 guilders from the poor table for carrying out work that helped the poor.[190] The citizens of Vianden and Diekirch had so much gratitude for the efforts of the Franciscan monks during the outbreak of 1668 that they voluntarily contributed to the foundation of a new church and convent.[191] Even where priests refused to help—as seen in the above-mentioned case from Haren—other local people stepped in to do the tasks such as acting as witnesses. Often these people were not elites but ordinary residents, and often women such as maids or *schrobsters*. And even when clerics were fearful, they still sometimes found solutions. In the burial register of 1666 for the small village of Keiem in coastal Flanders, a priest scaled a ladder to hear out of a window the last confession of a domestic maid who was dying of *contagione*.[192]

As we might expect, the narrative of epidemic-induced fears leading to widespread abandonment of family members is not always confirmed in the sources. For example, at Amersfoort in 1521, one man wrote a letter of explanation as to why he was not travelling, citing the fact that since his wife was dying of plague, he wanted to stay with her until she died.[193] Of course, there were cases where family members were not cared for—although this was rarely to do with fear of infection. Thus, in one letter from the plague year of 1636, we learn that one man, Christiaan Jan Fransz., wanted to pass off an infected family member to a Cornelis Jansz. Baerdt of Alkmaar on the grounds that he had more resources—perhaps so, given that Cornelis was the financial agent for Wollebrant Geleyns de Jongh, a trader and director of a trade post of the Dutch East India Company (*VOC*) in Gamron, Persia. Christiaan noted the costs of four guilders a week to pay to a plague keeper (*pestbewaarder*), and soon would have to move her to a pest house if the money ran out.[194] And it should be recognised that sometimes there was simply no alternative. Thus, after the severe epidemic outbreaks in Groningen in the 1660s and early 1670s—linked with the military exploits of the Bishop of Münster in the context of the Second Anglo-Dutch War—the orphanage was left with its highest ever number of children simply left parentless and without adult family members to pick up the burden.[195]

Epidemics, social responses, and the impact of industrialisation

Modern industrialisation in parts of the Low Countries started quite late from a western European perspective—not taking off until after 1800. As noted in Chapter 3, by the nineteenth century, the major disease threats had started to change somewhat—although moderate outbreaks continued in the countryside, many of the burdens were now recurring epidemics of cholera, tuberculosis, and smallpox, and often focused on cities and towns. Nevertheless, there is no sign that there was any kind of sharp deviation between a preindustrial and industrial or premodern and modern form of societal response to epidemic outbreaks in the Low Countries. In fact, much seemed to stay the same, despite the (slow and incomplete) uptake of germ theory ideas in the final third of the nineteenth century. Indeed, many of these collective mechanisms, including those mentioned above, were simply the same kinds of patterns of coping seen in non-epidemic times.[196]

Recent research has emphasised the expected patterns of behaviour in dealing with these anticipated and recurring outbreaks. For example, infectious diseases such as cholera and smallpox in the small town of Woerden in the nineteenth century were framed as a kind of managed risk rather than leading to any extreme or panicked measures.[197] A concept that has gained further ground is that of cultural resilience—the idea that individuals and communities in the Low Countries overcame potential adversity and hardships caused by epidemics such as cholera through moral and religious expression in the form of poetry, songs, sermons, novels, prints, and processions, using iconography and personification that on the one hand could spike fears but at the same time helped shape and solidify community through instructive emotions.[198] Likely, the spread of new technologies and mediums for widening access to this information only magnified further the scale of these collective responses—fostering links within communities but also between communities. Yet as in the preindustrial period, attempts by authorities to infringe upon collective expressions of solidarity and piety such as processions, dancing, and music, as seen during the cholera of 1866 in Antwerp, were met with popular resistance.[199]

Although epidemics in the preindustrial past were associated with some instances of charitable giving, perhaps one key difference between nineteenth-century responses and those further back in time was the closer link to charitable expression—and an expression this time not only born out of moral replenishment of the donor (very preindustrial) but genuine concern for the plight of the victims. This is very much in line with a recent analysis of the long-term temporal dynamics of disaster interpretation in western Europe, where the medieval frameworks of fear and wonder started to loosen and be gradually replaced by concepts of terror and pity.[200] Accordingly, we have evidence from various different contexts in Holland and Utrecht around the middle of the nineteenth century of the income received from cultural products—poems, published sermons, songs, and concerts—which was then given to those needy perceived as hard affected by cholera outbreaks.[201] Remarkably, the small town of Oud-Beijerland received a donation of 80 guilders from Grand Rapids in Michigan (which had many residents of Dutch origin) to support the community afflicted by smallpox.[202] As above, this transnational exchange was testament to the greater flows of epidemic information across wider areas, and the growing receptiveness to an interpretation of epidemics as products of something more than just localised phenomena in specific contextual conditions.[203]

We could also point to the emergence of new organisations concerned with the plight of families which had lost members of their household during an epidemic—such as the "cholera committees" (*De Commissie ter Ondersteuning van Nagelaten Betrekkingen van Choleralijders*) seen in Utrecht that ended up supporting activities such as soup kitchens (*volksvoeding*).[204] Although difficult to classify as bottom up or collective enterprises—most of the members were relatively well-to-do men active in social causes—they were voluntary and initiated entirely separate to the official city administration.[205] Nevertheless, and again, just like in the preindustrial period, charitable interventions during outbreaks of cholera were not wholly benevolent. For example, port towns such as Rotterdam and Antwerp in the late nineteenth- and early twentieth-century cholera outbreaks, taking in large numbers of migrants from different regions of eastern Europe, saw aid societies such as the Jewish Montefiore and Ezra take on paternalistic roles, emphasising hygiene in their "civilising" concerns over victims—with the related idea that this was necessary to prevent negative impacts on the status of Jews already settled and pre-existing in the cities.[206]

Conclusion

Whilst it would be an exaggeration to suggest that people in the preindustrial Low Countries did not fear falling sick during epidemic disease outbreaks or were not scared of epidemics occurring in other places spreading to their own communities, most anxiety that we observe was more connected to the restrictions and infringements devised by elites and authorities with power. Although much emphasis in the historiography has tended to be on the capacity of epidemics to serve as an instrument for repression or social control of citizens by administrations, with a disproportionate historiographical focus on the enactment of plague ordinances, the case of the Low Countries in the medieval and early modern period shows that people also resisted these regulations. Perceived agents of the administration or those involved in the disease economy were most likely to be subject to pushback, sometimes violent—even if those on the receiving end of this resistance, abuse, or violence were not always true representatives of the elite but vulnerable people themselves. Here, we have the paradox that while epidemics sometimes created extreme or disruptive social responses, often these responses were for the express purpose of maintaining customary practices and ordinary patterns of everyday life. Epidemic disease did not bring about revolutionary ideals or structural change—quite the opposite, these outbreaks stimulated conservative and reactionary tendencies based around maintaining a kind of lifestyle under threat.

The question we might then pose is why this was the case? Ultimately, beyond the obvious—being that preindustrial and early industrialising people tended to hold tightly to these customs and practices that bound communities together—first, we should note that although literature has usefully centred the importance of the common good (*bonum commune*) in the regulation of public health in the preindustrial Low Countries, the perception of who exactly belonged to the collective and what defined the common good varied between the different interests and layers of society.[207] The common good as defined by the city, town, or village administrations was very different to that defined by traders, farmers, and workers, and sometimes these definitions conflicted when faced with threat or pressure (such as through epidemic disease). The fact that abuse and violence were often perpetrated by ordinary citizens, rather than the powerful, should not surprise us—those elites with power tended to work with administrations or have economic interests that did not benefit from outright repression or conflict.

We should also note that epidemics likely produced this effect in the Low Countries because of their intrinsic characteristics. Scholars working on different parts of the Mediterranean have tended to emphasise how major plague outbreaks, for example, tended to be fewer and more severe than in central or northern Europe.[208] Although we might dispute the extent to which plagues such as that of 1630 in northern Italy really were so much more severe than those of 1636 in the Dutch Republic (see Chapter 3), we should at least acknowledge that Low Countries epidemic outbreaks were much more frequent and recurring over the long term. As seen in Chapter 3, consistently from the fourteenth century onwards we can reconstruct a significant outbreak every ten or fifteen years all the way up to the seventeenth century, and even after the final plague outbreak in the 1660s, epidemics still were highly recurring (but slightly less territorially pervasive) all the way into the nineteenth century. Industrialisation did not bring about much change in this regard. Put simply, people were used to epidemics regularly occurring and catered for them in their collective consciousness. Indeed, written documents and material culture show that people learned and adapted from previous outbreaks and certainly remembered them—to not remember was in fact explicitly moralised in a critical way. Hence, epidemics were not massive departures from the norm, even if they did cause burdens and hardships—they were part of the norm and therefore blurred the conceptual lines between epidemic and endemic. What we see next in Chapter 5 is that the consciousness of these pressures also helped dictate how communities and households managed their assets during epidemics under threat of redistribution.

Notes

1 Han and Curtis, *Infectious Inequalities*; Wald, *Contagious*.
2 On the transition from epidemic optimism to pessimism: Snowden, Emerging. On the new forms of anxiety from the 1980s: Sontag, *Illness*.
3 Barnes, Social Vulnerability.
4 For SARS: Person et al., Fear; Eichelberger, SARS. The COVID-19 literature is already too large to cite in full, but see Wikipedia's extensive list of incidents: https://en.wikipedia.org/wiki/Xenophobia_and_racism_related_to_the_COVID-19_pandemic.
5 Delumeau, *La peur*.
6 Naphy, *Plagues*; Ross, Syphilis; Monter, *Witchcraft*, 44, 47, 126; Bever, Witchcraft, 573; Andreski, The Syphilitic Shock.
7 McKinley, Foucault. For the original comments on sickness, health, and regulation: Foucault, *Discipline*, 195–200.
8 Bowsky, The Impact; Bowsky, The Medieval Commune; Bourdelais, *Les épidémies terrassées*, 27; Shirk, The Black Death, 357; Shirk, Violence; Horrox, ed., *The Black Death*, 43; Chiffoleau, La violence, 325–7. The Boccaccian narrative refers to the direct observations of Giovanni Boccaccio during the Black Death, who emphasised all these aspects of social breakdown in mid-fourteenth-century Florence.
9 Arnold, *Colonizing the Body*; Chandavarkar, Plague Panic; Bashford, Epidemics.
10 Remarkably, similar sentiments are visible even today. See, for example, on the issue of analysing the lives of women in the past, "we can reject a blanket insistence on quantifiable data, large sample sizes, corroborative sources": Lipscomb, How Can We Recover the Lost Lives of Women? 193.

11 On abandonment: Cohn, Plague Violence; and anti-Semitic violence: Cohn, The Black Death. For literature on Jewish persecution around the time of the Black Death in the Low Countries: Vanbossele, Egidius Li Muisis; Cluse, De Jodenvervolgingen. Charles of Luxembourg (who becomes Charles IV, Holy Roman Emperor in 1355) wrote a letter to the Luxembourg administration in July 1349, urging the Jews to be unharmed, followed by another in May 1350 to find ways to resettle Jews of the city—suggesting that expulsions had already taken place: Pauly, Pestepidemien, 56. Of course, it should be asserted that the Black Death was not the start of this persecution—upticks in blame for poisoning wells, for example, were already seen well before the mid-fourteenth century: Barzilay, *Poisoned Wells*; Nirenberg, *Communities*, 93–124.

12 Archambeau, Healing Options, 558–9; and for Jewish interpretations, in particular: Einbinder, *After the Black Death*. Some have downplayed excessive societal dislocation in the aftermath of the Black Death: Vargas, How a "Brood of Vipers" survived; Kelly Wray, *Communities*.

13 A narrative established in Cohn, *Epidemics*; Cohn, Pandemics. See, also, a range of outcomes presented in Jedwab et al., Epidemics.

14 Cohn and Kutalek, Historical Parallels; Cohn, Cholera Revolts.

15 Noordegraaf and Valk, *De gave Gods*, 221–4. And "the sources overflow with examples of all kinds of social disruption": Noordegraaf, Dearth, 56. Likewise, in Zwart-Kramer and Zwart, *Van pest*, 67: the 1636 plague "turned the functioning of the community totally on its head".

16 Noordegraaf, Calvinism. Of course, we should note that reverence for these religious weapons depended on context. Sometimes those associated with Catholicism, like the protective functions of St. Sebastian and St. Rochus, came to be rejected and mocked such as in 1570s and 1580s Antwerp: Coomans et al., Plague, 587. More generally in the literature of hazards and disasters in the preindustrial Low Countries, there has been emphasis on the importance of pious and spiritual rituals as a mode of coping: Duiveman, Praying; Duiveman, Breaking the Cycles.

17 The classic example posited being medics' tendency towards flight: Grell, Conflicting Duties.

18 Frijhoff, Gods gave afgewezen; Sundberg, *Natural Disasters*, 51–88, 212–50; Van Roosbroeck, Experts.

19 Rommes, Op het spoor; Rommes, Pest; Van Zalinge-Sporen, "Die contagieuse sieckte"; Klinkenberg, "Dye quade siecte". Nevertheless, we still occasionally see offhand statements such as "Plague, poverty and famine further undermined the traditional structure of many communities": Der Weduwe, *State Communication*, 58.

20 For the classic story of crackdowns from above: Lis and Soly, *Poverty*, 79; Naphy and Spicer, *The Black Death*, 80.

21 Curtis, Preserving.

22 For classic examples of cholera-induced rioting and resistance: Evans, Epidemics; Gill et al., Fear; Briggs, Cholera; Cohn, Cholera Revolts; Snowden, Cholera; Salomé, Le massacre. On the potential differences between plague and cholera riots: Cohn, Fear.

23 Murphy, Plague Ordinances, 142. We do have proclamations and bylaws announced by Tournai urban council as early as the Black Death of 1349–51 that attempt to bring together modest regulation of potentially corruptive activities but mainly accentuating continuities in daily social and economic practices: Billen and Boone, eds., *Bans*, 43–7. The originals were lost during the bombing of Tournai in 1940 but are based on fortunate discoveries of transcriptions by

nineteenth-century Tournai archivist, Frédéric Hennebert, in the University of Ghent library.

24 On post-Black Death flagellants: Jansen-Sieben, Ooggetuigen; De Cuyper, Egied van der Hoye; mentions via retrospective chroniclers: Joosting, ed., Cornelis Block's kroniek, 23; Van Bavel et al., eds., *De kroniek*, 21. An example in a year 1400 ordinance: Van Doorninck, ed., *Acten*, 28–9.

25 Curtis, Preserving, 284.

26 Coomans et al., Plague, 591.

27 Wassink, *Van stad en buitenie*, 259.

28 RHCE, Gemeentebestuur Gestel, 1620–1810, no. 336 [AO].

29 For dysentery ordinances in Groningen in December 1779: GA, Stadsbestuur van Groningen (2), 1594–1815, 1605, no. 805, 1143 [AO]; and also in Brabant in 1779: Van Asseldonk, *Veghel*, 307–9; and Guelders in 1779 and 1783: Christiaens and Evers, *Patriotse illusies*, 15.

30 Van Even, ed., Reglement, 135.

31 For the text: Anon., ed., *Annales*, XIII, 349–50.

32 Anon., ed., Ordonnantie Roermond.

33 Compare: Anon., ed., Ordonnantie Haarlem 1655, no. 4; with Anon., ed., Ordonnantie Leiden 1655, no. 2.

34 Coomans et al., Plague, 592.

35 Curtis, Where's the Disaster in Disaster Studies?

36 Beck, *Spiegel*, 200 [7/11/1624].

37 The need to collectively remember these outbreaks was something urged by contemporary authorities, and can be seen, for example, mirrored in the pamphlets and treatises written about flood events occurring in the early modern period and early phases of modern industrialisation: For the 1681/2 flood: Van Oudenhoven, *Antiquitates Cimbricae Renovatae*, 3; for the 1775 flood: Hendrik Hering, *Bespiegeling*, I, 46–7; for the 1825 flood: Thelwall, *Keert u Tot Hem Die Slaat*, 5–6.

38 SA, Archief van de Notarissen ter Standplaats Amsterdam, Afschriften van notariële acten in banden, 1612–1644, no. 96560 [AO].

39 Van Tielhof and van Dam, *Waterstaat*, 213, 341.

40 Graas, De verbeelding. According to the 1622 household census (*hoofdgeld*), Muiden had 891 residents. Thus, either the small town had almost entirely replenished its population in 20 years, or the death toll of the plague is overexaggerated: Ekamper, De summiere staat, 3.

41 Dippel, Kanttekening, 255.

42 Pollmann, Iconoclasts, 163.

43 Summaries of all these facets of epidemic administration through formal ordinances can be found in Van Veen, De pest; Van Andel, Pestepidemieën; De Backer, Maatregelen; Dupont, De bestrijding.

44 An ordinance in Groningen connecting plague, poverty, and begging, and making a distinction between the "real poor" and "work shy", and "our poor" and "foreign poor": Huisman, *Stadsbelang*, 23. The poor were explicitly paid to leave the city of Namur in the 1523 and 1530 outbreaks: Jacquet-Ladrier, Les épidémies, 131.

45 Coopmans, *De rechtstoestand*, 197.

46 Boterbergh, Burgers, sections 3.6 and 3.7.

47 Knibbe, Enkele Friese lonen, 102–4.

48 Seventeenth-century examples in this paragraph taken from Curtis, Preserving, 285–6.

49 Calculations from Leiden's seventeenth-century *Verpondingen*: Van Besouw et al., Epidemic Mortality.

50 This included the *stadsrekeningen* or *dorpsrekeningen* of Amsterdam, Besoijen, Breda, Den Bosch, Deventer, Grave, Hulst, Knollendam, Loon op Zand, Nijmegen, Sluis, Terneuzen, Utrecht, Venlo, Zutphen, and Zwolle: for the budgets, see Curtis, ed., Original Burials Data.
51 Ladan, *Gezondheidszorg*, 63.
52 Van Schevensteen, ed., *Documents*, I, 79–80, 153.
53 AEA, Stadsbestuur Amersfoort, 1300–1810, 0001.01, no. 18, fo. 9v [9/7/1599] [AO].
54 RHCE, Gemeentebestuur Gestel, 1620–1810, no. 336 [AO].
55 Riguelle, La police, 475.
56 RHCE, Gemeentebestuur Gestel, 1620–1810, no. 336 [AO].
57 HUA, Stadsbestuur van Utrecht 1122–1577, 701, Buurspraakboek of Luiboek, 1385–1391, 1396–1536, 1542–1555, 1560–1579, no. 16.17 [1490–99], fo. 75r [AO]. This original finding was made by Claire Weeda, Leiden University (pers. comms. 5 June 2020). On the uses of the *buurspraakboeken*: Coomans, *Community*, 115.
58 Ladan, *Gezondheidszorg*, 62–3.
59 Coomans, *Community*, 230. Although, it is not clear to which specific places and contexts this applied to, from the text.
60 Coomans, *Community*, 241.
61 Weeda, Doing the Dirty Work.
62 Hachez, Les fondations charitables, 189.
63 Huisman, *Stadsbelang*, 151.
64 Buursma, *"Dese bekommerlijke tijden"*, 79. Although, in line with the previous observation about fines above, this income was derived from numerous offences rather than the exceptional severity of the fine, since it was an offence also recorded outside of epidemic years and bringing an average of 150 to 200 guilders in.
65 ZAM, Godshuizen Middelburg, 1343–1812, 24.1, no. 19 [AO]; AEA, Stichting Armen de Poth te Amersfoort, 1342–1999, 0100, no. 571 [AO].
66 De Brouwer, "De aenclevende sieckte", 6.
67 Jacquet-Ladrier, Les épidémies, 134.
68 Janssens and Van den Branden, De pest, 43.
69 AEL, Archives de la Cité de Liège, 1434–1829, Registre aux enquêtes générales. 1634–1636, no. 10, fo. 36 [10/10/1634] [AO].
70 Nijssen, Zo ging dat.
71 Vanduynhoven, De jaren 1637 en 1668. The *burgemeester's* accounts in fact go on to show, besides ordinary salary payments, numerous extra expenses and services to be paid to the pest house master.
72 SB, Dekenaten Bergen op Zoom en Breda behorend tot Bisdom Antwerpen (1420) 1561–1802, ARC0007.3, no. 361. The document also refers explicitly to the dangerous contagion (*morbo contagioso periculose*).
73 Coomans, Making Good, 1062.
74 ELO, Stadsarchief van Leiden, (1253) 1574–1816 (1897), 0501A, no. 79, fo. 2v–3r.
75 Indeed, in one entry from the *kladresoluties*, it was noted that the *sieckenbesouckers* (visitors of the sick) had complained about the growing numbers of people going to the pest house creating hideous (*affschuwelick*) conditions: ELO, Stadsarchief van Leiden, (1253) 1574–1816 (1897), 0501A, no. 249 [5/7/1664].
76 Van Meeteren, *Op hoop van akkoord*, 35–6.
77 On this subject, see the series of criminal trials for Bologna spanning before, during, and after the Black Death: Dean, Plague; and followed up more generally for the early modern period in the same city: Rose, Plague.

78 Coomans, *Community*, 155–6.
79 Ladan, *Gezondheidszorg*, 62–3; Tamis, Ook zij slaat wel eens terug, 89.
80 Curtis, Preserving, 286.
81 In 1706, 1709/10, 1715, 1721, 1726, and 1728: Van den Heuvel, ed., Crimineel klachtboek, 42, 82, 117, 120, 394, 1027, 1438, 1447, 1667.
82 Viaene, Een woelige pestlijder.
83 These criminal records are digitally accessible via Anon., ed., Dataschurk; Anon., ed., Criminele sententies. In Den Bosch, these offences reappear in the city accounts, all with modest one guilder fines: one woman left the doors and windows open of her plague-infected house; one man did not hang straw out of his house after his wife was infected with *peste*; one man let the clothes of his dead daughter (from *peste*) out of his house: Van Zuijlen, *Inventaris*, I, 708.
84 Doedeijns, ed., Uitreksels, 63.
85 Doedeijns, ed., Uitreksels, 37, 236–7.
86 Doedeijns, ed., Uitreksels, 14–15, 24, 59.
87 Although highly nuanced for mountain communities of the western Alps in Naphy, *Plagues*. Formal persecutions based on perceived heretical religious practices have recently been investigated for the repeat epidemic outbreaks of 1523–32 on the Canary Islands: Geremia, Plague.
88 Dresen-Coenders, *Het verbond*, 227–65.
89 EAL, Huis Bergh, (828) 1227–1842, 0214, no. 7268, fo. 10v [AO]. On the exceptional nature of this case: Frijhoff, Satan, 397.
90 A well-known case from Den Bosch in 1595 involved the trial of Lyssen Thys, although the use of disease was ambiguous. A testifier against her spoke of how she used sorcery to give another woman, Aelken, *pokken* (likely, syphilis), while in her defence, Jan Wieringen told the court that he had stayed with his family in the house of Lyssen to escape from the raging *pest*: Harmeling, Het heksenproces.
91 Calculated from the appendix of Monballyu, *Van hekserij beschuldigd*. Some examples of convictions leading to burnings were recorded in 1468/9 based on accusations of causing *pest*: Monballyu, Schadelijke toverij, 267.
92 De Waardt, *Toverij*, 93–4.
93 Sharpe, Quantification.
94 Bogaers, Geleund, 341; Eisner, Long-Term Historical Trends, 126–8.
95 Coomans, Policing, 100–1; Coomans, *Community*, 155–6.
96 Van Besouw et al., Epidemic Mortality; Ladan, *De pest*; and Figure 3.13.
97 Especially Curtis, Preserving; and on the wider reception of epidemic knowledge produced by medics and clerics: Dekker, Coping; Dekker, God's Invisible Particles. For England: Williams, Urban Governance; for Tuscany: Henderson, Plague.
98 RAN, Brouwersgilde Nijmegen, 1562–1770, 300, Publikatie van de magistraat over de afgelasting van de kermis in verband met de pest en het verbod bier aan klanten van buiten de stad te leveren, no. 49 [AO]. Usefully accessible with a transcription at: https://watstaatdaer.nl/oefenen/complete-teksten/kermis-nijmegen-afgelast-vanwege-de-pest.
99 BHIC, Dorpsbestuur Veghel, 1310–1810 (1814), 7697, no. 65, fo. 21v [16/12/1664] [AO]; Van Asseldonk, *Veghel*, 308.
100 Coomans, *Community*, 235–6.
101 Der Weduwen, *State Communication*, 265. In 1670 in the *Oprechte Haerlemse Dingdaegse Courant*, it was noted that fewer people had been sick or died in Leiden than in the previous decade and nobody had been brought to the pest house in the previous two years.

102 On the importance attached to this duty: Den Boer, Naar een geschiedenis; Van Meeteren, *Op hoop van akkoord*, 32. Similarly, in London in 1637 it was noted in the aftermath of an outbreak that "[the poor] hold it a matter of conscience to visit their neighbours in any sickness, yea, though they know it to be the infection": Slack, *The Impact*, 232.

103 Temminck, Begraven. Although seemingly innocuous, the act of placing these items was very important. As mentioned above, authorities tended to crack down with strong punishments on elaborate decorations for burials of those who died from plague: Andel, Pestepidemieën, 1852. Nevertheless, people continued to do so. In the epidemic and famine of 1565, two women, Met and Geertgen Stoeldreijers, make *pellendwelen* (cloth products) for others to lay on their coffins as they are dying of *pest*. One of them forgets this item in their house: GAA, ORA Arnhem, 2003, no. 400, fo. 105v–6r [12/11/1565] [AO].

104 Klein-Hamming, Van burenplicht.

105 Van Breemen-Kruyt, De gave Gods, 48.

106 ELO, Stadsarchief van Leiden, (1253) 1574–1816 (1897), 0501A, no. 55, fo. 57r–8r [28/1/1624]. According to the General Ordinance of the Neighbourhoods (*Generale Ordonnantie op de Gebuurten*) in Leiden, the eight closest neighbours to the house where someone had died bore this obligation. The court (*Gerecht*) in the end decides to give this duty to a broader selection of residents and not only the eight closest houses.

107 Van der Weyde, Bijdrage, 3131. A regulation also seen for the Alexian brothers and sisters of Bergen op Zoom during the epidemic of 1577: WBA, Archief van de stad Bergen op Zoom, 1397–1810, 0005, no. 3112.

108 Bogaers, Geleund, 350; Rommes, Op het spoor, 114.

109 Helms van Eis, ed., Landpachters.

110 There are mentions of *pest* in the protocol of the civil affairs already in 1622, but it is unclear if this is in Groningen city or the surrounding region: GA, Hoge Justitiekamer en andere gewestelijke rechterlijke instellingen, 1444–1811, 136, no. 854, fo. 401.

111 GA, Rechterlijke Archieven III, a9 [22/6/1604]. As a sign of the pressures, a new cemetery (Nieuwe St. Walburgskerkhof) was opened in the north of the city specifically for plague victims: Schroor, *Rurale metropool*, 40.

112 Huisman, *Stadsbelang*, 153.

113 Huisman, *Stadsbelang*, 157. In some cases, in the seventeenth century, we see ten stuivers per corpse. For example, that was the amount paid to Hoeven Dircxzoon to take the plague dead and set them to rest in Wijk-bij-Duurstede, a village near Utrecht: Heijmans, ed., Nadere toegang, 250 [21/9/1603]. In other cases, we see fixed sums for work across a period—for example, 100 florins (guilders) for a year's work of helping carry and bury bodies connected to the *haestighe sieckte* in Breda: SB, Stadsbestuur Breda (oud administratief archief) 1280–1810, Stadsrekeningen, no. 554, fo. 122v [15/10/1604]. By the individual rate of corpse collection that would represent the collection of 200 bodies within the year by one person.

114 Lonsain, Een oproer, 57.

115 GA, Register Feith, 1291–1815, 2041, Ordonnantiën op het begraven van de aan de pest gestorven, no. 878, fo. 419 [5/5/1623 and 12/8/1623].

116 Deusing, *Twee Diepzinnige en heilzame onderzoekingen*, 49–51.

117 Viaene, Reeuwers; Devriese, Dood. The term *reeuwer* seems far more prevalent in Flanders than further north in the Low Countries where more general terms of *schrobber* and *schrobster* prevailed (see Chapters 5 and 6). It has, moreover, been suggested that the pejorative meaning of *reeuwer* tended to persist in parts of Flanders especially after the 1460s episodes—as revealed at Diksmuide where

they were said to harbour intentions of secretly taking items from vacant houses: Viaene, Reeuweghe, 317.

118 On this rhetorical effect: Mareel, Urban Literary Patronage, 50–2.

119 Huyghebaert, Reeuwers, 98, 100.

120 Roelens, Het sodom, 219–20.

121 Mercier, *La vauderie*, 7, 11–12, 19; Huyghebaert, Reeuwers, 99–100. However, recent work has pointed to links between the burning of Waldensians (a religious group founded in the twelfth century and known for their frugality and sobriety) in and around Arras in 1459/60 and persecution of *reeuwers* described as "lower-order plague workers": Reinhardt, *Plague Workers*, 30–41. As stated by Reinhardt, more work is possible and needed on this topic.

122 Beijers, ed., Meierijse schoutsrekeningen, no. 12996, fo. 229, 233, 241–2, 248, 258 [last accessed April 2025]. More information on these cleaners and their position within society is addressed in Chapters 5 and 6. Verifying these kinds of punishments, the bailiff of the Land van Breda wrote to Prince Willem of Orange about the horrifying crimes occurring in the villages of Oosterhout and Zundert in 1558, and a case of a man who was found guilty of spreading *pest* and put to death in a way "never seen before" in the Barony: Kappelhof, ed., Kroniek, 43–4.

123 BHIC, Schepenprotocol Lith, 7323, no. 41, fo. 21 [3/10/1557] [AO].

124 Van der Wiel and Ekamper, Kromme sikkel, 88–9.

125 Coomans et al., Plague, 593, 595, 603.

126 Van Honacker, Résistance locale, 46–7.

127 Breuer and Lesger, *Dood*, 86, 90.

128 Coomans et al., Plague, 597.

129 Geltner, Rural Policing.

130 De Brouwer, "De aenclevende sieckte", 6.

131 BHIC, Notarieel protocol Den Dungen, 5115, no. 3, fo. 85 [21/11/1646] [AO].

132 Janssens and Van den Branden, De pest, 57.

133 Also mentioned, the huts in the forest on the edges of Braine-le-Comte: Matthieu, ed., Mesures réglementaires, 246.

134 For this case: Vera, *"dat men het goed van den ongeboornen niet mag verkoopen"*, 81. For disputes on the commons in the Campine and surrounding areas in Brabant: De Keyzer, Access Versus Influence.

135 Ladan, *Gezondheidszorg*, 63.

136 Nijboer, De Slaande Ingel, 73.

137 Anon., ed., Een geplunderde woning.

138 HUA, Notarissen in de stad Utrecht 1560–1905, no. 181 [24/10/1636] [AO].

139 Pauly, Pestepidemien, 64. Collective action sometimes encouraging rather than restricting contact during epidemics: Ogilvie, *Controlling Contagion*, 201.

140 Huisman, *Stadsbelang*, 27. Later, it was noted in 1576 that after the death of the bishop from *pest*, nobody would dare stay in his house (*fraterhuys*): Formsma and van Royen, eds., *Diarium*, 355 [22/10/1576].

141 Pannier, From Crisis Management to a Mediterranean Model? 41.

142 SB, Stadsbestuur Breda (oud administratief archief) 1280–1810, Stadsrekeningen, no. 619, fo. 98.

143 TRESOAR, Familie Van Sminia, 327, Afschrift van een brief van Assuerus van Vierssen d.d. 1656 gericht aan zijn kinderen onder de indruk van de te Leeuwarden heersende pest, no. 596 [AO].

144 Alink, ed., Getuigenissen, no. 685, fo. 177v [20/5/1519].

145 Franquinet, ed., Eene verordening, 142.

146 ELO, Stadsarchief van Leiden, (1253) 1574–1816 (1897), 0501A, no. 49, fo. 323v–4v [2/10/1603].

147 Alink, ed., Getuigenissen, no. 1019, fo. 259 [4/7/1520].

148 SR, Archieven van de Notarissen te Rotterdam en daarin opgegane gemeenten, 18, no. 588, akte no. 53, fo. 96–7.
149 EAL, Huis Bergh, 1227–1842, 0124, no. 1128 [8/7/1530] [AO]. Steven van Delen, a priest, sends to the *drost* of the Achterhoek villages of Etten and Gaanderen a cure he prepared himself, on account of the *pestilentie*. In 1598, several self-prescribed substances and drinks were prepared by brother Jan, a *cellebroeder* at Hasselt (Limburg), which were described as very good *voor die peste*: Gessler, Remediën.
150 Kayser, Le phénomène épidémique, 73.
151 Mentink, De rode loop, 138.
152 Rutten, *De vreselijkste aller harpijen*, 190.
153 Beyerman, De (tweede) pokkenepidemie, 11–12.
154 Mentink, De rode loop, 140.
155 Franken, De uitbarsting, 150–4.
156 Noordegraaf and Valk, *De gave Gods*, 99.
157 EAL, Stadsbestuur Groenlo, 1273–1811 (1852), 0138, no. 658 [AO].
158 For the Black Death and antisemitic violence in parts of Hainaut, Liege, Limburg, and Brabant, perpetuated by local and municipal authorities: Cluse, De Jodenvervolgingen. For the lessening severity of epidemic-related antisemitic violence over time: Cohn, *Epidemics*, 126–31; although Cohn concedes that Jews still continued to be blamed for disease in certain contexts in the early modern period.
159 Van den Heuvel, ed., Crimineel klachtboek, 117 [13/11/1726]. The same term found in notarial records from Rotterdam in 1652: SR, Archieven van de Notarissen te Rotterdam en daarin opgegane gemeenten, 18, no. 669, akte no. 56, fo. 78.
160 Jacquet-Ladrier, Les épidémies, 130.
161 GS, Stad Steenwijk tot ca. 1811, 14, no. 151 [AO]. See Chapter 5 for more details.
162 Van Zuijlen, ed., *Inventaris*, II, 1323; SA, Archief van Burgemeesters: Stadsrekeningen, 5014, no. 125, fo. 422 [AO]. It cost money to ring these bells when someone had died.
163 AEA, Stadsbestuur Amersfoort, 1300–1810, 0001.01, no. 21, fo. 68 [18/10/1617] [AO].
164 As seen in other contexts in early modern Italy: Coccoli, The Moral Economy, 143.
165 Reimann, Hospitality, 376–9.
166 RAZU, Wijk-bij-Duurstede, Stadsgerecht Rhenen, 066, no. 18 [28/1/1668] [AO].
167 Van Zalinge-Spooren, "Die contagieuse sieckte", 71.
168 AEL, Archives de la Cité de Liège, 1434–1829, Registre aux enquêtes générales. 1634–1636, no. 10, fo. 36v [10/10/1634] [AO]; Pauly, Pestepidemien, 60.
169 Mardaga, ed., *La patrimoine monumental*, 294.
170 Pauly, Pestepidemien, 62.
171 One woman had worked in a plague-infected house in the village of Cothen near Utrecht in 1615 and had smuggled out furniture for her husband to sell (the urban administration of Amersfoort thus forbade her return to the city): AEA, Stadsbestuur Amersfoort, 1300–1810, 0001.01, no. 20, fo. 479v [27/12/1615] [AO].
172 BHIC, Schepenprotocol Dinther, 7603, no. 11, fo. 221r [6/3/1637]; no. 12, fo. 48v [AO].
173 Van Meeteren, *Op hoop van akkoord*, 50.
174 RHCE, Gemeentebestuur Gestel, 1620–1810, no. 336 [AO].
175 Mentink, De rode loop, 140.
176 Jacquet-Ladrier, Les épidémies, 134–5.

177 Jacquet-Ladrier, Les épidémies, 134.
178 Nijssen, Zo ging dat, 49.
179 Lejeune, *Mémoire historique*, 156–7.
180 GAA, Hertogelijk Archief, Financieel beheer Rekeningen C1492–1543, no. 1332.209, fo. 242v. This original finding was kindly provided by Remi van Schaïk. The nuns of Reyde were originally from the Dominican monastery of Oosterreide, but upon the flooding of the Dollard in 1508/9 (with repeat flooding problems thereafter) had to move to the western part of rural Groningen in Lucaswolde in 1528. On this flood and resettlement: Curtis, Danger.
181 Van der Wiel and Ekamper, Kromme sikkel, 76–7.
182 Noordegraaf and Valk, *De gave Gods*, 124.
183 BHIC, Schepenenprotocol Sint-Michielsgestel, 5121, no. 43, fo. 215r [17-5-1561] [AO].
184 De Brouwer, "De aenclevende sieckte", 12.
185 See the references above to the Zwartzusters of Breda in 1596, and Sister Elisabeth Strouven journeying from Hasselt to Maastricht in 1633.
186 Jacquet-Ladrier, Les épidémies, 132.
187 WBA, Archief van de stad Bergen op Zoom, 1397–1810, 0005, no. 6, fo. 252r–4v.
188 Hildebrand, Hollandsche Kapucijnen, 98.
189 Van Beurden, ed., *De handelingen*, 74.
190 Boeren, Een cellebroeder, 35–6.
191 Pauly, Pestepidemien, 62.
192 Keiem burial register, 1642–99, accessible at https://agatha.arch.be/data/images/513/513_9000_000_00396_000/0_0213, fo. 213r: "*9 augusti sepulta est in coemeterio de octe, quia contagione obierat, Maria ancilla Jacobi Maes sine aliquo officio, audita eius confessione cum scalis per fenestram*". The interpretation of this event in a previous publication is incorrect: Curtis, The Female Experience, 5–6, 18. With thanks to Jan Van Acker, Abdijmuseum Ten Duinen, for this correction, pers. comms. [1/10/2020].
193 AEA, Stadsgerecht Amersfoort, 1435–1811, 0012, no. 436-02, fo. 137v [13/11/1521] [AO].
194 RAA, Collectie Wollebrand Gelijnsz de Jonghe, no. 53, letter 17 [6/8/1636] [AO].
195 On the epidemics and war situation: Ufkes, De verzorging; for the orphanage findings: Westerholt, Genoeg voor een heel weeshuis? 98.
196 Tanis, *An Epidemic*, 66.
197 Walhout and Beekink, Just Another Crisis? 76.
198 Jensen, Cultural Resilience, 123, 130.
199 Bruyndonckx, *Een cultuurgeschiedenis*, 48.
200 Labbé, Aux origines.
201 Jensen, Cultural Resilience, 132–3; 't Hart, *Utrecht*, 239–40.
202 Beyerman, De (tweede) pokkenepidemie, 6.
203 Harrison, Pandemics, 130–3.
204 't Hart, *Utrecht*, 235.
205 Tanis, *An Epidemic*, 28; De Graaf, "Dat een ieder zich beijvert zijn zwakke krachten in te spannen", 296–7.
206 Reimann, Hospitality, 373–6.
207 Weeda, The Porous City, 116.
208 Alfani, Plague; Blažina Tomić and Blažina, *Expelling the Plague*, 224.

5 The redistributive powers of epidemics

Wealth, resources, and inequality

The economic impact of disease is a subject with long historiographical roots—how the Black Death shaped agrarian economies in western Europe was something already considered in literature of the late nineteenth century.[1] Although its impact was downplayed by scholars in the early decades of the twentieth century, since then various economic effects of the Black Death have been considered—assessing its posited impact on the transition from arable to pastoral farming; on the weakening of serfdom and other forms of feudal relations; on rural-urban migration patterns; on access to land and the land market; on micro-demographic behaviour and the ages of marriage; on the types of employment available and the wages earned; on living standards and diets; and much more. In more recent times, building on prior work, scholars have also suggested that the Black Death had an important role to play in stimulating divergent patterns of economic development across regions—interacting with pre-existing economic, demographic, and institutional conditions—and leading to relative economic disparities between different areas of Europe, and more grandly, between select parts of western Europe and the rest of the world.[2] And while Robert Brenner once stated that these different social and economic outcomes seen across Europe "proceeded from similar demographic trends", the Black Death's mortality impact across regions was anything but standardised—creating even further sources of variation.[3]

What stood out in the previous Black Death literature was the lack of systematic attention given to its capacity to redistribute wealth and property—severely lacking behind studies into real wages, for example. This is perhaps understandable given the paucity of quantifiable information we have to establish distribution markers before and after the Black Death in even relatively straightforward-to-measure resources such as land (straightforward in that it physically exists).[4] Even today, our most convincing information on Black Death-induced wealth redistribution comes from a few limited villages in parts of northern Italy, Tuscany, and the Kingdom of Valencia, and one small town in Germany and Catalonia.[5] More feasible would be to look outside the confines of the Black Death, and secure empirical information on the distribution effects of other epidemic outbreaks in better documented periods. Still, however, in the specific domains of wealth and property, the

DOI: 10.4324/9781003694908-5

number of empirical cases we can call upon as evidence is quite limited.[6] Clearly, this is testament to the high demands required of the source material—it simply takes a long time to reconstruct all the information from these types of original manuscripts. Furthermore, to make any kind of causal claim for the impact of an epidemic disease on redistribution of wealth or property, we would have to have markers of distribution for years both shortly before, during, and after an outbreak—and then place any redistribution seen in relative perspective with a long-term run of distributive markers.[7] Yet, most information of this kind comes from fiscal registers and other kinds of censuses, which tend to appear rather randomly in particular years, often with substantial gaps, and rarely part of a long consecutive series. Hence, most of the highly valuable scholarship we have today on the long-term trends of wealth inequality comes from places furnishing datapoints that are separated by many years in time—quite acceptable for reconstructing long-term dynamics, and perhaps also for making cautious inferences about potential effects of stand-out epidemics, but not useful enough for tight systematic analysis of individual epidemic episodes.[8]

Despite the lack of empirical material necessary for the task, this has not stopped scholars first offering a generalised view on what the "usual" redistributive effect of an epidemic has been throughout history, and second, some of the reasons or logic behind this. Walter Scheidel, for example, has suggested that significant epidemic outbreaks in the past have tended to serve as one of his four identified "violent levellers" (the others being mass mobilisation warfare, revolution, and state failure)—even if the distribution markers that he uses are not consistent but often shift from wealth, to housing, to property, to wages, and so on, and the scales that he operates at drift from the individual community to more macro areas containing numerous communities, sometimes whole countries.[9] For Scheidel, like many other scholars, the egalitarian impact of an epidemic tends to be based on what has been modelled on what is known about (mainly) western European societies' experiences of the Black Death—even though we have been warned that the economic effects of the Black Death cannot be seen as representative of broader epidemic-economy interaction.[10] Large amounts of death ultimately mean that the cards are stacked a little less in the hands of those with capital, and a little bit more in the hands of those surviving labourers.[11] Of course, such an emphasis on changing ratios between population levels and available resources is hardly new—it was at the very core of the Malthus- and Ricardo-inspired empirical approaches to the high- and late-medieval economy established by M.M. Postan already beginning in the 1930s.[12]

However, in those scarce cases where we do have quantitative information at the level spatially and temporally refined enough to directly link up with individual epidemic outbreaks, rather than the substantial structural redistributive impact of disease, these studies tend to suggest that (a) much of the downward deviations in measurements such as Gini Coefficients are entirely modest (for example, a reduction of 0.02 in Ivrea during the 1630 plague), and (b) temporary blips in the broader scheme of things (for example, in Ivrea, the Gini Coefficient stabilising at a higher level than before the 1630 plague already from 1632 onwards).[13] Indeed, in the early modern period before industrialisation, these epidemics were apparently tiny downticks in the general trend towards incrementally higher inequality seen in most parts of western Europe.[14] In fact, what appears to be more interesting is not how epidemics act as great levellers of wealth, but how, despite population-resources logic and potential splintering of property, they often failed to do so—or rather failed to do so to a significant and lasting degree. The big story is not epidemics as destructive levellers but how societies, or certain interest groups within those societies, have worked out ways over time to stop this from happening.

Thus, scholars have suggested that institutions were developed to mitigate this kind of redistribution from taking place. During the early modern period in many parts of western Europe, impartible inheritance practices started to be strengthened, which prevented estates from becoming overly fragmented,[15] or, as in the case of the Republic of Venice and Bavaria, for example, other institutional restrictions on subdivision of property or narrower definitions of lineage such as the *fideicommissum* or *in solido* inheritance were developed that helped the wealthy or privileged (especially aristocrats and ecclesiastical institutions) to shield their larger assets from the threat of splintering or transferring out of the family or institution altogether.[16] In the Kingdom of Naples, for example, it has been shown that especially propertied families tended to prevent their daughters from getting married for this purpose—instead sending them off to convents, nunneries, and other religious institutions as lifetime single women.[17] In Japan, other institutional mechanisms were involved such as widespread adoption of non-inheriting sons into childless (or son-less) households (which were more likely after epidemics)—achieving the same kind of stability in wealth and landowning structure as in the European examples, but instead entrenching equality rather than inequality.[18]

Nevertheless, while this might be a sufficient institutional explanation for a lack of redistributive impact from epidemics in impartible conditions, we currently do not have much empirical evidence on the redistributive impact of epidemics in societies exhibiting strong partible inheritance practices. This is an issue given that partible inheritance practices were still strong in many parts of early modern Europe,[19] and given further importance because it is unclear in which direction redistribution would go after epidemics—would fragmentation of assets result in access to property for a wider range of people, or simply limit accumulation possibilities for the poorer strata, or leave smallholders susceptible to being outcompeted in land markets?[20] It is also an important consideration for the explicit case of the Low Countries, which exhibited in both medieval and early modern periods very diverse inheritance characteristics between small regions very close together—ranging from the most inegalitarian impartible inheritance practices among eldest sons in rural

Groningen to highly egalitarian and partible inheritance practices among men and women, and wives and children (with numerous variations) in parts of Holland and Brabant, for example.[21]

Chapter 5 examines the economic redistribution of wealth and property during and after episodes of epidemic mortality, situating this process within the broader prevailing institutional conditions that shaped asset transfer in the Low Countries. The chapter is organised into three coherent sections. The first explores the general economic effects of epidemic outbreaks—what pressures and burdens, and incentives and opportunities they generated. The second presents empirical evidence on redistribution of wealth and property—drawing on recent findings from my research team in both urban and rural contexts, with particular attention to contexts where partible inheritance dominated. The third section investigates a less frequently addressed dimension of epidemic-economy interaction—the direct economic costs of epidemic disease at the micro-level, offering a nuanced perspective on prevailing assumptions about redistribution driven by epidemics.

General economic effects of epidemic disease: Pressures, burdens, and incentives

As mentioned already in the book's introduction, epidemic disease has not formed a substantial role in the major historiographies concerning social and economic change in the preindustrial Low Countries. It is clear, however, that epidemics did create different kinds of economic pressures, burdens, and incentives for communities. Although, as noted above, inheritance practice could impact upon the direction of redistribution provoked by epidemics, epidemics also placed direct pressures on the practice of inheritance itself. Indeed, the notion of heirs' greed or avariciousness was a constant theme in the book, *De gave Gods*, although it is sometimes difficult to unpick this from rhetorical and moralising observations of contemporaries and their assumptions about certain categories of people and their likely behaviour.[22]

Disagreements are certainly plentiful in the notarial records. In the Brabant village of Sint Michielsgestel in 1566, a long family dispute was brought before the magistrates that was set off by the sudden death of someone infected with the *gave Gods*.[23] A comparable situation was brought to the magistrates of Asse, near Brussels, by a group of individuals demanding compensation for caring for the deceased during their plague sickness in 1576.[24] A similar exceptionally long-drawn-out battle over inheritance in the wake of multiple deaths within a family has been well elaborated upon for Tilburg in the aftermath of an epidemic in 1625.[25] Here, the death of an entire family—father, mother, and children—meant that the vacant estate was fought over by relatives of two surviving grandmothers, one of whom was angered by the other's decision to quickly sell off part of the estate before an agreement was reached on the division. The whole process was brought before the local magistrates of Tilburg, and a final verdict was only made two and a half years later.

The death of one or more claimants on a resource, and the sudden timing involved, meant that different kinds of arrangements were drawn up in anticipation of this problem occurring in the future. In the villages of Chaam and Alphen, near Breda, the contraction of disease was already written into a 1549 contract over land use rights—where it was agreed that the use of property between two parties had to be based on the contingency that neither of the two parties got afflicted with a "contagious infectious" disease.[26] Sometimes the sudden nature of the death preceded formal writing down of where assets were meant to go—especially to those outside the family. Thus, a few years later in 1559, returning to Sint Michielsgestel, one man had to go to the magistrates to obtain a forced declaration to confirm that he had previously acted as a cleaner (*schrobber*) in another person's house who had been suffering with (and eventually died of) plague and had already been promised 12 guilders and their best cow.[27]

Sometimes notarial documents were explicit in the conditions behind a sale or transfer of property involving the presence of epidemic disease. At Tilburg in 1533, for example, a piece of land was explicitly sold off to pay plague-induced debts.[28] In another example from the aforementioned Sint Michielsgestel in 1639, one man was left complaining that since his wife had died of plague and some of the (rights to the) property had passed to the children, given the strict adherence to partible inheritance practices in the region, he was simply saddled with all the debts from those pieces of land that were bought when the wife was alive.[29] Similarly, during an outbreak at the Campine village of Gierle in 1668, the deaths of some children's parents led to a sale of numerous assets in order to come up with the capital to pay the new guardians of the minors.[30] Often disease acted as a stimulant for very quick action. At Veghel in 1615, a transport act noted that a husband and wife were so fearing death from the *sieckte der pestilentie* that they were already arranging transfer of half of their meadow (*hoeijbeempt*) to another party.[31] At Oss in 1636, a couple that were infected with the *contagieuse sieckte der peste* immediately drew up a testament to announce distribution of properties and lands.[32]

Financial burdens within communities could be substantial, although authorities did try to step in to cover some costs. Occasionally, and especially for areas of sixteenth-century Flanders such as in Roeselare, Ypres, and Geraardsbergen, urban administrations paid quite substantial amounts—in Roeselare, an infected woman was given seven Flemish pounds and three *schellingen* (roughly equivalent to 43 guilders).[33] Sometimes, however, these payments by administrations were accompanied by other self-interested concerns. Thus, in Namur in 1523 and 1530, the poor were simply paid to leave the city during the plague outbreaks, out of fear that they were both the source of and likely to further spread the affliction, while an alternative strategy during the later outbreak of 1558 was to provide public aid to make sure those confined to their houses remained there.[34] Furthermore, later, as we move into the seventeenth century, the sums paid seem to be increasingly smaller. For example, at Breda in 1604, the city government paid several tiny sums including 31 stuivers to a wife of a soldier who had died of *de peste* and was left with four children.[35] This was the equivalent of roughly half a week's work for an unskilled male day labourer in Breda at the time.[36] In 1665, the Amsterdam city government just covered the costs of ringing the church bells for the propertyless (*onvermogende*) families of the deceased who had died of the *contagieuse sieckte*.[37] At Namur in 1668, the local government gave an allowance of six sous per adult and four sous per child, which was narrowly enough to cover the cheapest kind of burial costs.[38]

Overall, these were inconsequential amounts for the recipients but also for the distributors. The total proportion of the city budget (expenses) paid out during the plague of 1666 in Breda on explicitly plague-related issues (wages, concessions, medications, and relief) came to just over two per cent, and for 1667 nearly two and a half per cent, and thus easily absorbed within the long-term flexible public finances.[39] Indeed, what is evident from the case of seventeenth-century Breda (Figure 5.1) is that epidemics did not create too many lasting effects on the city budget. The most significant period of budgetary pressure came with the impact of the siege of 1637 and its aftermath, but most of the epidemics that occurred separate to war activity such as in the late 1660s or in the dysentery of 1676 were even occasions where urban incomes exceeded expenditures—emphasising starkly the lack of governmental resources that were thrown at these issues. Indeed, it has already been mentioned in Chapter 4 how the administration in Groningen managed to secure record income derived from high quantities of fines imposed during the plague of 1665/6—using the epidemic as a source of resilience and vulnerability—urban finances were flexible, adaptive, and hence resilient, where expenses and incomes tracked together, while those experiencing the epidemics experienced hardships and suffering with minimal protection.[40]

Filling the vacuum, and especially in rural communities, local poor tables often stepped in to provide some help, although again this was often limited in nature. At the village of Geervliet, south of Rotterdam, in 1573/4, small payments were made for potions said to cure two children *van de pest*, and similar findings have been found for the poor table at Tilburg in the same years.[41] At Zutphen in 1576, the church master distributed three sums of money to the plague afflicted—15 stuivers for a bed in a pest house; three *witten* (type of coin similar in value to the stuiver) for a woman to look after her infected child; and a little more than a stuiver to a woman for a measure of wine said to have curative properties against the plague.[42] Such payments are perhaps expected given that poor relief in the sixteenth- and seventeenth-century Low Countries tended to be structurally set up to protect needy women more than men—the early modern manifestation of the deserving poor concept often applied to the nineteenth century.[43] It was not an absolute rule, however. For example, in the village of Abbenbroek, 10 kilometres

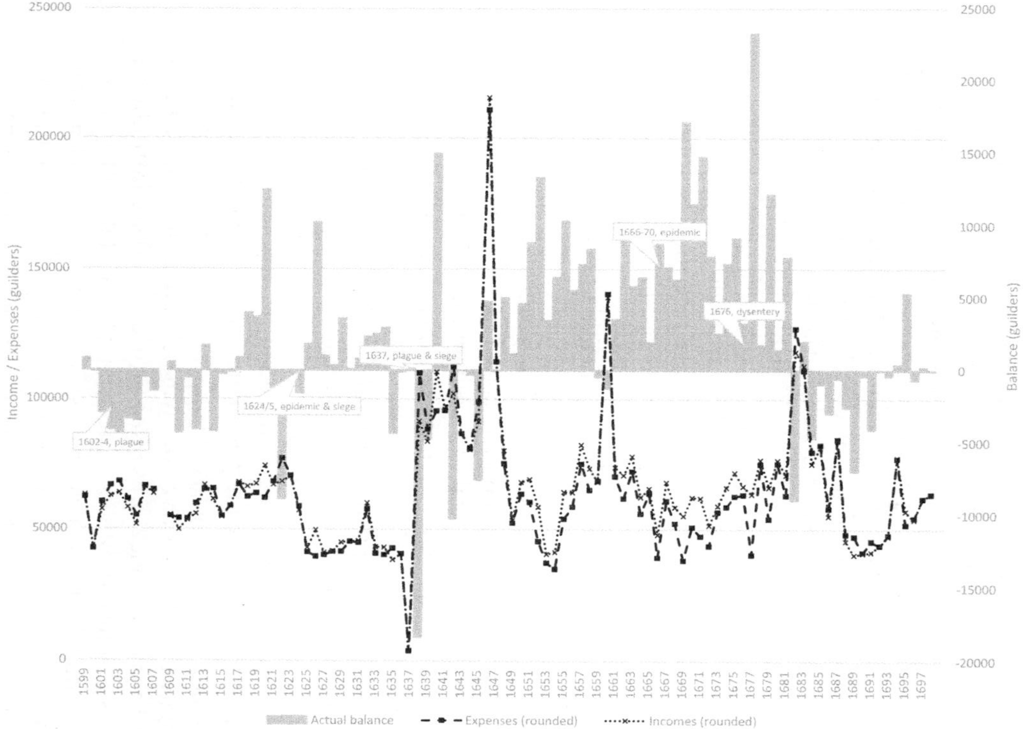

Figure 5.1 City financial accounts, Breda, 1599–1698

Source: SB, Stadsbestuur Breda (oud administratief archief) 1280–1810, Stadsrekeningen, nos. 549–647. Years represent March to March: Hence, 1599 is the equivalent of March 1599 to February 1600. Plague years 1602–4 identified through burial records and plague workers in the source: no. 554, fo. 122, 198r, 203–4. We know that the years of 1624/5 included a terrible siege at Breda, and in the burial records 1625 is the sharpest increase in mortality year of the seventeenth century. The impact of the general plague outbreak in 1636 is difficult to discern in Breda through missing administration, although an epidemic occurred in 1637 together with a siege of 1637, with lingering mortality in 1638/9. From 1666 to 1670, there are explicit mentions of epidemic-related expenses every year in the *stadsrekeningen*: no. 615, fo. 114; no. 616, fo. 102–5; no. 617, fo. 100–2; no. 6178, fo. 98–9. The dysentery outbreak of 1676 is mentioned every year of the *stadsrekeningen* up to 1683, nos. 626–32.

southwest of Rotterdam, one man received 36 stuivers while his wife was said to be on her deathbed with the *gave Gods*.[44]

Frequently, these kinds of local-level institutions were restricted in what they could do, simply because pressure points such as epidemics affected the amount that could be given to them in the first place.[45] Nevertheless, donations to poor tables, hospitals, and orphanages, especially from the privileged in society, helped with the very excessive costs derived from sudden outbreaks.[46] One woman gave money to the St. Geertruiden hospital in Deventer in 1596 with the express instruction to be used for the "wretched poor, infected with plague".[47] Sometimes these cash gifts were substantial. One widow, a Leiden cloth worker (*servietwercker*), gave 150 guilders to the pest house in her will—perhaps with the knowledge that a new one was planned to be constructed (finished in 1661).[48] A private deed was drawn up in 1631 by a couple who arranged for rights over one morgen (0.85 hectares) of land in the Betuwe village of Elst to be handed over to the Arnhem orphanage on account of the prevailing plague (*heersende pest*).[49] Gifts such as these might have been small tracts of surface area but were important as they represented structural long-term income for the receiving institutions. In the Drenthe village of Vledder, it appears that the plague of 1400/1 was the stimulant behind the foundation of a vicarage in 1402 with numerous gifts of tracts of land from the villagers explicitly attributable to the great mortality (*groter sterfte*).[50]

Patients directly afflicted also gave parts of their inheritance up. Indeed, the masters of the Amersfoort pest house declared in 1610 that those who were sick and ended up in the hospital often relinquished their goods to the institution, and the Groot Gasthuis of Den Bosch explicitly mentioned receipt of gold, rings and jewels, and clothing from the infected.[51] One skipper from Rotterdam rewrote his testament to give a third of his silver cups he had kept in the pest house to that institution in recognition of their expenses.[52] Another plague-infected woman (*aan de peste krank was*) gave 12 guilders to her local priest during her last confession, and instructed him to give it to St. Pieters hospital, Arnhem, where the priest confirmed it would be spent on the poor there.[53] It is also interesting that when we have fuller last testaments of those with plague that did not have surviving children, more substantial inheritance (larger sums of money) was often provided to these institutions, and surviving direct family (brothers, sisters, and their children) received less economically valuable items such as dresses or cutlery.[54] As seen from Figure 5.2 looking at the case of the wooden pest house constructed during the severe epidemic of 1635 in Leiden, annual income in normal years was often structurally higher than the costs, but in times of epidemics, when costs started to quadruple over the normal rate, as in the aftermath of the plague of 1655, for example, exceptional forms of income helped manage the burden—mainly achieved through capital loans or gifts from individuals. Again, then, institutional resilience during these outbreaks was quite high.

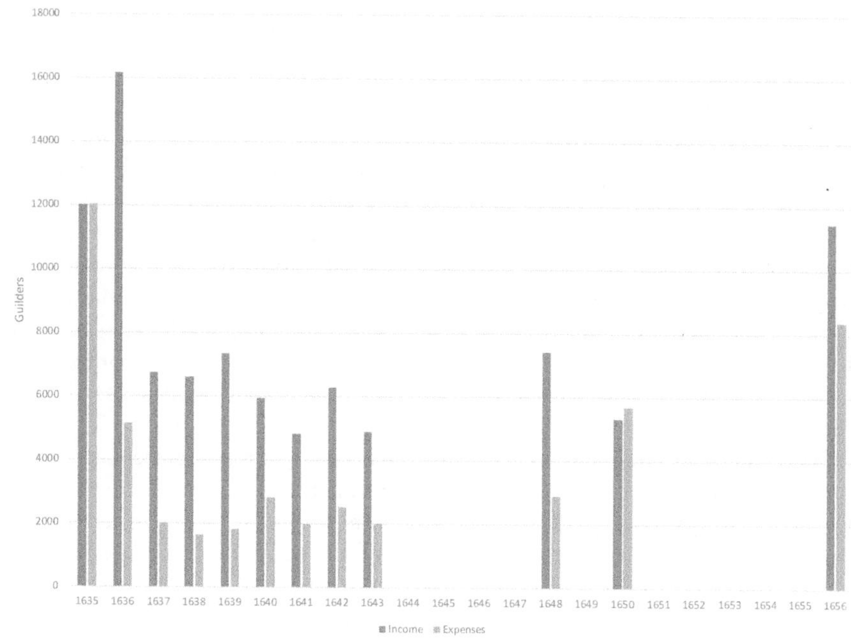

Figure 5.2 Income and expenditure at the Leiden pest house, 1635–56

Source: ELO, Archieven van de Gasthuizen, 1311–1873, 0504, no. 1696. The income is that derived from within the year by subtracting the balance carried over.

Local lordships also can be found offering support on occasion—in line with recent literature emphasising paternalistic forms of protection offered by seigneuries, or the use of seigneurial institutions by peasant communities for their own interests.[55] In the aristocratic Huis Bergh family archive, we have a letter explaining receipt of rye and oats as compensation for feeding boarders during the previous *pest* outbreak.[56] Of course, institutions that received funding from private individuals often did so with the acceptance of certain conditions. Thus, at Arnhem in 1602, one Johan Roeloffsen and his wife declared in a letter that if they were to die of the ongoing "pestilential gift from God" (*godelijke gave der pestilentie*), then, according to an agreement of 1588, the annual fee paid to the orphanage was enough to ensure that their own children would be taken in by the same institution.[57] In a similar fashion, guilds sometimes gave money to institutions such as pest houses as a way of reserving places for their members, as seen during the epidemic of 1624/5 in Schiedam, and demonstrating that pest houses were not as widely rejected and resisted as perhaps assumed.[58]

Probably one of the most important formal interventions that governments could make was to offer concessions to afflicted communities or people. We have several cases where city or village authorities would reduce taxes on account of the demographic damage caused by an epidemic outbreak.[59] In Mons, the annual urban "perception" taxes on goods such as beer and wine were simply not collected in 1615 or 1616 on grounds of the *maladie contagieuse*.[60] Exemptions were made for certain people badly affected by population losses such as millers who were reliant on people coming specifically to their mill.[61] Wine producers received a remission of their debts in The Hague, after the neighbourhoods and guilds had banned the consumption of wine through the ongoing epidemic in 1665.[62] One man in 1554 was able to secure a reduction of the tax on entry (*weggeld*) for temporary visitors to his village, Helmond, since he was not able to travel to other places to market his goods.[63] Occasionally, we hear of cases where travel restrictions placed on infected households were reconsidered on the grounds of the economic damage that could occur, as seen in the case of a wine trader from Maastricht in 1669.[64]

Nevertheless, these cases are outnumbered by those references where authorities were petitioned by residents citing the disastrous effects of an epidemic—and yet we rarely hear whether these petitions were successful.[65] One of the most detailed reconstructions of the economic damage inflicted by disease can be seen in the village administration of the Brabant village, Schijndel, in 1637. In one five-page document detailing witness declarations from surviving residents to the magistrates of Den Bosch, it was noted that the village had been severely damaged by *pestilentiale sieckte* across the period 1633–7. *Schrobbers* and *bewaerders* (guardians) had to be paid over the period, where the wages were said to collectively reach 18,000 guilders—an exorbitant sum and far more than the rates paid to these plague workers individually (see below, and Chapter 6). The plague that raged from May 1636 to Carnival 1637 was so severe, it was said, that a third of the inhabitants had died—but also the animals had died of hunger, and those that survived were severely indebted.[66]

It is well known that periods of hardship because of harvest failures or high food prices, causing "crises of subsistence", tended to lead to raised mortality not via the mechanism of direct outright starvation but indirectly through a wide range of different disease afflictions caused by malnutrition, movement and migration, or consuming items not generally regarded as edible or drinkable. The subject of plague and famine, however, has had little resolution. Although some have suggested a close association between the two, the temporal dynamics are unclear.[67] When we look to the northern parts of the Low Countries in the late Middle Ages from the Black Death to the middle of the fifteenth century, few of the plague outbreaks occurred closely during or after grain price spikes—with the only exception being the major epidemic of 1439.[68] Instead, if there was any association at all, most periods of food crisis tended to come after the mortality spike connected to the epidemic outbreak. Similarly, in the southern Netherlands, it has been recently observed that "grain prices only peaked during or after these waves of pestilence, but in no case did this happen in the period before the plague".[69] That leads us to tentatively conclude that rather than famine driving epidemic mortality, epidemic mortality also drove agricultural production and distribution problems, pointing to mechanisms such as a reduced labour force able to gather harvests, disruption to trade relations, and general fears and restrictions that accompanied the outbreaks. The most important recent work that might support this line of thinking has shown, for the outbreaks of the Black Death, *pestis secunda*, and that of 1368/9, that in the aftermath of all three, the percentage of household budgets of unskilled labourers needed to buy the minimum amount of bread (for survival) in cities of Flanders and Cambrai went above the "food security thresholds" of 60 and 80 per cent.[70] Epidemics created economic difficulties rather than were caused by economic difficulties.[71]

We can even see evidence to this effect directly mentioned in the sources in the aftermath of the Black Death. In one statute from 12 December 1351 (see Figure 5.3), it is noted that through the times of mortality in 1350 (*temporalibus propter mortalitatem*), the isolated monastery of Zwartewater (13 kilometres north of Zwolle) was in a neglected condition, and their possessions and fields by "whose fruits they were sustained" remained "unproductive and uncultivated" (*infructuosi et inculti remanent*).[72] Two further charters have recently been found that also mention post-Black Death cultivation issues on the lands of the deanery of St. Pieter at Utrecht. The first, written in May

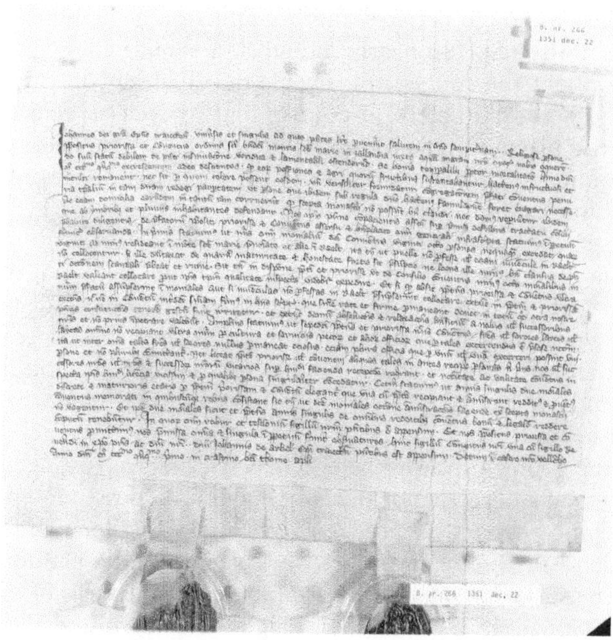

Figure 5.3 Statute from Bishop Jan van Arkel to Mariënberg monastery, Zwartewater, 1351

Source: HUA, Bisschoppen van Utrecht, 218-1, no. 170 [AO].

1352, noted the lack of income from the lands due to high mortality, and the second, written in September 1353, noted substantial deaths of tenants, the lands laying vacant and abandoned, and falling susceptible to plunder from roving bands of men.[73] Similar examples have long been known in parts of Flanders. The abbot of the St.-Martin abbey in Tournai, Gilles li Muisit, described how severe mortality in the years 1349/50 left farms and vineyards uncultivated due to a contracted labour force.[74]

These problems recurred over time. Thus, during the outbreak of plague in 1575, Wouter Jacobsz, the prior of the Stein monastery close to Gouda, heard from someone from Amsterdam who had been to the village of Vianen (near Utrecht) that the plague had "savaged" the arable areas, with much land simply lying bare (*veel schoender coornlant in die conterey woest, dreest ende onbebout bleve liggen*).[75] At Bergh, a letter from the local lordship noted the difficulties of taking in the corn tithes through the raging *pest*.[76] Indeed, at Tilburg during the plague outbreak of 1600, one farmer was so afflicted by the *gave Gods* that he had not been able to pay his debts, and therefore had not sown any grain.[77] The city administration of Breda declared in 1627 that the land around the village of Zevenbergen had been left unworked through the deaths of many inhabitants through dysentery (*rode loop*) in 1620 and *pest* in 1624/5.[78] In rural Hapert, another farmer simply could not afford the lease price for his farm between 1658 and 1659, citing the effects of the plague—although perhaps another affliction as he noted his animals had also been affected.[79] In nearby Lommel, a similar complaint was made a year later about the *contagieuse sieckte* that had left the farmer in great poverty.[80] It should be noted, of course, that as well as epidemics among humans, cattle plagues and sheep scabs destroyed whole herds and created extreme economic losses for farmers. In the Drenthe villages of Beilen and Ruinerwold, for example, the infestation of cattle plague in 1673/4 led to no yielded imposts on horned cattle in those years (i.e., the death of the whole cattle population)—the first time between 1620 and 1805 that this had ever happened.[81] At Leiden, the brackish water that led to the epidemic outbreak of a disease which might have been a form of cholera (blue speckling on the skin was noted) in 1669 was also said by the farmers around the Aar and Rijn rivers to have led to reduced dairy yields from the cows that drank the same water in 1668.[82]

One of the problems, nevertheless, is being able to distinguish between multiple pressures occurring at once—demographic losses to epidemics did not happen in a vacuum. Hence, at the villages of Gulpen and Margraten, in the Landen van Overmaas (today, Dutch Limburg), a petition was made to exempt the surviving inhabitants from taxes on the basis of mass mortality through *pest* in 1579 but also through mass flight and the damage to the village through siege conditions (*belegering*), which had led to the lands being uncultivated for four or five years.[83] A similar petition was made in the Brabant villages of Hoge and Lage Mierde where, through the combination of military excesses and the *pest*, more than half the residents were said to have died in 1636, leaving the lands fallow until 1639, and those that were cultivated on the sandy soils producing only "frugal rewards" (*sobere vruchten*).[84]

Of course, it was also possible to directly earn from epidemic outbreaks in a disease economy, as shown in Table 5.1. Those involved in registering transactions connected to deaths such as notaries, found their workload raised considerably.[85] Salaries and wages, and the conditions

Table 5.1 Examples of earnings from epidemic disease-related economic activities

Year	*Locality*	*Activity*	*Wage*
1567	Groningen	Cleaning waterways & burning plague-infected material	15 rijder 3 stuivers per activity
1598	Roermond	Visiting the *pest* infected	6 stuivers per day [*m/f*]
1598	Roermond	Burying infected corpses	6 stuivers per corpse
1599	Amersfoort	Carrying & burying infected corpses	6 months' work, 6 guilders per month. + per corpse: 1 guilder per rich with coffin; 0.75 guilder per rich w/o coffin; 0.5 guilder per ordinary person; the poor for free
1603	Wijk-bij-Duurstede	Bringing corpses from houses & burying	10 stuivers per corpse
1604	Breda	Burying infected corpses	100 florins for 1 year's work [*m*]
1604	Breda	Carrying & burying infected corpses	75 florins for 1 year's work [*m*]
1604	Breda	Visiting the *pest* infected	150 florins for 1 year's work [*m*]
1606	Den Bosch	Caring for infected pregnant women	50 guilders for 1 year's work [*f*]
1617	Amersfoort	Bringing corpses from houses & burying	10 stuivers per corpse
1623	Herk-de-Stad	*Pestmeester* tasks	100 guilders, 2 pattacons, food, drink, board: 2 months' work
1632	Antwerp	*Pestmeester* tasks	600 guilders per year [*m*]
1637	Dinther	*Schrobber*	42 guilders for 6 weeks 5 days' work [*m*]
1637	Dinther	*Schrobster*	6 guilders 15 stuivers for 6 weeks' work [*f*]
1637	Dinther	*Schrobster*	60 guilders 16 stuivers for 7 weeks' work [*f*]
1637	Dinther	*Schrobster*	50 guilders for 7 weeks' work [*f*]
1637	Dinther	*Schrobster*	83 guilders for 8 weeks' work [*f*]
1637	Lille (BE)	*Schrobber*	20 guilders for 20 days' work [*m*]
1644	Den Bosch	Visiting the infected	350 guilders per year [*m*]

(*Continued*)

Table 5.1 (Continued)

Year	*Locality*	*Activity*	*Wage*
1655	Turnhout	Pest doctor	½ ducat a day, food & drink [*m*]
1664	Leiden	Pest house helper	150 guilders for 3 months' work [*m*]
1664	Leiden	*Pestmeester* tasks	300 guilders for 6 months' work [*m*]
1666	Leerdam	Bringing corpses from houses & burying	12 stuivers per corpse [*m*]
1666	Breda	Surgeon	500 florins per year during plague; 200 florins non-plague [*m*]
1666	Breda	General help	3 florins 3 stuivers per activity [*m/f*]
1666	Breda	Bringing corpses from houses & burying	6 florins per activity [*m*]
1667	Breda	Transporting *pestmeester* furniture	40 florins from Heusden to Breda [*m*]
1668	Breda	*Schrobster* for barracks	10 guilders for 4 weeks' work [*f*]
1668	Mons	Surgeon	1,300 florins per year [*m*]
1669	Breda	Bringing corpses from houses & burying	73 guilders for 1 year's work [*m*]
1669	Breda	Bringing corpses from houses & burying	312 guilders for 1 year's work [*m*]
1669	Breda	Bringing corpses from houses & burying	16 florins 10 stuivers for 22 corpses [*m*]

Sources: Van Beurden, ed., *De handelingen*, 23–4; Huisman, *Stadsbelang*, 27; Heijmans, ed., Nadere toegang, 250 [21/9/1603]; SB, Stadsbestuur Breda (oud administratief archief) 1280–1810, Stadsrekeningen, no. 554, fo. 122; no. 615, fo. 114v–16v; no. 616, fo. 102r; no. 617, fo. 100v; no. 618, fo. 98v–9r; Van Zuijlen, ed., *Inventaris*, II, no. 1167; AEA, Stadsbestuur Amersfoort, 1300–1810, 0001.01, no. 17, fo. 655v; no. 21, fo. 68 [AO]; Nijssen, Zo ging dat, 49; Van Schevensteen, ed., Les traités, 189; BHIC, Schepenprotocol Dinther, 7603, no. 11, fo. 419; no. 12, fo. 33r, 35r, 70r, 110 [AO]; Janssens and Van den Branden, De pest, 27; BHIC, Resoluties van State, 178, no. 186, fo. 245 [6/9/1644] [AO]; Adriaensen, Turnhout, 26; ELO, Stadsarchief van Leiden, (1253) 1574–1816 (1897), 0501A, no. 249 [*kladsresoluties*: 5/7/1664, 19/7/1664]; De Veer, De pest; Hachez, Les fondations, 190–1 [16/6/1668].

involved, varied greatly, however, and were often renegotiated.[86] Long-term structurally contracted work in the domain of plague, for example, was rare, despite the recognition of its repeatable and recurring nature. Administrations tended to pay for necessary labour when the threat of an epidemic was coming or already upon them and likely reflected financial limitations. Although some pesthouse masters were paid an annual salary for several years, as at Antwerp from 1632 to 1637, most were short-term arrangements—sometimes as much as a year, but usually for a few months. Some of the temporary work was financially highly lucrative. Just three months' work as a helper in the Leiden pest house (newly constructed from stone) in 1664 earned one man enough to pay for three years' rent of a moderate house in a decent neighbourhood of the city—and hence epidemics were surely the only time that (certain types of) physical labour was so highly valued in preindustrial communities to quickly change the fortunes of an individual.[87]

Nevertheless, earning from disease was also not always straightforward. Thus, while city surgeons and physicians could earn subsidised housing and clothing for residing in a town during a plague, they also had other restrictions sometimes written into their contracts—reaffirming their duty to routinely care for the infected poor and limiting their movements.[88] Sometimes payments were delayed. At the west Brabant village of Wouw during the dangerous contagion (*morbo contagioso periculose*) of 1625, for example, it was noted that the heirs of Cornelis van Roije had to deliver a large sum of 84 guilders to the local *pestmeester* on account of Cornelis' debts for prior services (likely in the pest house).[89] Given the dangers and hardships associated with much of the work, some epidemic workers also complained about their pay. Hence, the city accounts of Breda in 1667 show that both the disease comforter (*sieckentrooster*) and the carriers of corpses (*pestdraghers*) were unhappy at not receiving enough for tasks they regarded as heavy burdens (*lastte zware*).[90] Clearly, earning through epidemics could come at the cost of substantial personal harm. In 1644, a request was made by one Cornelis Janssen of Eindhoven that as a comforter of the sick in Den Bosch, and having performed his job in difficult circumstances for the past 15 years, he had lost his own wife and six children to disease, and now demanded a higher fee than the 350 guilders a year to support him.[91] The same man was mentioned again during an epidemic of 1656 at Den Bosch, and his personal damages by 1657 were clear—he had lost another daughter and his shop on account of treating infecting soldiers.[92] These personal losses were recognised with a 200 guilders one-off payment. Sometimes certain dangers were written into the conditions of the working contract. The new master of the pest house during the plague of 1664 at Leiden was employed for six months at 50 guilders a month, but with 150 guilders payable to his widow if he died.[93]

Furthermore, the epidemic economy also brought with it new forms of inequality in earning potential—and sometimes visible spatially through urban environments. Indeed, recent analysis of a plague outbreak in the 1570s in Antwerp—a period marked by a temporary transition from Catholic to Calvinist governance in the period 1577–85—showed how inhabitants' ability to participate in social and economic life often was dictated by intersecting categories of class, socio-economic status, and religious identity.[94] In this valuable recent analysis, poorer Catholics found themselves (a) more likely to be subject to official domestic closures of their houses by being demarcated as infected and locked in, and (b) less likely to obtain health passes as certification of their ability to continue to trade. Authorities unevenly applied institutional restrictions and institutional vehicles of mobility—allowing groups such as more affluent Protestant merchants to reap rewards over others in the case of Antwerp.

Redistribution of wealth

Given that epidemic diseases in the preindustrial Low Countries created different sorts of contextualised economic pressures, burdens, and incentives, it is quite logical that they would also lead to redistribution of economic resources. Originally, quite a disproportionate amount of attention was paid by economic historians to the impact of epidemics on wages, and especially the Black Death. Not only were wages easier to collect in serial form going back into the past, but it was easier to link developments to a kind of standard Malthusian logic where population decreased, and resources stayed the same, thus real wages would rise as the value of labour to capital increased. The bargaining position of ordinary labourers was said to be strengthened in relation to elites with power and resources, and further demonstrated in declining returns to safe assets for different outbreaks.[95] Recent scholarship, especially from the southern Low Countries, has tended to nuance this so-called "golden age of labour", however—building on already long-known issues with "sticky" wages to demonstrate difficulties for certain groups in purchasing power and food security.[96]

When we place developments in an even broader context, social and economic historians have moved even further away from the idealised view resting on population-resources or labour-capital redistribution. First, it has not been clear that the increase in real wages seen in certain parts of western Europe after the Black Death (and now nuanced in its extent and timing) was ever replicated in contexts of high mortality during other epidemics in the preindustrial period. Two large plague outbreaks in the seventeenth century (on the relative severity, see Chapter 3), for example—1630 in northern and central Italy and 1656–8 in the Papal States and the Kingdom of Naples—did not have comparable effects on real wages.[97] In fact, wages, on occasion, could be driven down by overall aggregate contractions of the economy, decreasing demand for labour.[98] And in some cases, cities were replenished by migrants too quickly to have any structural realignment of factor prices.[99] Second, as noted in the introduction to this chapter, more scholarship is starting to think more explicitly about distribution and redistribution of wealth and property as opposed to a fixation on wages. This is important, since land, property, and wealth are almost universal building blocks of historical and modern societies, whereas wages are not.[100] Even in the highly commercialised and urbanised Low Countries, wages rarely comprised more than 50 per cent of preindustrial household income—and were, of course, frequently lower than that in most places.[101] Nevertheless, while we have more and more empirical evidence for wealth distribution in preindustrial (disproportionately western European) societies, the number of case studies explicitly looking at systematic links between clearly identified epidemic disease outbreaks and redistribution of wealth or property is limited. This section attempts to provide some of the most up-to-date work from the Low Countries on the subject.

Up to a few years ago, there was effectively no information that linked mortality spikes caused by epidemics and wealth or income redistribution. This is because the first attempts to systematically collect both sets of information across long periods of time were only made within the past decade or so, although with no integration of the two types of series.[102] At best, it has been observed on the basis of a reconstruction of income inequality in early modern Den Bosch that the decline in the Gini Coefficient in 1636 might have been attributed to the simultaneous plague that occurred in the same year.[103] Others have tentatively pointed to modest equitable redistribution in Antwerp in a context of sharp demographic decline in 1584–6, although not specifically connected to epidemic disease.[104]

More systematic work is now being developed on the subject, however. One ongoing case study focuses on the impact of epidemic mortality on the redistribution of housing wealth within the city of Leiden in the period 1632–68—exploiting the spatial variation in deaths across neighbourhoods and streets of the city. To do this, we bring together a highly complete, annual burial series for the city, where deaths can be attributable to (consolidated) streets, and the social distribution of housing ownership, highly detailed and geo-located to streets, across four points in time (1632, 1644, 1657, and 1668; interspersed by three epidemic outbreaks of different magnitudes in 1635, 1655, and 1664).[105] The case study is valuable because while other literature across Europe has examined epidemic mortality and economic redistribution but with the confounding factor of simultaneous warfare-induced destruction, Leiden was unusual in that the three outbreaks occurred in an environment where armies and soldiers were nowhere present.[106]

Figure 5.4 shows that on an aggregate level, epidemic mortality in the city of Leiden barely shifted the distribution of housing wealth as measured through a Gini Coefficient. One might consider this remarkable—especially given that between the indicator years of 1632 and 1644, more than a third of the population had died during the outbreak of 1635. It is also strange when we look deeper into more refined spatial aspects of the results. Indeed, what we show in Figure 5.5 is that not only did epidemic mortality tend to increase turnover between housing owners—higher shares of turnover in streets with high epidemic mortality, as one might expect—but this also occurred in specific housing sectors. Indeed, what we show is that the normal or non-epidemic pattern of housing transfer tended to be between moderate wealth housing owners who were owner-occupiers—living in the house they owned—and that epidemics shifted turnover more towards poorer streets which were often characterised by consolidated ownership, meaning that one person owned several houses in these streets and thus was an investor in real estate.

The shift in turnover in these areas might be expected given that epidemics in seventeenth-century Leiden tended to afflict poorer areas more severely,

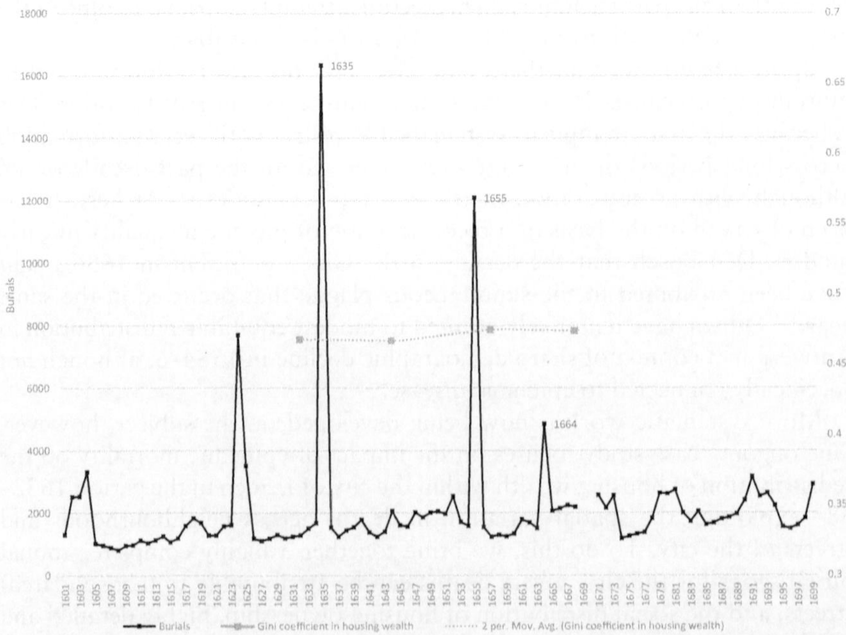

Figure 5.4 Epidemic mortality and aggregate distribution of housing wealth, Leiden, 1632–68

Sources: Burials: Curtis, From One Mortality Regime to Another?; housing wealth: Van Besouw et al., Epidemic Mortality. Dataset built from original manuscripts: ELO, Stadsarchief van Leiden, (1253) 1574–1816 (1897), 0501A, nos. 3529–34.

as mentioned in Chapter 3. However, given that these houses were often rented to poor tenants, turnover was not stimulated through the direct mortality effects of death of owners, but deliberate retreat by investors from this market.[107] Owners used epidemics as a reason to get rid of parts of their housing portfolio. Rent payments were often disrupted by the death of tenants—and delayed or unpredictable payment and vacancies were a major preoccupation of urban real estate landlords in the early modern period all across Europe.[108] And this is understandable given what we know about plague regulations and renting in the city, mirroring findings for other cities in the Dutch Republic.[109] For example, in 1664, neighbourhood officials in Leiden were instructed to make sure the floors of houses in which someone had died of plague remained closed for 14 days, that renting of these houses and rooms did not take place until eight weeks after the previous death, and that inheritance decisions relating to the property did not occur until two months had passed.[110] Epidemics made this kind of housing wealth unattractive, and this was exacerbated by the pull of other investment opportunities such as government bonds. Previous research into the fortunes at death of a sample of the main Leiden regents showed that housing as a share of their wealth

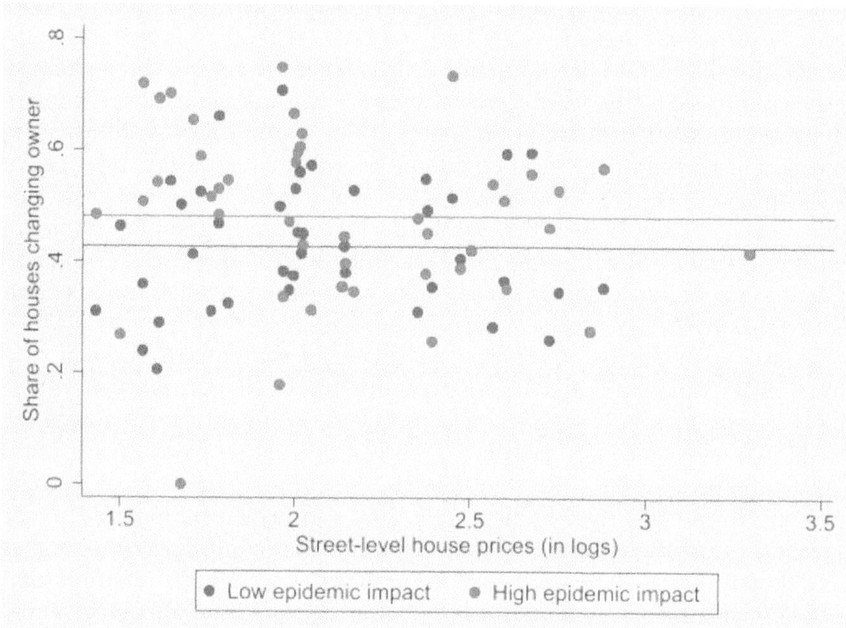

Figure 5.5 Turnover of houses in streets with low and high epidemic mortality conditions, Leiden, 1632–68

Source: Based on data used in Van Besouw et al., Epidemic Mortality. In ordinary conditions, that is "low epidemic impact", houses tend to change owner more in the lower-middle range of values. In "high epidemic impact" conditions, this trend shifts more to the lowest value houses and the most valuable houses.

portfolios dropped from more than 40 per cent in the seventeenth century to less than five per cent a century later.[111]

Still, of course, it brings us back to the puzzle—how can we square so little aggregate change in housing wealth distribution with substantial extents and different forms of epidemic-induced housing turnover? Overall, in recent literature, we have shown that this turnover could not affect the aggregate figures because (a) extra turnover was concentrated in houses of little value; (b) the new owners taking on the vacant houses were just as wealthy as previous ones (i.e., it was not a new market for poorer types); and (c) these new owners were not "new"—they already owned houses in Leiden. Consequently, our work reminds us that simply using aggregate indicators such as Gini Coefficients can hide or obscure a lot of significant developments occurring under the surface that only emerge after decomposing the data.[112]

Currently, however, there is a much greater pool of empirical evidence produced for the dynamics of distribution and redistribution in urban contexts than rural areas, where much of the focus has instead been on unequal relationships between city and countryside, or unequal development paths between different rural areas.[113] That notion is magnified even further on the specific subject of epidemics and their capacity to redistribute resources in the countryside—there are few examples we can call upon. Some scholars have tried to quantify distributions of wealth or a segment of wealth such as land within preindustrial rural communities using an aggregate figure such as a Gini Coefficient.[114] However, this is usually static and taken from singular years in time, largely because we lack temporally granular empirical distribution markers within the same localities across a long series—in turn, affecting our ability to draw causal links between epidemic outbreaks and redistribution.[115]

To deal with this issue, we have made use of the unusual survival of a land register (known as the *Veldboeken*) for the large west Brabant village of Oudenbosch, which, with some gaps, provides annual figures across the whole of the seventeenth century.[116] This allows us to create distribution markers before, during, directly after, and in the long term after a specific epidemic outbreak—thus linking mortality and redistribution in a more explicit way. Although land does not represent total wealth, previous studies have shown that it often comprised more than 80 per cent of wealth within preindustrial rural communities—and of course, more generally, represented the means of achieving subsistence but also was used for surplus extraction, collateral, and asserting social status.[117] Further added value to our source material is that the *Veldboeken* allow us to distinguish between distribution at the owner level and user level (see Figure 5.6), or more simply, across those that owned the land (rentier owners and those farming their own land) and those that worked the land (those farming their own land and those leasing from others). This is important because for preindustrial rural societies, access to resources was often just as valuable as owning resources (with the lines between the two blurred), and although scholars have long suggested that the proliferation of leasehold was an important factor in rural economic development (and inequality), we rarely have any quantitative insights into the proportion of land that was devoted to leasing, how this changed from year to year, and how this related to epidemic mortality.[118]

A precondition to understanding the redistributive impact of epidemics in a particular community is to know when these outbreaks took place. Unfortunately, Oudenbosch does not provide particularly useful burial registers for the seventeenth century—only a short series from 1634 to 1660 which misses the likely significant years of 1637/8.[119] In a recent paper, we used a variety of different evidence to show seventeenth-century outbreaks in Oudenbosch in 1604, 1625, 1636 (with lingering mortality to 1637/8), 1662, and 1666—although in this part of west Brabant, the epidemic of 1625 was clearly the most severe, and likely linked to the effects of a terrible siege at Breda in 1624/5.[120] Thus, for example, we have explicit references to long periods in 1625 where no lessons were given at the Oudenbosch school as a result of the outbreak.[121] Marriages in the village ramp up in 1626 to 36

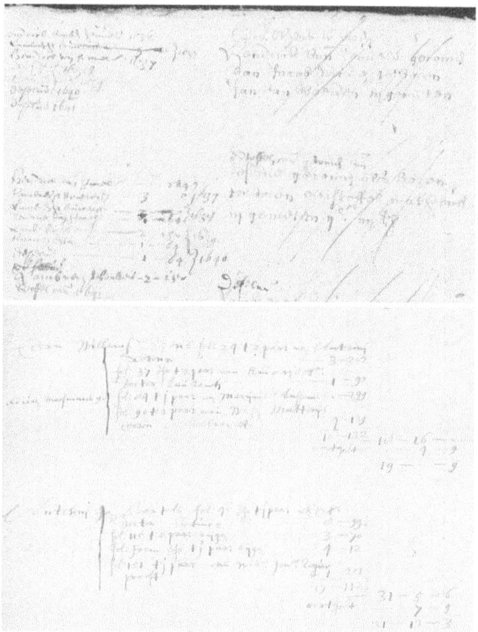

Figure 5.6 Examples of the *Veldboek* formats up to 1649 and from 1661

Source: WBA, Dorpsbestuur Oudenbosch, 0300, nos. 0918–29, 0960–8. The above example shows land users on the left-hand side and landowners on the right and is organised by plot of land. The bottom example shows land users on the left-hand side, with all the plots attributable to them, while owners (if present) are listed per plot.

compared to an annual average of 7—a common sign seen in the aftermath of spiked mortality.[122] This is corroborated by direct references to the *contagieuse sieckte der peste* in a personal financial account from the nearby town of Bergen op Zoom, and the even closer village of Wouw, where the dangerous contagion (*morbo contagioso periculose*) of 1625 is mentioned.[123] In the nearby village of Roosendaal, 108 people are explicitly mentioned as dying with *peste* in 1625, and burials spike up in the neighbouring village of Oud Gastel.[124] In the town of Bergen op Zoom, the *gasthuis* saw its expenses spike up to a higher level in 1625 (4,000 guilders) than seen at any other point in the seventeenth century.[125]

In Figure 5.7, based on the *Veldboeken* database, we show the proportions of land in Oudenbosch that changed hands from year to year. In previous literature, the annual average rate of land turnover (percentage of total surface area transferring to new hands through the land market) calculated for other areas of the early modern Low Countries and northwest Europe is anything up to two per cent—but frequently less than that.[126] In Oudenbosch, this average was much higher at around six per cent of the total, and a median of 4.4 per cent where exceptional years drive up the mean—indicative of the

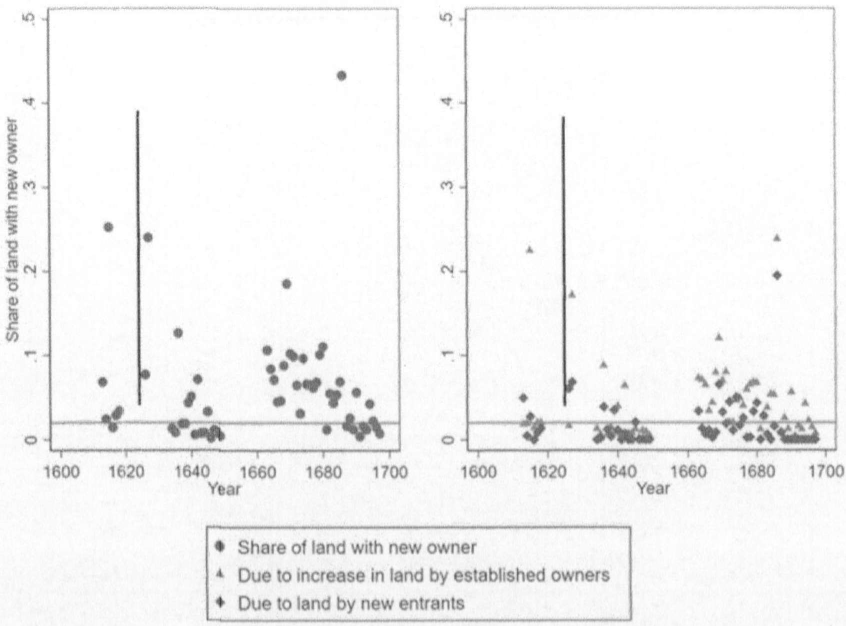

Figure 5.7 Turnover in landownership, Oudenbosch, 1606–97

Source: Curtis and van Besouw, Lifecycle. The vertical lines represent the severe epidemic outbreak in 1625.

capacity for redistributive change—but also spiked up considerably in certain years such as in the aftermath of the 1625 epidemic where around a quarter of the land fell into new hands.[127]

For those that died during this epidemic, the land would often have been redistributed into many different hands—fragmented into several portions as the inheritance practice seen in this part of rural west Brabant was highly egalitarian with both surviving partners and male and female children able to inherit portions.[128] Accordingly, this is how we can understand the aggregate distribution figures presented as Gini Coefficients in Figure 5.8. After the epidemic outbreak of 1625, which created substantial excess mortality, the deaths of landowners and land users meant a raised tendency towards land turnover and a downward tick in the Gini Coefficients as estates ended up being fragmented among heirs (with some lag in the recording process, as these changes only became visible in 1627) and farms taken on by different people or left vacant.

However, despite the substantial decline in the Gini Coefficient after the epidemic of 1625—around 0.05 for ownership and a massive 0.1 for land use to 1627—the most interesting part of this process, and in line with what was recorded by Alfani for the urban context of Ivrea during the plague of 1630, is the very rapid rebound of the previous distribution level, followed

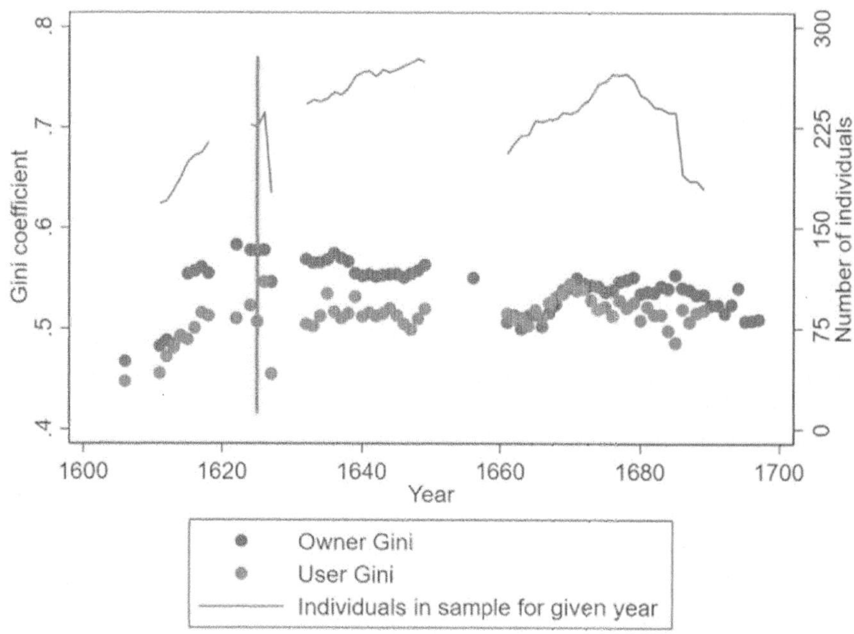

Figure 5.8 Land distribution among effective owners and users, Oudenbosch, 1606–97

Sources: Curtis and van Besouw, Lifecycle. No land use figures are available for 1656 or from 1689 onwards. The epidemic of 1625 is marked by the vertical line.

by persistence and stability over the long term of the seventeenth century, notwithstanding minor flickers.[129]

The question remains, then, what is driving this rebound of the land distribution to previous levels within the matter of a few years? By performing a more detailed lifecycle analysis of the land acquisition strategies of all those landowners and land users in seventeenth-century Oudenbosch, we have shown that much has to do with the lack of incentive to keep hold of large quantities of land beyond a perceived optimum—a process of lifecycle decumulation rather than accumulation.[130] As shown in Figure 5.9, for the least wealthy three-quarters of Oudenbosch society (i.e., the majority of inhabitants), the most land ever owned or worked by households was in the initial phases when they received land and became "independent" landowners or users. In fact, most of these people in Oudenbosch spent most of their lives getting rid of land over the medium or long term—achieving an optimal size of farm in line with availability of labour, capital, and commercial potential of the land itself. Hence, we might understand that in periods when land transfer was heightened such as after the epidemic of 1625, many new people saw themselves become independent landowners and land users

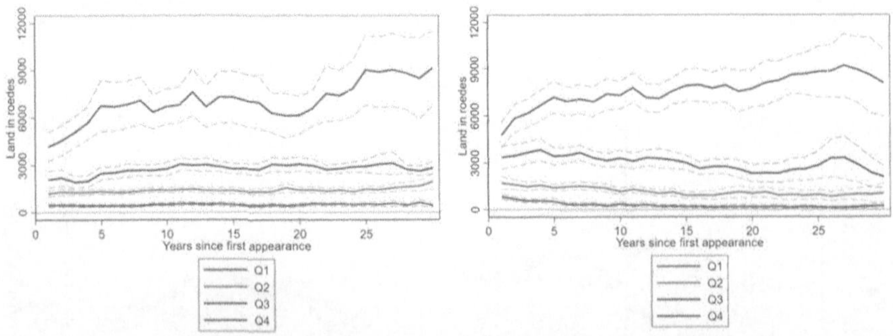

Figure 5.9 Average lifecycle landownership and land use per quartile of wealth, Oudenbosch, seventeenth century

Sources: Curtis and van Besouw, Lifecycle. The graph on the left shows lifecycle landownership and the graph on the right shows lifecycle land use. Q1 (the trend line at the bottom of both graphs) represents 25 per cent of landowners or land users with the least amount of land owned or used, and Q4 represents 25 per cent of landowners or land users with the most. The maximum amount of land owned (used) by an individual at any point in their life defines their position within a quartile. We go up to 30 years as few landowners and land users had independent landholding careers beyond this amount if we consider that men acquired their farms around their early or mid-twenties and average life expectancy was around the mid-fifties.

for the first time—driving down aggregate inequality as measured by Gini Coefficients—but these Ginis quickly rebounded as heirs got rid of this property. Epidemics, then, accentuated a general existing social logic. Some of this property was reincorporated into the hands of wealthier groups—although not to an excessive degree as even the wealthiest quartile did not tend to accumulate too much after the initial five years.

What is clear from the above case of Oudenbosch is that the extent to which a society valued an asset affected the epidemic-induced redistribution of the same asset—and this societal value changed over time and across context. Interestingly, a parallel has also been drawn in other recent work on land redistribution in a seventeenth-century village in the Rijnland area of Holland, which was more commercially vibrant than west Brabant. What has been shown is that after the epidemic outbreak of 1655/6 in Hazerswoude, smallholders were able to gain access to tiny fragments of land, courtesy of the strict principles of partible inheritance, but this did not prove to have an egalitarian or equitable effect because many poor or modest households simply had acquired an asset of depreciating value—and a value which went further downward within these inheritors' lifetimes (potentially, also, as peat as a resource became depleted).[131]

Of course, not all resources were owned and accessed privately by households and institutions in the medieval and early modern period.[132] A large portion of communities' wealth was tied up in collective institutions—and access to these collectively pooled resources was never equal, even among members, and could be subject to redistributive change through endogenous reform and external pressures.[133] These collective institutions could take many forms, some more well known than others, although two of the most important in the preindustrial Low Countries were guilds (usually, although not exclusively, in cities and towns, and with exceptional diversity) and different types of common land in some parts of the countryside.[134] Especially rural commons were subject to the strong pressures associated with changes in population numbers, although most focus has remained on the challenges of too many people wanting access to the common—population increases, in tandem with other factors, creating too many free-riders that lead to the inevitable depletion of the common resources.[135] Indeed, the formalisation and structural reorganisation of many commons in the Low Countries came in the twelfth and thirteenth centuries under conditions of strong population growth and conflict over rights of use.[136] Most historical work on the subject, therefore, has tended to disprove the inevitability of this so-called "tragedy of the commons"—not least through the malleability and flexibility of the institutions themselves—but still, it should be said, that greater attention has been paid to the subject of too many people impacting upon a common rather than too few.[137] One question that has not had too much clear resolution yet, or at least very little empirical historical evidence, is what happens when there are suddenly too few members of a collective—such as through an epidemic disease outbreak?[138] Is that a problem? How does that affect access and distribution to the collective resource? Indeed, it has been suggested that too many people created pressures, but at the same time these institutions often functioned well at optimal levels of participation with members paying into the system through money, pre-existing private wealth, labour, and service. This kind of issue can be highlighted by the recognition that over time, the proportions of active and passive commoners could change.[139]

From the Low Countries, we have only fragmentary insights, sometimes indirect. Scholars have recognised the potential redistributive consequences of disruptive events but not elaborated further.[140] It has been shown, for example, that due to low levels of participation in 1709, non-members and outsiders were invited by the inland Flanders communities of Assebroek and Oedelem to temporarily graze their livestock on the abundant pastures.[141] This was likely linked to the deaths of animals through extreme winter cold (the great frost) of 1708/9 and the ensuing famine fevers that reduced the rural populations substantially in this period through raised mortality.[142] This kind of issue did not lead to any structural redistribution of collective resources, however—they were temporary interventions to maintain the functioning of the institution.

Perhaps the most explicit work has been performed on the commons (*Marken*) in the rural region of Westerwolde, Groningen, in a paper that remains unpublished.[143] For the effective functioning of the commons here, their institutional resilience rested upon the continuous presence of "original" peasant farmers with rights to the commons (*eigenerfden*) in the local villages—*Marken* that were formalised in the first place under conditions of thirteenth-century population pressure on resources.[144] Accordingly, it was, of course, a major challenge when repeat incidences of damaging warfare and epidemics (especially in 1568, the early 1590s, 1623/4, and 1665–7) occurred, reducing inhabitants and creating inheritance and succession problems.[145] Despite this, however, Adriaenssen and 't Hart show that transfer of farms with common rights—and thus instability in the commons themselves—was not inevitable in most of the villages. In fact, the various village *Marken* in this region of the northern Netherlands, at least in the sixteenth and seventeenth centuries, dealt with periods of excessive mortality by actively seeking out insiders who could be trusted to take on the management of these farms and shares in the commons temporarily, until the surviving minors could come of age. Only as a very last resort were farms sold to outsiders, when all institutional adaptations had been exhausted, and local lords worked with the peasant communities to ensure this.[146] Of course, this fits neatly with the understanding of how localised collective institutions worked in other areas of preindustrial western Europe—where one of the most important recurring characteristics was to maintain internal cohesion and prevent access to perceived outsiders.[147]

Direct costs of epidemics at the household level

A final aspect of epidemic-induced redistribution to be considered is absolute financial ruination. Already mentioned above, we have numerous cases of modest intervention from various institutions and individuals to ease the burden of those in need—especially for those men or women who had lost a partner. In Zutphen, for example, we learn from the city's financial accounts of 1598 that one man's death from the *pest* had led his surviving wife and children into a descent into poverty.[148] In the village of De Meern, close to Utrecht, the plague of 1663 had led a schoolmaster's family into a cycle of debt, as restrictions were imposed on his students—forcing his wife to start working as a cleaner in infected houses, and eventually being evicted from their home.[149] Yet, as noted earlier in this chapter, the payments often made to those in need were derisory, and rather than true welfare provision, barely covered basic costs of the burials of deceased or soon-to-be deceased family members, let alone compensation for *schrobbers* and *schrobsters*, medicines, guardianship, the cessation of trade or farming, or extra costs associated with environmental infringements and precautions.[150] Indeed, while a large amount of literature on the redistributive impact of epidemics has tended to focus on the balance between people and resources, or capital and labour, with the idea that epidemics killed people but left resources untouched, this was far from the case.[151]

The intention of this section is to gain some initial insights into how burdensome these costs were at the micro level of the individual household. What were these expenses that ordinary people faced when experiencing epidemic diseases? These can be well illustrated by zooming in on household lists of assets and debts that had to be paid after a death in the family during an outbreak. Illuminating examples of these *momboirrekeningen* are found for the Brabant village of Dinther in the rural Meierij of Den Bosch. In two households examined in very close detail, I reveal the income and costs connected to families that were badly hit by the severe plague of 1636—losing both adults (husband and wife) and some children, while leaving several (minor) children behind as heirs of the final estate.

From the two households examined in detail (Table 5.2), we can see that the impact of plague within the family carries great implications for the transfer of assets to the next generation. Indeed, although in the literature we often see epidemic disease as a potential vehicle for earlier social mobility—young adults potentially receiving their inheritance sooner—what we see in these two cases is that plague destroys the life chances of the children that are heirs of the estates, albeit to different degrees.[152] In the case of the heirs of plague-stricken Jan Bernaert, the surviving children effectively have no estate to speak of—indeed, they are saved from substantial debt simply by the widespread sale of goods and especially land from the property portfolio. In the case of Stoffel Lambert's child heirs, with fewer assets to get rid of, the eventual costs and expenses were so great that they inherit a debt, which starts to accrue interest. In both cases, the presence of costs explicitly related to dealing with and experiencing plague reduces the capacity of both households to transfer a substantial estate—leaving them with nothing or less than nothing. This can be contrasted with other entries in the *momboirrekeningen* where the death of the head of household was not associated with an outbreak of epidemic disease, and the capacity for keeping a coherent estate in transfer was greater. For example, Jacomina, daughter of Jan Jan Adriaens, ended up with 1,942 stuivers (just over 97 guilders) passed onto her heir, which was her surviving husband Dierck Diercxen van der Boer.[153] Indeed, epidemic outbreaks increased the likelihood of both parents dying—and it was the greater vulnerability of the surviving children (often minors) that was behind some of the rapid disappearance of the estate, as explained below.

So, what were these plague-related costs that so clearly affected the transfer of coherent assets for these two rural households? First, as mentioned above, plague costs represented a greater share of the burden for Stoffel Lambert's household compared to that of Jan Bernaert. Although both households had equivalent levels of expense after the deaths of the two husband-and-wife couples through plague, Jan Bernaert had fewer plague expenses, but more ordinary costs relating to higher levels of indebtedness he had accumulated during his lifetime. For Stoffel Lamberts, the financial costs of having plague enter his household were enormous. Almost a third of his estate was wiped out simply through employing *schrobbers* and *schrobsters* to clean and perform duties in his house, and included tasks such as looking after the children for seven weeks, likely over the period when the house needed to be locked down, purifying the house with a special smoke, and the process of travelling to other local places such as Rosmalen and Den Bosch in search

Table 5.2 Income and expenses of two households in Dinther (post 1636 plague)

Overall				
	Heirs of Jan Bernaert		*Heirs of Stoffel Lamberts*	
Income/assets	8,912		4,978	
Costs/expenses	8,798		8,050.25	
Total estate	114		(3,072.25)	
Costs created through plague				
	Heirs of Jan Bernaert		*Heirs of Stoffel Lamberts*	
Plague costs	2,718.5		6,502	
Non-plague costs	6,079.5		1,548.25	
Categories of costs				
	Heirs of Jan Bernaert		*Heirs of Stoffel Lamberts*	
	Stuivers	*% of total*	*Stuivers*	*% of total*
Non-plague costs				
Registration of deeds/documents	226.5	2.6	156	1.9
Unpaid debts	5,821.5	66.2	1,371.25	17
Mostly plague costs				
Travel	3.5	0.1	26.25	0.3
General services in infected house	346	3.9	286.25	3.6
Medicines, foods, drink, or other products consumed in infected house	538	6.1	778.75	9.7
Medical costs	0	0	63	0.8
Plague costs				
Getting rid of, transporting, or selling furniture from infected house	21	0.2	115	1.4
Registering, leasing, & selling of land	50	0.6	334	4.2
Maintaining animals while infected	57	0.7	0	0
Schrobber/schrobster *services*	1,024	11.6	2,635.25	32.7
Maintaining children while infected	416.5	4.7	833.5	10.4
Funeral costs	240.5	2.7	1,451	18
Maintaining land while infected	53.5	0.6	0	0

Source: BHIC, Schepenprotocol Dinther, 7603, no. 12, fo. 32r–7r, 47r–55r [AO]. The transcribed data can be consulted at Curtis, ed., Original Burials Data. All figures converted to stuivers for comparison. My calculated totals do not correspond exactly with the accounting and sums made by the scribe of the consulted books. For Jan Bernaert, my expenses come to 8,798 stuivers, whereas 8,810 stuivers are listed in the book total. For Stoffel Lamberts, my expenses come to 8,050.25 stuivers, whereas 8,058 stuivers are listed in the book total; and my income comes to 4,978 stuivers, whereas 5,092 stuivers are listed in the book total. These discrepancies might be because some of the individual items listed in the accounts are missing a precise value. These small discrepancies do not change the magnitude or direction of the overall findings. The categories of costs classified as "mostly plague" are those where usually it is related to the disease, but occasionally they list individual costs borne by the deceased in their life prior to becoming infected. For example, Stoffel Lamberts had medical costs relating to the services of a surgeon earlier in his life.

of candidates willing to work in the infected house—again reinforcing the point made earlier in Chapter 4 that finding household cleaners in rural areas was not easy. Furthermore, when we add these costs to those of more general one-off tasks performed in the plague-infected house—for example, using lime as a fumigator, or constructing a door to keep one room "pure" (*suijver*)—and the costs associated with all the food, drink, medicines, and other products delivered to the locked-down house and for the use of the children after the death of the parents, then these specific plague-related expenses (some of the most direct kinds) came to nearly half of the total costs. Funeral expenses were also substantial, although they could deviate sharply. The Stoffel Lamberts household spent about five times as much on this domain, which seems to be connected to a more lavish funeral conducted over two days for Stoffel and his wife, Emken—potentially an expression of his status as a local "significant".[154] This contrasts somewhat with the official view of authorities which tried to make plague funerals short and modest affairs (again, mentioned in Chapter 4). Here, in a more isolated rural village, outside the supervisory control of authorities, local people continued to cling to their usual customs and reverence for the dead, irrespective of a feared disease. This was similarly seen in a probate register of another couple dying of *pest* in the Over-Betuwe village of Bemmel in 1636, where numerous labour and materials costs were listed for their funeral—and provisions for the neighbours to participate in the wakes (food and beer), despite the oft-cited attempts of authorities to restrict this aspect of social life.[155]

Epidemics heightened the risk of both parents dying, and with sub-adult or minor-age children inheriting the estate, this also created redistributive problems. First, there were the direct costs of looking after the children. One of the tasks of the *schrobsters* employed in the infected and locked-down household was to take care of the children, a large expense, but this was exacerbated by the numerous individual costs that came up. Children had to be supplied with various clothes, bedsheets, shoes, and clogs, and received their own care when sick. But second, and perhaps more importantly, there were several indirect plague-induced costs connected to the deaths of both adult parents. Many of the decisions concerning the estate hinged on the actions of close-by guardians and other local officials such as magistrates and secretaries. In both cases presented above, children who could not look after the land saw parcels sold—to which they received money but also had to pay those individuals who arranged these sales. In fact, any transfer led to these kinds of payments—inheriting children were found paying those adults charged with selling the children's furniture (from the infected house) at auction, paying adults to do basic agricultural tasks on their lands such as ploughing, harrowing, and weeding, and paying those helping supervise and protect the lands from thieves or those likely to encroach. Some might have been clear transactions, but it is easy to see in the records how this could easily slip into exploitation of the vulnerable. Officials and neighbours were, for example, paid sums to convene at their houses when making transactions and signing documents in the children's names—with the children footing the bill for food consumed, and beer and wine drunk.

It should also be noted that it was not just the nature of the plague-related costs that ate into the estate that could be passed on to potential heirs—it was also the sudden timing of the deaths involved. People tended to acquire debts for products, services, and credits from a variety of parties, and planned to pay these back over an extended period. Sudden deaths during epidemics disrupted these intentions, and family members often had to take on the burden. For example, Trijn Dircx van Hoorn, who ended up in the Leiden pest house during the epidemic of 1655, left an account detailing all her debts upon dying in the institution.[156] Over the previous years she had compiled debts to various people, including from her own family—the delivery of food, cloth, tin, shoes, and wine, as well as substantial capital loans made out seven years previously—eventually coming to a sum of 120 guilders 18 stuivers. The account notes that a search was made to find and account for those still owed money (in Hoorn) by her sister—and perhaps the likely candidate who had to absorb these debts.

Conclusion

Although there is still more work to be done, empirical evidence compiled so far on the redistributive impact of epidemic disease in the preindustrial Low Countries suggests, first and foremost, that these outbreaks created the theoretical means for changes in the distribution of wealth, property, or assets, simply by creating conditions for increased turnover. Qualitative sources are plentiful in the different kinds of inheritance disputes that occurred in the aftermath of mass deaths, and quantitatively we see all kinds of different properties shifting from urban housing stocks to landownership in commercial and less commercialised rural areas. Accordingly, we often (though not always) see small declines in the Gini Coefficients measuring distribution of these assets—and yet, as with previous pioneering works, often proving to be temporary and modest declines.[157] While Alfani and co-authors have tended to emphasise the importance of shielding institutional mechanisms that stopped estate fragmentation in conditions of impartible or quasi-impartible inheritance—preventing long-term structural change—the fact that the same outcomes occurred in the Low Countries in conditions of extreme partible inheritance practice suggests that the primacy of this factor should be questioned, or at least only working contextually in tandem with other factors.[158]

More philosophically, Chapter 5 has shown that the lack of structural change was not solely in the temporary nature of the redistribution but the fact that any downward flickers of the distribution hardly represented greater egalitarianism in principle. Housing wealth redistribution in the city of Leiden tended to be in sectors of poor housing owned by wealthy investors, which ended up in the hands of similar investors. In rural areas, many households got access to land that they either did not want or was depreciating in value. In fact, while the appearance of *The Great Leveler* in 2017 might have been the high point for the view linking epidemics and equitable distribution outcomes, subsequent work, and certainly the evidence compiled so far in this book, suggests that any redistribution was simply entrenching existing inequalities.[159] Initial insights into the direct economic damages that epidemics could create at the micro level potentially affirm that—given that it is highly plausible that the direct economic damages disproportionately bore a toll on the poorest within society.

Notes

1 Gasquet, *The Black Death*; Seebohm, The Black Death.

2 Pamuk, The Black Death; Pamuk and Shatzmiller, Plagues; Bailey, *After the Black Death*, 283–325; Álvarez-Nogal and Prados de la Escosura, The Rise; Van Bavel and van Zanden, The Jump-Start; Epstein, Cities; Hatcher, England; Jedwab et al., The Economic Impact; Voigtländer and Voth, The Three Horsemen; Belich, *The World the Plague Made*.

3 Brenner, Agrarian Class Structure, 39. For variation in Black Death mortality: Izdebski et al., Palaeoecological Data; with a conversation about the implications of the methods employed: Curtis, Reduction; Izdebski et al., Reply. The impact of the Black Death on nuptiality and fertility across different regions, furthermore, is poorly understood at present, due to the lack of demographic evidence collected before 1350. Hence, the importance of studies such as Bennett, Wretched Girls; Bennett, Married.

4 Pioneering work was focused on reconstructing relative sizes of landholdings before and after the Black Death, but often for two dates widely separated in time. For England: Raftis, *Tenure*, 19–20; Hilton, Reasons, 279–80; for France: Le Roy Ladurie, *Les paysans*, I, 151–2; Bois, *Crise*, 140–1; for Italy: Herlihy, Santa Maria Impruneta, 259–60; Herlihy, *Medieval*, 181–3. Most of this early work is characterised by emphasising the rise of a kind of "middling peasantry", but it is unclear whether we can interpret that process as increasing inequality or increasing equality.

5 Alfani, Economic Inequality in Northwestern Italy; Alfani and Ammannati, Long-Term Trends; Ammannati, La Peste Nera; Almenar Fernández, Wealth Inequality; Miquel Milian and Morelló Baget, Economic Inequalities. The German town of Quedlingburg has markers from 30 years before the Black Death and 175 years after it: Alfani et al., Economic Inequality, 17–18. Even when we have distribution markers for individual localities before the Black Death in places well furnished with source material such as central Italy, many of these localities either do not have distribution markers after the Black Death, or more often, have distribution markers that cannot be compared as they measure something else entirely or have different rates of exclusion: Ammannati, La disuguaglianza economica, 44–6.

6 Observed already in Curtis, All Equal in the Presence of Death? 125.

7 One of the most important empirical contributions that conforms to this narrow criterion is still the study on Ivrea during the 1630 plague: Alfani, The Effects. We also have literature with at least one wealth distribution indicator (roughly) ten years either side of an epidemic for early modern Augsburg, Padua, Bergamo, and Barcelona: Scheidel, *The Great Leveler*, 336–8; Alfani and Di Tullio, *The Lion's Share*, 116–19; Brea-Martínez and Pujadas-Mora, Estimating, 407–9. For

the case of Augsburg, it is difficult to separate out war and epidemic effects, while for the case of Barcelona, no potential causal epidemic-induced mechanisms are elaborated upon in any detail. On a related note, while recent literature has been rather celebratory of our increased capacity to store, organise, and analyse ever increasing amounts of digital (big) data from the past—for example, Ruggles, The Revival—the tight temporal and contextual demands on having two or more sets of data to integrate remain a key barrier, not least when combining mortality and economic outcome variables.

8 Three summaries of this vast literature: Alfani, Epidemics; Alfani, Economic Inequality in Preindustrial Times; Alfani, *As Gods Among Men*, 36–65.

9 For the epidemic-related sections: Scheidel, *The Great Leveler*, 289–342.

10 Alfani and Murphy, Plague, 331. That the Black Death should not be seen as a model should be obvious given that epidemics of the past 1,000 years had wildly differing levels of socio-economic and demographic selectivity in mortality, but also occurred simultaneously with other confounding processes such as warfare or famine. Some scholars point to levelling effects of warfare caused by direct destruction of capital goods: Alfani et al., Economic Inequality; while others point to the unequal effects of army impositions on rural communities and regressive forms of taxation, which often increased during wars: Van Besouw and Curtis, Estimating; Alfani and Di Tullio, *The Lion's Share*, 174–80; Schaff, Warfare. Food crises apparently had no redeeming egalitarian qualities—either encouraging the rich to speculate or the poor to sell off the last of their property out of desperation: Campbell, *The Great Transition*, 196; although peasants selling off movables such as animals first: Sales i Favà, Leasing, 183–5.

11 Scheidel, *The Great Leveler*, 304–5. See, also, at the heart of an entire thesis on the Black Death and global disparities in economic development the argument that "the Black Death not only halved populations, but also doubled the average amount per person of everything…Plague inverted the balance not just between labour and capital, but also between people and all kinds of goods and resources, and gave common folk among the survivors a taste of a materially better life": Belich, *The World the Plague Made*, 448. A large literature has already discussed the notion of improved living standards for peasants and labourers after the Black Death, well-summarised in Bailey, *After the Black Death*, 251–4; Campbell, *The Great Transition*, 373–86; Dyer, *Standards*, 296–317. Such a view rests on the acknowledgement that many western European societies prior to the Black Death were poor with high pressures on resources. See the wide-ranging recent volumes: Benito i Monclus et al., eds., *Économies*; Cristoferi, ed., *Socio-Economic Inequalities*; Bourin et al., eds., *Les disettes*.

12 The most important essays republished in 1973 within Postan, *Essays*.

13 Alfani, The Effects, 63. Of course, 0.02 might represent a significant reduction, but this is not contextualised or relativised, so we have no way of knowing. Its rapid reversal suggests not. Further, it should be noted that the 1630 plague in Ivrea, as in other parts of Piedmont, was quite modest in impact, with a death rate of less than eight per cent: Alfani, 62. One wonders what the redistribution would have looked like in one of the localities in the heart of Po Valley which had 40 per cent death rates: Alfani, Plague, 418. Recent literature has examined epidemic-induced redistribution (or, as it turns out, the lack of redistribution) for localities in the Republic of Venice after the 1630 plague, where this outbreak was much more severe: Alfani et al. Wealth Inequality and Epidemics.

14 However, to be sure, this stylised fact of incrementally increasing inequality across the long term from the fifteenth century onwards has only been suggested through empirical evidence taken from different parts of Italy and the Low Countries: Ryckbosch, Economic Inequality; Alfani, Economic Inequality in

Preindustrial Times; and as soon as we get markers from different parts of Eurasia across the long term such as in Iberia or Germany, the standardised incremental increases are not quite as visible or consistent: Alfani et al., Economic Inequality; Álvarez-Nogal and Prados de la Escosura, The Rise; Brea-Martínez and Pujadas-Mora, Estimating; Reis, Deviant Behaviour?; Canbakal and Filiztekin, Wealth Inequality; Pfister, Economic Inequality; Kumon, Adoption.

15 Alfani, The Effects, 67–70. It has been argued that, before the Black Death, societies in western Europe were much more likely to follow the pious logic of liquidating their estates to bestow to different beneficiaries, but after the Black Death, there was a greater attachment to the perpetuation of material things across generations: Cohn, Renaissance Attachment. Research from nineteenth-century Hesse (Germany) has shown that persistent practices of impartible inheritance can be linked to higher levels of landholding inequality: Wegge, Inheritance Institutions; with the argument further developed to link the maintenance or persistence of historical partible inheritance with contemporary egalitarian outcomes: Hager and Hilbig, Do Inheritance Customs Affect Political and Social Inequality?

16 Van Bavel, *The Invisible Hand?* 138; Alfani and Di Tullio, *The Lion's Share*, 84–5; Hurwich, Inheritance Practices.

17 Curtis, An Agro-Town Bias? 704. Although this was regionally diverse—with the greatest adherence to this practice seen in Principato Citra (today Campania).

18 Kumon, Adoption.

19 Berkner and Mendels, Inheritance Systems; Cooper, Patterns; and persisting into the nineteenth century: Wegge, Inheritance Institutions.

20 Fertig et al., Introduction, 2–3.

21 On this regional diversity in inheritance practices: De Haan and Hoppenbrouwers, Intergenerational Transfer, 345; Van Bavel, *Manors*, 246, 285; Paping and Karel, The Rural Succession Myth, 46.

22 Noordegraaf and Valk, *De gave Gods*, 177.

23 BHIC, Schepenenprotocol Sint-Michielsgestel, 5121, no. 43, fo. 416v [25/5/1566] [AO].

24 RtL, Archief van de schepenbank van Asse, 94, no. 842 [AO].

25 De Brouwer, Erfenisperikelen.

26 SB, Vestbrieven, no. 765, fo. 193–4 [26/3/1549].

27 BHIC, Schepenenprotocol Sint-Michielsgestel, 5121, no. 43, fo. 119v [17/3/1559] [AO].

28 De Brouwer, "De aenclevende sieckte", 5.

29 BHIC, Schepenenprotocol Sint-Michielsgestel, 5121, no. 47 [AO]. On partible inheritance in the hinterlands of Den Bosch: Vermeer, Testamentary Practices, 483–4.

30 Sas, Die Swaerigheyt, 120.

31 BHIC, Schepenprotocol Veghel, 7700, no. 41 [116], fo. 122–3 [4/4/1615] [AO].

32 BHIC, Schepenprotocol Oss, 7365, no. 65, fo. 360–1 [7/5/1636] [AO].

33 Viaene, Smette, 317.

34 Jacquet-Ladrier, Les épidémies, 131.

35 SB, Stadsbestuur Breda (oud administratief archief) 1280–1810, Stadsrekeningen, no. 554, fo. 204r.

36 For the wages conversion: De Vries, An Inquiry, 82–3.

37 SA, Archief van Burgemeesters: Stadsrekeningen, 5014, no. 125, fo. 422 [AO].

38 Jacquet-Ladrier, Les épidémies, 127–8. At this time, the magistrate also required all foreigners to show a clean bill of health if they wanted to enter the town. One sou is the equivalent of a stuiver.

39 SB, Stadsbestuur Breda (oud administratief archief) 1280–1810, Stadsrekeningen, nos. 615–16.
40 On this concept but for flooding: Soens, Resilient Societies; the concept reused for grain shortages: Van Onacker, Social Vulnerability.
41 SVP, Rekeningen Heilige Geest, no. 750, Geervliet uitgaven [AO]; De Brouwer, “De aenclevende sieckte”, 5.
42 RAZ, Archief van de Kerkmeesters van de Hervormde Gemeente te Zutphen. Rekening van kerkmeester Derrick van Thyll (buiten), 1576, no. 292 [AO].
43 Pot, *Arm Leiden*, 263–4; Van der Vlis, *Leven*, 64–5; where poor relief institutions sometimes became fearful that certain women would continually prove a burden on the system: Muurling et al., Unwed Mothers, 24.
44 SVP, Rekeningen Heilige Geest, no. 750, Abbenbroek uitgaven [18/11/1603] [AO].
45 Thus, a letter written in February 1640 notes that the St. Pieters *gasthuis* at Culemborg had been burdened with so many expenses on account of the great death *vanden pestilentiale siecte* that had raged for almost three years in the town: RAR, Tiel, Archief van het stadsbestuur van Culemborg, 1318–1813, 0826, no. 1596 [AO].
46 On this issue, especially in rural areas: Van Onacker and Masure, Unity, 79–80; where it is shown that in places with greater inequalities such as larger landlords or tenants in coastal Flanders, gifts were more common and played a symbolic function of dominance. More positive on the solid financial basis of poor relief institutions in Holland: Dijkman, Bread.
47 SD, Sint Geertruiden Gasthuis, 0794, no. 23 [14/9/1596] [AO].
48 ELO, Archieven van de Gasthuizen, 1311–1873, 0504, no. 1711 [17/5/1658].
49 GAA, Burgerweeshuis te Arnhem, 2090, no. 490 [AO].
50 Blok et al., eds., *Oorkondenboek*, II, no. 1130 [11/11/1402].
51 AEA, Stadsbestuur Amersfoort, 1300–1810, 0001, no. 19, fo. 610v [5/5/1610] [AO]; Coopmans, *De rechtstoestand*, 198.
52 SR, Archieven van de Notarissen te Rotterdam en daarin opgegane gemeenten, 18, no. 4, fo. 10–13 [28/10/1648].
53 GAA, ORA Arnhem, 2003, no. 399, fo. 86 [23/09/1596] [AO].
54 GAA, ORA Arnhem, 2003, no. 412, fo. 170v–1r [19/11/1605] [AO].
55 Buylaert et al., The Political Economy.
56 EAL, Huis Bergh, 1227–1842, 0214, no. 2734 [AO].
57 GAA, ORA Arnhem, 2003, no. 411, fo. 211v–12r [29/9/1602] [AO].
58 Schmitz, Schiedam, 132.
59 At Steenwijk, west Brabant, in 1569, for example: GS, Stad Steenwijk tot ca. 1811, 14, no. 151 [AO]; or at Groningen in 1666 with the remittance of lease sums: Schroor, *Rurale metropool*, 61.
60 AEM, Archives de la ville de Mons. Section ancienne, 1200–1836, Registres annuels de perception. 1496–1632, no. 1359, fo. 488 [AO]. Note, this is the digital scan folio number.
61 For example, at the coastal village of Rockanje, on the South Holland island of Voorne-Putten, in 1604: Auwerda-Berghout, ed., Voorne, no. 163, fn. 225.
62 Wagenaar, *“Dat de regeringe niet”*, 28.
63 Van Zalinge-Spooren, “Die contagieuse sieckte”, 63.
64 Klinkenberg, “Dye quade siecte”, 282–3.
65 At Turnhout in 1572, the leasers of mills requested a reduction in rents on the grounds of epidemic-induced depopulation which had led to fewer users of their services: Adriaensen, ed., Turnhout [21/1/1572]. A letter was written in 1575 requesting lighter fiscal demands for the village of Kesteren, where the plague was said to rage: EAL, Huis Bergh, 1227–1842, 0214, no. 1676 [15/9/1575]

[AO]. A similar request was made in 1581 by the residents of Oldebroek that they should not be taxed too highly given the effects of the plague: EAL, Huis Bergh, no. 445 [27/12/1581] [AO]. A petition for lower taxes was made by the Campine village of Lille in 1607 on account of mass mortality through *contsieuse zieckte der peste*: Janssens and Van den Branden, De pest, 43. The *contagieuse sieckten* of 1666 in the village of Vught prompted the inhabitants to request a third off their leases, as consumption of produce had fallen greatly through the epidemic: BHIC, Resoluties Raad van State, 178, no 209, fo. 1261v [27/11/1666] [AO]. The masters of Veenendaal appealed for some years without tax because of the twin damages of fire and *pestilentie* in 1667: RAZU, Stadsbestuur Rhenen, 152, no. 843 [27/1/1668] [AO].

66 BHIC, Dorpsbestuur Schijndel, 1312–1811, 5016, no. 32 [AO].

67 Initial work for the early modern Low Countries linked the two: Noordegraaf, Dearth, 61, 65; although this is more applicable for the sixteenth century than the seventeenth century: Curtis and Dijkman, The Escape. In the wider literature, others tend to doubt the causal association. See, for example, "the plague was an autonomous cause of high mortality, decoupled from the great fluctuations of economic and social life": Slack, *The Impact*, 76–8; and "the commonplace 'first famine then fever' will not bear historical scrutiny…Famines and epidemics are not invariably linked in historical records": Carmichael, Infection, 52. Earlier literature strangely tended to downplay epidemics as the main cause of mortality in preindustrial societies; for example, for a nearby region of northern France: Goubert, *Beauvais*, 75.

68 Curtis, Plague, 91–5.

69 Espeel, *Prices*, 223. Similarly shown for Cambrai in earlier literature, although less clearly: Neveux, La mortalité, 86. The temporal link between harvest failures as shown through yields in tithe records and epidemic outbreaks is a little tighter in the southern Low Countries, although this might also reflect the complex relationships between medieval harvest and price information: Soens, No Second Lord, 87–90.

70 Espeel, Plague, 354, 356–7.

71 A line of argumentation put forward in Curtis, Plague.

72 Huiting, *Domeinen*, 163; Curtis, Plague, 79–80.

73 Huiting, *Domeinen*, 163; The existence of the first charter was mentioned in De Boer, *Graaf*, 34.

74 Espeel, Plague, 355. Potentially exacerbated by heavy rains and localised flooding in areas close to the Scheldt River.

75 Van Eeghen, ed., *Dagboek*, I, 537. Also, referred to in Noordegraaf and Valk, *De gave Gods*, 48.

76 EAL, Huis Bergh, 1227–1842, 0214, no. 445 [11/8/1582] [AO].

77 De Brouwer, "De aenclevende sieckte", 11–12.

78 Kappelhof, ed., Kroniek, 65–6.

79 BHIC, Resoluties Raad van State, 178, no. 202, fo. 523 [22/11/1660] [AO].

80 BHIC, Resoluties Raad van State, 178, no. 202, fo. 207v [1/5/1660] [AO].

81 Bieleman, Rural Change, 116. Similar economic damages suggested for Warneton in southern Flanders during the most severe eighteenth-century outbreaks: De Herdt, La peste bovine.

82 Van Tielhof and van Dam, *Waterstaat*, 213, 341.

83 HCL, Landen van Overmars, 01.075, no. 8677 [AO].

84 BHIC, Raad en Rentmeester-Generaal Domeinen, 9, no. 18, fo. 10r–11r [15/3/1639] [25/3/1639] [AO].

85 Moquette, Pestepidemieën, 35.

86 Druwé, Pest, 1282.

87 Conversion of earnings to house values based on our 1632–68 *Verpondingen* database: Van Besouw et al., Epidemic Mortality.
88 Coomans, *Community*, 243.
89 SB, Dekenaten Bergen op Zoom en Breda behorend tot Bisdom Antwerpen (1420) 1561–1802, ARC0007.3, no. 361.
90 SB, Stadsbestuur Breda (oud administratief archief) 1280–1810, Stadsrekeningen, no. 616, fo. 104v.
91 BHIC, Resoluties Raad van State, 178, no. 186, fo. 245 [6/9/1644] [AO].
92 BHIC, Resoluties Raad van State, 178, no. 198, fo. 255v [18/5/1656]; no. 199, fo. 202 [8/5/1657] [AO].
93 ELO, Stadsarchief van Leiden, (1253) 1574–1816 (1897), 0501A, no. 249 [*kladresolutie*: 19/7/1664].
94 Coomans et al., Plague.
95 As suggested recently: Jordà et al., Longer-Run. However, the method of separating out epidemic and war-related variables in this study is highly questionable given the lack of proper consideration to the nuances of measuring warfare. These issues about questionable warfare datasets for the preindustrial past are addressed in Van Besouw and Curtis, Estimating.
96 Geens, *A Golden Age*, 23–9; Espeel, Plague. An important nuance of a similar nature focusing on the nature of remuneration has been made for England: Claridge et al., (In-Kind) Wages.
97 Alfani and Percoco, Plague; Rota and Weisdorf, Italy.
98 Fochesato, Origins. With a broader point made that by the early modern period in many parts of western Europe, wages were more stable in the face of mortality spikes through higher productivity thresholds: Fochesato, Origins, 109.
99 Francke and Korevaar, Housing Markets.
100 Variations on this critique are everywhere in Hatcher and Stephenson, eds., *Seven Centuries*. Thus, for Qing China, even recent attempts to upwardly revise the prevalence of wage labour make straightforward concessions such as "wages were not the main source of earnings in rural China" and "full-time wage earners may have been a minority": Liu, Wages, 3. This is without even going into a discussion of the complexities of what remuneration really meant for preindustrial societies: Caferro, Petrarch's War; Claridge et al., (In-Kind) Wages.
101 Geens and Blondé, An Apology, 22–3.
102 The first attempt to collect large amounts of mortality evidence over a long period: Curtis, Was Plague an Exclusively Urban Phenomenon?; and for a non-exhaustive list of income, wealth, and land inequality markers from different sources and forms in the Low Countries: Ryckbosch, Economic Inequality; Hanus, Real Inequality; Van Zanden, Tracing; Van Zanden and Soltow, *Income*; Curtis, Danger; Curtis, *Coping*, 147–80; Hilkens, *Living*; McCants, Inequality; Dombrecht and Ryckbosch, Wealth Inequality; Lambrecht and Ryckbosch, Economic Inequality.
103 For the income inequality figures: Hanus, Real Inequality, 750. For the observation: Hilkens, *Living*.
104 Kooten, Levelling.
105 More refined details of the precise dimensions of the case, the sources, the data, and the methodology are found in Van Besouw et al., Epidemic Mortality.
106 An example of epidemics, warfare, and redistribution together: Alfani et al., Economic Inequality. On the limited nature of military activity in seventeenth-century Holland: Van Besouw and Curtis, Estimating.
107 Investors came to dominate the housing market in Leiden towards the later phases of the sixteenth century in line with the rise of the textile industry: Van Steensel et al., Housing Inequality.

108 Lesger, *Huur*; Baer, Landlords; Drelichman and Agudo, Housing.
109 In Haarlem during the outbreak of 1635/6, it was remarked that "now the houses and residences lost their inhabitants and often stood empty"; while contemporaries in Leiden in 1642 specifically related decreases in rents to "deaths which have followed and exposed the city": Noordegraaf and Valk, *De gave Gods*, 139. Rental prices declined after seventeenth-century epidemics in Amsterdam, although they recovered quickly: Francke and Korevaar, Housing Markets.
110 ELO, Stadsarchief van Leiden, (1253) 1574–1816 (1897), 0501A, no. 79, fo. 2v–3r.
111 De Vries and van der Woude, *The First Modern Economy*, 592; Prak, *Gezeten burgers*, 125, 132.
112 Further elaboration of the full results can be found in Van Besouw et al., Epidemic Mortality.
113 't Hart, *Oorlog*, 105–24. For a relevant critique: Hilkens, Verschillende ongelijkheden? 85–6.
114 For rural wealth: Alfani and Ammannati, Long-Term Trends; Alfani, Economic Inequality in Northwestern Italy; Yates, Change, 624–5; Bengtsson and Svensson, The Wealth. For distributions of land: Curtis, *Coping*, 91, 137–8, 170–1, 203, 247–50; Curtis, Danger, 126–30; Martinez-Galarraga and Prat, Inequality, 30; Almenar Fernández, Wealth Inequality; Furió, Economic Inequalities.
115 Curtis, All Equal, 125. Fiscal and property registers, a major source for reconstructing distribution, do not appear serially but in random individual years. An alternative approach has linked demographic information to sources that reveal an individual's recorded wealth at death, although not used for establishing changes in asset distribution in rural communities over time: Cummins, Marital Fertility. Even literature on nineteenth- and early-twentieth-century rural distribution rarely shows temporally high-resolution dynamics across years: For example, see Lust, Prospering.
116 WBA, Dorpsbestuur Oudenbosch, 0300, nos. 0918–29, 0960–8. Our fuller study on long-term land accumulation and decumulation introduces the specific contextual case of Oudenbosch: Curtis and van Besouw, Lifecycle.
117 For the 80 per cent figure: Martinez-Galarraga and Prat, Inequality, 30. Nevertheless, it is clear that this is contextually variable, and other scholars, especially for the late Middle Ages, have suggested that inequalities derived directly from distributions of land might over-exaggerate impoverishment. On this, see the exceptional recent volume incorporating material culture: Jervis et al., *The Material Culture*.
118 On the blurring of the lines: Curtis, *Coping*, 23–62. On leasehold and development: Van Bavel, *Manors*, 170–7; Van Bavel, *The Invisible Hand?* 171–3; Bailey, *After the Black Death*, 301–7; Whittle, *Agrarian Capitalism*, 314–15.
119 WBA, Doop-, trouw- en begraafboeken Oudenbosch, 1609–1811, 0302, no. 3. A product of instability in the religious denominations which were present. After the Peace of Westphalia in 1648, the Catholics had to give up their church in the village.
120 For these other epidemics, see the Supporting Documents provided in Curtis and van Besouw, Lifecycle. The impact of the Siege of Breda in 1624/5 was much more demanding on the surrounding rural hinterlands than that of 1637. See the earlier maps of Figure 3.6 for the minimal impact of the 1636 plague in west Brabant, but the localised uptick of mortality in 1638.
121 Goyarts, De pest, 34.
122 WBA, Doop-, trouw- en begraafboeken Oudenbosch, 1609–1811, 0302, no. 1.

123 WBA, Notaris Wouter de Witte, Minuutakten van andere akten, 1625–7, 0050, no. 64, fo. 127v–30v [act no. 69]; SB, Dekenaten Bergen op Zoom en Breda behorend tot Bisdom Antwerpen (1420) 1561–1802, ARC0007.3, no. 361.
124 All data obtainable in Curtis, ed., Original Burials Data.
125 Huffmeijer, Op weg, 37.
126 Van Onacker, Bedrijvige boeren? 53; Van Bavel, The Land Market, 135–6; Sabean, *Property*, 355–70.
127 Although this seems high, another village in the Middle Rhine Valley area of Germany saw more than a third of inhabitants involved in a case of land transfer to a new owner in a single year: Schäfer, Land Transactions, 39.
128 As seen directly in the *Veldboeken* themselves. But also, more generally for west Brabant: De Haan and Hoppenbrouwers, Intergenerational Transfer, 345; Hoppenbrouwers, Doorgifte, 92.
129 Alfani, Effects. Although we say urban context of Ivrea, this was a population of around 2,500 and thus only around double the size of Oudenbosch village.
130 Further detail on the methods involved is in Curtis and van Besouw, Lifecycle.
131 Hilkens, Mortality. See, also, the work in a broader context of land distribution and use: Hilkens, *Living*. On the declining rewards for central Holland peat villages across the period in question: Tielhof and van Dam, *Waterstaat*, 222–6.
132 As emphasised in the critique on the recent inequality literature: Van Bavel, Wealth Inequality.
133 Curtis, Did the Commons?
134 For the different forms that appeared in the preindustrial Low Countries: De Moor, *The Dilemma*. For the rural distribution of rights of common to arable, pasture, woodlands, and marshes in the Low Countries: Hoppenbrouwers, The Use; De Moor, Common Land; De Moor, *The Dilemma*, 61–99.
135 The original thesis associated with Hardin, The Tragedy of the Commons. Later critiqued in Ostrom, *Governing*.
136 De Moor, The Silent Revolution, 186. A similar argument was made almost 70 years earlier in Slicher van Bath, *Een samenleving*, 22–4. To be sure, collective organisation of agriculture occurred in some parts of Europe well before this time with lines of continuity going back into antiquity (which are also subject to debate over characteristics and chronology): Oosthuizen, *Tradition*. However, structural formalisation is different from absolute origins and is why the twelfth and thirteenth centuries are important.
137 All the historical work that has gone into disproving the tragedy of the commons theory is well-summarised now in De Moor, *The Dilemma*, 11–13, 158–61. For a similar observation of the over-focus on population pressure rather than underuse: Miyanaga and Shimada, "The Tragedy of the Commons".
138 Surely a more relevant question to address in contemporary societies characterised by high levels of collectively pooled resources given global trends of rural migration towards cities, leaving rural societies depleted of people: Berge and McKean, On the Commons.
139 De Moor, *The Dilemma*, 125.
140 Van Zanden, The Paradox, 136.
141 De Moor, *The Dilemma*, 144–5.
142 Lachiver, *Les années*, 274; Devos and Van Rossem, Oud, 42, 44.
143 Adriaenssen and 't Hart, Farming Communities. The paper was previously freely accessible on the personal website of the late Leo Adriaenssen but is now out of use. It is a paper I previously used and cited in previous work: Curtis, *Coping*, 213.
144 Groenendijk and van Schaïk, Isolated, 314.

145 These issues were already recognisable in the Middle Ages. A charter referred to by the above-mentioned Groenendijk and van Schaïk produced in 1484 refers to the shifting and placing of boundary markers (*scheidpalen*) between Ter Apel monastery and the Marke of Lauwede in "the current times of pestilence" (*der teghenwordiger tydt der pestilencien*). Manuscript accessible at http://www.cartago.nl/nl/oorkonde/kta061a.xml. Issues of inheritance after multiple deaths, and where the rights descended to, are found in some of the earliest lists of rights and obligations (*willekeuren*) for the commons: For example, at Langewold, Drenthe, in 1282: Blok et al., eds., *Oorkondenboek*, I, no. 157, rules 23–4 [18/6/1282].
146 Adriaenssen and 't Hart, Farming Communities, 23–4.
147 Di Tullio, Cooperating; Casari, Emergence; Lana Berasain, From Equilibrium.
148 RAZ, Oud archief van de stad Zutphen (1206–1815), 0001, Rekeningen van Johan Ruter, 1598–1599, no. 1159, fo. 6 [AO].
149 Polak-de-Booy, Dansen.
150 Sas, Die Swaerigheyt, 120–3. During epidemics, tasks such as carrying away dung heaps were made daily—financial burdens passed on to ordinary tradespeople and workers: Coomans, *Community*, 227. For a broader quantitative assessment of what welfare provision in the northern Low Countries represented in the early modern period: Van Bavel and Rijpma, How Important?
151 Curtis, Trade, 5.
152 On the early inheritance-social mobility angle: Benedictow, *The Black Death, 1346–1353*, 261.
153 BHIC, Schepenprotocol Dinther, 7603, no. 12, fo. 106v [AO].
154 BHIC, Schepenprotocol Dinther, 7603, no. 12, fo. 169r [AO]. In another magistrate's act, Stoffel Lamberts was noted as having carried out the duties of the village *burgemeester* in 1633, shortly before his death.
155 GAA, Huizen Nettelhorst en De Heest, 0418, no. 312, fo. 4 [AO].
156 ELO, Archieven van de Gasthuizen, 1311–1873, 0504, no. 1615A.
157 Alfani, The Effects, 63.
158 Alfani and Di Tullio, *The Lion's Share*, 84–5.
159 Scheidel, *The Great Leveler*.

6 Women's experiences of epidemics

Opportunities, burdens, and narratives

Like research into female experiences of environmental hazards such as floods, droughts, and earthquakes,[1] recent experiences of epidemic diseases such as HIV and AIDS, Ebola, Zika, and COVID-19 have suggested that women and girls experience these outbreaks differently from men—although analyses have often been hindered by a lack of data disaggregated down the lines of sex and gender.[2] Meanwhile, gendered analyses of COVID-19 have taken off in these past years, but potentially have the twin flaws of entrenching myopia (a privileging of COVID and diseases that behave like it such as influenza) and becoming itemised lists of all the ways women are said to be more negatively affected compared to men.

More productive, instead, would be to pose the issue as an actual problem to be solved—why epidemics have mainly created restrictions and burdens for women in some contexts (elements of vulnerability) and elsewhere have been vehicles through which female agency has led to women's opportunities and adaptation (elements of resilience). This is not easy to unravel, however, not least because the causal and confounding variables are so numerous, including differences in the characteristics of the epidemics; differences between societies where women's position was often very different; and differences within societies where gender intersected with other categories including age or socio-economic status, among others. Furthermore, the outcomes for women are not straightforward either. For example, although immediate or short-term suffering or burdens can be severe, they can sometimes change or even disappear over time. Hence, we require a view from history—not least to be able to separate out short-term hardships and opportunities for women from structural changes to women's lives. This insight is further important because historical literature has suggested that while women have often responded in dynamic ways to mega-shifts in circumstances, over time men have sometimes reined in those gains.[3]

As mentioned in Chapter 5, historical research into the redistributive consequences of epidemics has taken off in recent years, although the differing impacts of these outbreaks between women and men have had little consideration in this literature.[4] Indeed, how valuable are arguments that epidemics had "levelling" qualities, for example, if we leave out half of the adult population?[5] And in recent times, scholars have been preoccupied with aspects of

DOI: 10.4324/9781003694908-6

sex-selective epidemic mortality, as mentioned in Chapter 3, but less on the welfare and fortunes of the surviving women in the aftermath of outbreaks.

Furthermore, historical research into women and epidemics is polarised between two sub-fields. Economic historians have tended to privilege women's wages, like the general epidemic-redistribution literature mentioned in Chapter 5, but the paucity and difficult-to-interpret nature of the evidence have led to wide differences in views.[6] Thus, some have suggested that women (or rather certain statuses of women) did not gain from the posited "golden age of labour" said to occur in some places after the Black Death of the mid-fourteenth century which saw potentially advantageous conditions for peasants and labourers,[7] while others have argued that in certain historical contexts women benefitted from general labour shortages.[8] One of the issues is that this topic tends to essentialise questions such as "did women benefit from the Black Death", when a more appropriate question, similar to above, would be "why did women benefit from the Black Death in certain contexts over others?" But perhaps more fundamentally, wages are not straightforward welfare indicators.[9] Wages only remain relevant in wage-earning societies, and even in those societies, women did not always perform wage labour. Historically, and even in some places today, women have often contributed more to household economies and participated in informal markets.[10] Furthermore, the extent to which women's wages were responsive to demographic and market conditions—or instead set by gendered values or institutional restrictions—is still debated, and thus of clear relevance when we try to consider the impact of epidemic outbreaks.[11]

Women could survive diseases and take on new post-epidemic forms of employment and financial remuneration, but of course simultaneously experience other forms of prejudice, restriction, and persecution.[12] Hence, social and cultural historians have usefully provided evidence for this development but often via individual cases that employ a diverse array of qualitative evidence for a brief snapshot in time—i.e., during one epidemic outbreak.[13] Although Chapter 6 does not offer a systematic comparative research approach—still there is room for a large-scale research project focused on this issue—the discussion is moved forward somewhat by (a) looking at outcomes for women in a variety of cases across a long period of time, and (b) incorporating a wider range of indicators of impact on women, some economic, some socio-cultural, and including tangible assets such as possessions and conceptual assets such as identities, roles, and representation of women.

Adaptations to social and economic roles

In recent literature, especially on the early modern Low Countries, social and economic historians have tended to foreground concepts such as female agency and independence—often pointing to features such as high numbers of single (never married) women, late ages of marriage for those women that did take husbands, high levels of female involvement in lifecycle service, and high levels of female participation in varied economic activities both within and outside the confines of the domestic household.[14] Interestingly, this situation also seemed to be in stark contrast to the male breadwinner economic model that was, like other places such as England, said to characterise many parts of the industrialising Low Countries in the nineteenth century, where women were more confined to their domestic environments.[15] Furthermore, women's physical presence out in public and communal settings is said to have been very clear already by the fifteenth century in much of the Low Countries.[16] Scholars have focused on widespread competencies in women's numeracy and literacy by the early modern period, and in turn, their cultural, literary, and artistic contributions.[17] Women also benefitted from an inheritance system that was both partible and highly equitable in many (but certainly not all) parts of the Low Countries such as Holland and Brabant, where male and female often inherited equal shares, and widows inherited portions of estates or rights to estates alongside children.[18]

When we look to the preindustrial period, however, we also should recognise that concepts such as female agency have epistemological nuances which complicate their application within certain historical settings.[19] That is to say, we should at least be aware of the dangers of reliance on normative indicators that might make sense in the twentieth and twenty-first centuries, but do not necessarily mean the same things to people living in, for example, sixteenth-century Ostend. In my view, some of these inconsistencies or contradictions can be brought to the surface by zooming in on how preindustrial women fared during certain pressure periods such as epidemic disease outbreaks.[20] As mentioned in Chapter 3 above, together with colleagues, I have made some progress in recent times with sources that do not appear to structurally under-record women, showing that during medieval and early modern epidemics, women tended to die in greater degrees than men, when compared to the ratios in normal or non-epidemic times. This is based on the largest pool of sex-disaggregated adult mortality estimates that we currently have for anywhere in the preindustrial world.

Although biological or physiological principles tend to suggest women should out-survive men during epidemics and famines, what my findings have suggested is that certain societal conditions can conspire in certain historical contexts to reduce, eliminate, or even reverse this female mortality advantage (more on this concept in Chapter 3). It remains to be seen, however, to what extent this is borne out of gender inequalities in access to resources, welfare, and protection, or is instead a product of differences in exposure to vectors or points of contagion connected to distinct gendered roles. My sex-selective epidemic mortality findings also fit uneasily with the recent narratives of female agency and independence in the medieval or early modern Low Countries mentioned above, or perhaps more reasonably that female agency and independence, if accepted empirically, did not necessarily lead to favourable health outcomes during pressure points such as epidemic outbreaks. In this section, then, I suggest some of the reasons behind these unfavourable outcomes for women, focusing on the changes in some of the economic and social roles that women took on during epidemics, and how they, at least partially or to a degree, differed from those of men.

One thing that has been shown recently is that late-medieval and early modern outbreaks of plague, dysentery, or typhus, for example, tended to cluster spatially and temporally at the household level. In other words, when one person was sick or infected within a household, by either sharing experiences of the same conditions or vectors, or through the contagious nature of the disease itself, there was a high chance that others from the same household also would experience the same fate.[21] These are highly relevant observations when we consider that women likely spent more time in the domestic household, and likely were also responsible for a disproportionate role in the provision of ordinary care tasks (of children, for example) but also medical care within the house.[22] Women often made key decisions regarding family health decisions concerning epidemics.[23] The dangers of infecting other family members at close quarters were something already recognised and creating concern in the seventeenth century. One infected woman from Utrecht, Cunera Adriaens, decided during the plague outbreak of 1604 to get a local pest house master to throw her own sister, Neeltgen, out of the house "for scientific reasons that...Cunera has in her pestilence" (*voor redenen van wetenschap dat...Cunera in haar pestilentiale sieckte heeft*).[24]

Sources from the Low Countries reveal some of the difficult decisions that women sometimes faced within their own households if they themselves fell sick. Witnesses noted on 14 February 1520 during an epidemic outbreak in the town of Kampen that a maid had left a baby on the steps of another house because her mistress was too sick to take care of it any longer. Nevertheless, although the baby was taken in, it was also likely infected, as it already died some three days later.[25] Later in the sixteenth century, at the fort of Schenkenschanz, Cleves, in 1599, the multiple deaths from *pest* of a military corporal, his wife, and five of their children meant that the young two-year-old daughter, Anneken, was left alone. Eventually, a midshipman took pity on her and promised to bring up the child with every virtue (*alle deugd*)—yet this burden was left to his wife, since it was also noted that if the wife died before the child was articulate, she would then be sent away to distant relatives.[26] Women played an important role in taking in children without guardians due to sudden losses of parents through epidemic mortality. In the small town of Zierikzee, Zeeland, several examples have been found of women taking in young girls, some of them even sick themselves, during epidemics in 1568 and 1573.[27]

Although (especially medieval) medical historians of the past three decades have done much to emphasise that women played a bigger role in health care than previously thought, largely because tasks were carried out domestically, we should also recognise that during epidemic outbreaks, women's care burdens often extended outside of households to other public health institutions. For example, during the plague of 1515 at Mons, the local government decided on 9 May to install several women in the St. Nicolas hospital to treat those afflicted.[28] And as indicated in Chapter 5, it was possible to earn from these roles. At Harderwijk in 1525, on the edge of the Zuiderzee, a woman called Lene was paid in sums of peat, wood, and rye for her role as guardian (*bewaarster*) of those suffering from *pest* and other infectious sicknesses (*besmettelijke ziekten*) in the isolated hospital constructed from wood on the periphery of the town.[29] Fortunately for her, this did not seem to affect her life expectancy as she was found in the same role 22 years later.[30] Elsewhere, women sometimes were paid to tend to infected soldiers housed in temporary institutions, working alongside male surgeons, as seen in the series of outbreaks in the 1660s and 1670s in Groningen connected to the military incursions of the Bishop of Munster.[31] Similarly, poor women could find paid work as fumigators of premises considered infected such as schools, orphanages, barracks, and streets, often making use of smoke or lime to tackle the perceived corrupted airs and vapours.[32]

Temporary or permanent employment of women in public health settings can be seen as additional to the efforts of women working in ecclesiastical institutions that were also tasked with treating the sick. For example, a group of four "devout" women were given the role of tending to the sick in Rotterdam during the *pestilentietijden* of 1485.[33] The Zwarte Zusters of the Molenstraat, Breda, treated a young boy who was afflicted with dysentery in 1596—giving him bread, butter, eggs, and herbs.[34] Later, in Namur in 1638, two religious women, Jeanne Anceau and Marguerite Verlée, suddenly put themselves at the service of the infected by treating strangers in the guardhouse, praying for them, and asking for nothing in compensation.[35] Single women in beguinages have also been recorded as helping out in different hospitals across the southern Low Countries during epidemics.[36] Of course, this was not without problems. For example, a midwife named Lycken Dolcx from Leiden complained in 1538 that her reputation had been negatively affected in the community because she had treated pregnant women who were infected with plague.[37]

Given that women were prominently placed in public institutions to help cope with the demands of disease, it is perhaps no surprise that women were also disproportionately found to receive care within these same institutions.[38] Partially this might be explained by the fact that most public health institutions such as pest houses and hospitals set up to deal with an intake of those suffering from an affliction during an epidemic were situated in urban environments, and by the sixteenth and seventeenth centuries at least, these cities and towns were home to more women than men. Thus, for example, by 1614, the Catharinagasthuis in Leiden reserved five rooms for women and yet only two for men, while the Elisabethgasthuis did not take in men at all.[39] Some scholars have suggested that greater levels of female migration to early modern cities such as Amsterdam was stimulated largely by the improved chances of receiving, among other things, medical provisions.[40] Perhaps so for the larger cities, although when looking at the incoming patients in another hospital in Middelburg in the years 1659–61 (a sample of almost 1,000 people), this is not so clearly demonstrated—41.8 per cent of patients were female.[41] When considering epidemic disease, however, we should also be aware that many ordinary hospitals did not take in those suffering from an infectious disease (as well as children or pregnant women), as other institutions from the sixteenth century onwards were seen as better equipped for those issues—linked to the specialisation of institutional care processes described in Chapter 2.[42] Nevertheless, some hospitals such as at Bergen op Zoom in 1525 and Den Bosch in 1606 introduced special services for certain categories of women such as those that were suffering from the plague (*haestige siecte*) and were at the same time pregnant.[43] And like ordinary hospitals, pest houses were also spatially divided between men and women. In Leiden, the pest house had three rooms for women and two for men.[44] Some women were desperate to enter these institutions. At Rotterdam during the outbreak of 1635, for example, a midwife with a child threatened a pest house official with a knife to be admitted—though apparently rejected three days later on the grounds of not being afflicted with the disease.[45] Yet, not all women shared this same desire, as demonstrated by those who tried to escape these places and continue their social lives. In Delft in 1665, for example, two women were punished and sent to a house of correction (*tuchthuis*) because, upon previously being confined to a pest house, they had tried to escape to visit others, and then could only be taken in as fugitives.[46] As mentioned in Chapter 4, pest house confinement severely conflicted with deeply held desires for continued sociability.

Still, one of the most important care-related roles that women often played during preindustrial epidemics was not limited to their own households but providing this service to other non-kin-connected households with one or more infected members. It is not entirely clear when the phenomenon began to take hold in the Low Countries, but at best we can say at some point in the fifteenth century, when considering the timing of the shift to more formal institutionalised forms of epidemic-related healthcare.[47] Indeed, as mentioned in Chapter 5, people in houses that were identified as having plague or a related disease came to rely on paid outsiders to provide a range of services connected to care, cleaning, and other forms of administration such as fetching food and goods for the house, witnessing testaments, carrying and codifying corpses, and tending to children, animals, and crops—in Dutch *schrobbers* or *schrobsters* and in French *héridesses*. Although it is clear that men could do this task, in the early modern Low Countries context at least, it seems as though more female examples could be found than male.[48] As a subject of initial study, this group of workers—one of the most important in managing epidemics at the micro level—has been relatively neglected, which is unfortunate as they provide a window into the lives of the often poor women weakly represented in the historical record.[49] Some fragments of information can be found that suggest the women and men who did do this job were indeed of low financial means. In one *momboirrekening* (financial accounts of a guardian) for the Brabant village of Dinther in 1580, for example, it was noted that a man was to be paid for baking bread for both "the poor and the *schrobbers*" (*voor de armen en voor de schrobbers brood gebakken*).[50]

On the one hand, women (and girls) could gain financially from performing these care tasks in other people's houses—possibly important if there had been a loss of earnings from the death of other adults in their own household during the outbreak. And as mentioned already in Chapters 4 and 5, this kind of work was highly needed—infected households in smaller communities often needing to hire in willing personnel from other places far away such was the sudden spiked demand for these services. Hence, while officials tried to enforce limitations on earnings—the plague ordinance of Breda from 1535, repeated in 1575, limited wages to four stuivers for a day and night's work as a cleaner—most of the time we see payments well above that.[51] Indeed, women in some contexts earned enough to purchase items from the households of the deceased made available at auction. One *schrobster* named Grietken bought a boiler (*ketel*) for two guilders and an apron (*schort*) for 30 stuivers, for example, while Catharina, noted as a nurse (*pleegster*), bought some butter for one guilder and was helped through an advance on her payment of ten stuivers.[52] At Schijndel in 1605, one *schrobster* named Lijsken van Gessen could only be paid her 15 guilders after the sale of the infected household's furniture.[53]

Nevertheless, women—and especially younger women and girls—tended to earn much smaller amounts than men for doing the same kind of work. A good example can be seen from in Figure 6.1 taken from the *momboirrekeningen* of the village of Dinther during the plague years of 1636/7, already introduced in Chapter 5. Here, we see in this case that a male *schrobber* and a female *schrobster* worked in the same house of Jan Bernaert, infected *metter peste*, for a similar amount of time (six weeks and five days, and six weeks, respectively), and yet the male *schrobber*, Hanrick Huijberts, earned more than six times the amount of the *schrobster*, Anneken. In addition, Anneken saw that sum paid to her father—suggesting a young woman or girl was doing this job, which is different from the older profile of searchers noted for London.[54] Factors such as the age of the female *schrobster* or the wealth of the family household in which they worked likely drove differences in earnings across contexts. Indeed, another woman, Elizabeth Jacobs van Vilvoirden, for seven weeks' work in Stoffel Lambert's house in the same village of Dinther during the same plague, earned much more than both young Anneken and Hanrick Huijberts—60 guilders and 16 stuivers.[55]

These inequalities in earning potential were not restricted to domestic *schrobsters* but were mirrored in cases of women working in institutions. The previously mentioned woman employed to care for pregnant plague-afflicted women in the Den Bosch hospital in 1606, for example, earned 50 guilders for the year's work—roughly a twelfth of other male wages for work done in pest houses and hospitals, and only narrowly more than the one-off task of transporting furniture from Heusden to Breda (the return journey

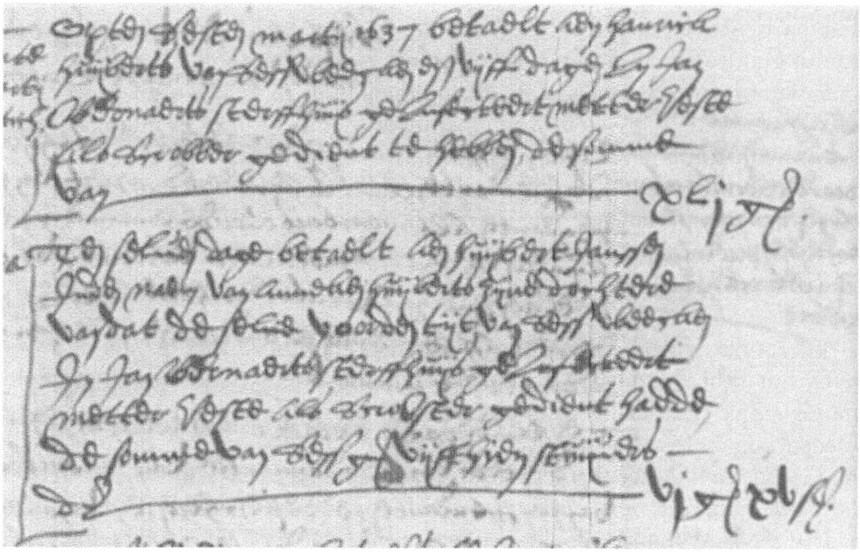

Figure 6.1 Payments to plague cleaners, Dinther, 1636/7

Source: BHIC, Schepenprotocol Dinther, 7603, no. 12, fo. 51v [AO]. *Translation*: "On 6 March 1637 paid to Hanrick Huijberts for 6 weeks and 5 days in the deathhouse of Jan Bernaerts infected with plague, as a cleaner, the sum of 41 guilders...On the same day paid to Huijbert Janssen in the name of Anneken Huijberts his daughter for the same time of 6 weeks in the deathhouse of Jan Bernaerts infected with plague, as a cleaner, the sum of 6 guilders 15 stuijvers".

would take less than a week) in 1667 for the incumbent pest house master (see Table 5.1 from earlier).

In addition to the inequalities in financial rewards from the role of *schrobster*, women who took on these care-giving roles not only exposed themselves to sickness but also could be subject to various forms of abuse. This is perhaps predictable given that the connection between the respective parties—care-providers and the recipients of this care—was not one of kinship or even friendship, but frequently a financial arrangement between strangers, and thus potentially leading to mutual suspicions.[56] For example, in the small Brabant towns of Oisterwijk and Oirschot in 1523, several women working as *schrobsters* were found in the magistrates' accounts accused of plague spreading through supposed deliberate contamination of doors and handles in the houses of those under their care.[57] The magistrate went further and suggested that these *schrobsters* had even tried to gain more business by smearing excrement of the infected on the door handles of the rich.[58] In another case just seven years later, a bailiff took into his custody a *schrobster*, Neelken Claesdr., who had been accused by her own husband of deliberately killing off those infected with plague, and furthermore, had used sorcery (*toverien*) to bring the infection into other houses on the street.[59] In this particular case, the accused woman was set free and the husband was found guilty of making false accusations, but we have other situations—at Nieuwpoort in coastal Flanders during the plague of 1601–4, for example—of women being convicted of witchcraft during a chain of events that often began with something innocuous such as the verbal cursing of another person with *pestilentie*.[60] *Schrobsters* also had the dubious misfortune of having to get involved in delicate inheritance disputes between the kin of those that they worked for—one woman who served in an epidemic-afflicted household in Tilburg in 1625 had to stand before a court and declare as a witness the exact order of the deaths within the family.[61]

Of course, it was not just plague cleaners that faced these kinds of problems but other women working in domestic contexts such as household maids employed during disease times. Thus, in the Brabant village of Sint Oedenrode in 1485, a man was fined ten guilders for binding the feet of his maid and leaving her in the house—at the time she was said to be infected (*sieck was van der pestilentien*)—while he went out drinking.[62] Women providing medical support could also experience dangers. During one localised outbreak in Gouda, likely in 1629 or 1630 given the date of conviction, one female healer (*genezeres*) named Marritgen was given a bloody nose and beaten "black and blue" (*bont en blauw geslagen*) by the wife of a man who had initially employed her.[63]

Epidemics sometimes got in the way of women performing their work—disrupting their usual income. One widowed woman from Amsterdam named Elske saw her usual role as a chair setter (*stoelenzetser*) for church services ended by the plague of 1636, and although she received 12 guilders in compensation, a little while later she was frequently found inebriated, fighting with neighbours, and banned from the special evening meals (*avondmaal*).[64] Perhaps one of the most interesting cases of downward spiralling of fortunes can be found from the village of De Meern, just to the west of Utrecht, during the seventeenth century. Plague in 1663 hit a local schoolmaster's family hard, and they lost four children to the epidemic. His wife was also apparently sick but survived. Given the usual restrictions on mobility, together with the numerous deaths of children, the schoolmaster, Segemundus Muller, struggled to keep his school going.[65] Accordingly, his (second) wife, Marrigje Stevens van Gulik, from nearby IJsselstein, was forced to go into work as a *schrobster*—cleaning in other people's houses. The loss of four children and mounting debts were devastating burdens to carry. The church council remarked on the fact that she had now consigned herself to drink, and later she was found in a pest house, and said to be dancing on the coffins that lay outside. In the end, this was enough to lose her job and be ejected from their house—later found looking for work and housing in Utrecht.[66]

Furthermore, women working in disease-infected houses were not only subject to specific dangers on the job but often had difficulties in receiving payment or the inheritance promised in the event of death of the care recipient. Thus, in Amersfoort, commissioners were brought in on November

1599 during an outbreak of plague to mediate a disagreement between one man, Gerrit van de Dashorst, over payment to his *schrobster*.[67] Elsewhere, in nearby Utrecht during the plague of 1636, a remuneration dispute even broke out between two step-sisters.[68] As noted in Chapter 5, controlling the direction of where assets and property should end up after severe epidemic outbreaks was not particularly straightforward—and women often were disproportionately affected by this. For some women, the sudden death of another family member could mean that they no longer had the means to hold on to a particular type of property such as land. Thus, on 22 October 1521 in Breda, one young daughter who saw the death of her mother to plague (*haestiger siecte der pestilentie*) simply had to sell the copyhold or ground lease (*erfpacht*) to another wealthier widow because of the debts incurred.[69] In Utrecht in 1637, one woman, Sara de Dayle, lost her husband and two children to plague, and through her own health issues, was in no position to maintain the family business—eventually selling it all to a male distant relative from Dordrecht.[70] Not all arrangements were distrustful and involved excessive conflict, however. At the small Brabant village of Berlicum in 1630, a woman who was infected with the "contagious pestilential sickness" (*contagieuse sijecte der pestilentien*) gave the sum of 50 guilders to her domestic maid in recognition of all her trusted service (*getrouwen dijenst*) that she continued to perform, even during her sickness.[71] The maid's services might have rendered it unnecessary to employ an outside plague cleaner. Furthermore, women with resources could, like men, financially benefit during epidemics. During the 1625 outbreak at Leiden, for example, one woman with a large garden outside the city was paid 12 florins to temporarily provide an isolation area for infected orphans.[72]

Women accessing property

Literature on female access to property such as land in preindustrial western Europe has tended to emphasise cultural norms that were antithetical to the notion of women cultivating land independently (outside of marriage)—even though women clearly were often farmers in the sense that agricultural tasks required the labour of an entire family.[73] Accordingly, although mortality crises provoked by epidemics should technically have brought more land into the hands of widowed women, most of the scholarship on the Black Death (mainly in England, it should be noted) has tended to suggest that this inheritance was very temporary—and overall, women's independent landownership remained persistently low across the long term.[74] This should not be seen as an inevitability, however, since while women perhaps did not often farm land independently (quantitatively speaking, as a proportion of total amount of land or total number of farmers), they could reap the rewards of it indirectly, for example, through various leasing arrangements or as security for other investments.[75] Indeed, in many parts of the preindustrial rural Low

Countries, access to resources via leases was often more important or valuable than ownership.[76]

My own research into epidemics and women's landownership in seventeenth-century Oudenbosch, west Brabant (previously mentioned in Chapter 5), tends to support the story of the temporary nature of women's landed gains after epidemic mortality but with some nuances too. Figure 6.2 shows that in this rural community, where equitable principles of partible inheritance gave women the plausible opportunity to own or work land independent of marriage, single women (usually widowed, but occasionally never-married) tended to own around ten per cent (or less) of the total surface area in the village, but after the two major epidemic spikes seen in 1625 and 1636/7, this almost doubled to a fifth of the land. These changes, however, were not persistent structural ones. Within a space of a decade or less, the level of land owned independently by women fell back to the original markers. The same could be said of land use strategies. After epidemics, more of the land was directly farmed independently by women themselves—but

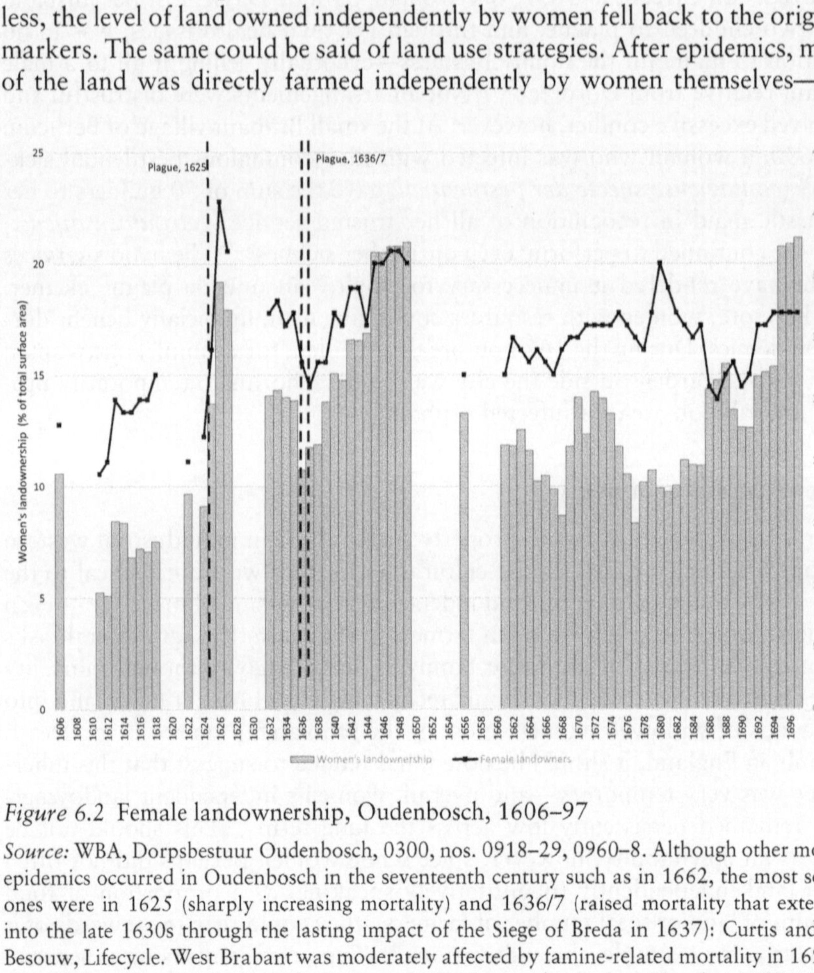

Figure 6.2 Female landownership, Oudenbosch, 1606–97

Source: WBA, Dorpsbestuur Oudenbosch, 0300, nos. 0918–29, 0960–8. Although other modest epidemics occurred in Oudenbosch in the seventeenth century such as in 1662, the most severe ones were in 1625 (sharply increasing mortality) and 1636/7 (raised mortality that extended into the late 1630s through the lasting impact of the Siege of Breda in 1637): Curtis and van Besouw, Lifecycle. West Brabant was moderately affected by famine-related mortality in 1693/4, potentially accounting for the spikes in women's landownership in the mid-to-late 1690s: Curtis and Dijkman, The Escape.

these were mere temporary deviations from usual strategies of indirectly exploiting the land, where usually more than three-quarters of female landownership was leased out to a tenant who was usually male.[77] Was this the case of women simply unable to hold onto epidemic-induced gains under pressure from patriarchal attitudes and institutions, or did women use these gains to trade in for other perceived benefits, perhaps in the form of financial instruments, favourable marriages, or care arrangements?

Only further systematic research can shine more light on the meaning and interpretation of these trends. Not least, because different rural contexts might show up alternative developments. Recent work on female landownership in some villages in the central Rijnland area of Holland between the sixteenth and early eighteenth centuries, a more commercialised and market integrated context than Oudenbosch, saw similar average women's landownership rates of ten per cent of the surface area, although not always responding as sharply to epidemic mortality (never reaching a fifth of the total landownership, for example).[78] Figure 6.3 shows three different trajectories in three villages. Koudekerk roughly followed the model shown above for Oudenbosch—raised levels of female landownership in the major epidemic periods followed by a return to a structurally lower level. Warmond saw very temporary

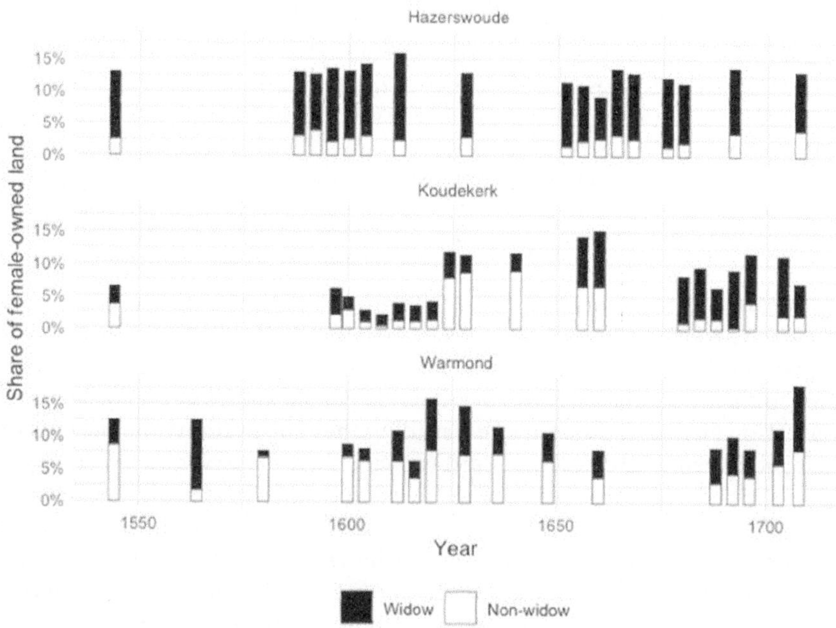

Figure 6.3 Female landownership in three Rijnland villages, central Holland, 1544–1708

Source: Hilkens, *Living.* The most significant epidemics coinciding with periods covered with land distribution data include 1624/5, 1636, and 1655/6.

increases in female landownership in the mid-1620s, but which quickly dropped off and was not receptive to later outbreaks in 1636 and 1655.[79] Hazerswoude just had very stable levels of female landownership over the long term regardless of demographic changes. At the very least, we can see that although creating the potential for female landownership in a context of very strictly egalitarian and partible inheritance, this was not always realised in practice.

Restrictions, punishments, and social controls

As noted in Chapter 4, epidemics have sometimes exploded into different expressions of violence—either by authorities towards targeted groups, or by groups from below against authorities. Scholars are now starting to devote more attention to women's role in this process. On the one hand, it is reasonable to expect that with widespread historical inequalities in access to wealth, rights, and resources, women might have been put in situations where they were more susceptible to persecution or violence during and after epidemics. The term the "colonised body", already now more than 30 years old, was used to refer to the ways in which authorities—in this case British colonial medical elites in late nineteenth- and early twentieth-century India—instrumentalised diseases such as plague to gain institutional control over women's lives and physical dominion over female bodies.[80] Other literature on colonial contexts tends to refer to the scourge of domestic violence in isolation situations during epidemics, and we have a host of different individual examples from early modern Italy where women were physically abused and publicly shamed.[81]

Yet, at the same time, other literature has also noted that women were participants in epidemic-related violence—resisting male authorities and officials and also targeting other women of certain perceived status.[82] This should not surprise us given that women have been important instigators of or participants in other kinds of violent protests throughout history, in particular, food riots and those related to arbitrary taxation, and specifically in the Low Countries.[83] Furthermore, women who were officially confined to their households through city-wide plague and epidemic ordinances, were also capable of avoiding and evading these institutional limitations on their movement.[84] Accordingly, in line with these observations, in this section I show that epidemics in the medieval and early modern Low Countries brought with them new ways for authorities to impose different types of social controls, and even coercive punishments—and although there were great differences in experiences within communities, epidemics did overall tend to create greater restrictions for women than men. Nevertheless, on occasion, women were found using epidemics to resist authorities themselves—indeed, where communities were threatened from outside, women's stronger informal networks and solidarity relationships came to the fore.[85]

One of the most visible ways in which authorities tried to restrict women during epidemic disease outbreaks in the Low Countries was through the regulation of social interactions during events, and especially clamping down on the problems of excesses connected to eating, drinking, and fighting.[86] This became much more explicit from the sixteenth century onwards, and thus especially female presence at funerals became something tightly controlled. More moderate interventions were simply the spatial separation of women from the men. We can see this from a plan of a cemetery in Groningen in Figure 6.4. The Nieuwe Kerkhof of St. Walburg was a cemetery constructed on the northern periphery of the city in response to the raised mortality caused by an ongoing plague outbreak in 1623, and we can see clearly that the mourning women, visible through demarcation by clothing, were drawn at a physical distance from the men. Whether this map reflected spatial realities or not is irrelevant because it reflects a gendered way of thinking about funeral space.

On more extreme occasions, however, women were banned from attending funerals entirely.[87] Urban authorities feared sociability amongst poorer citizens, even outside of epidemic periods, but social contact and mixing of large numbers of people during disease outbreaks also tended to

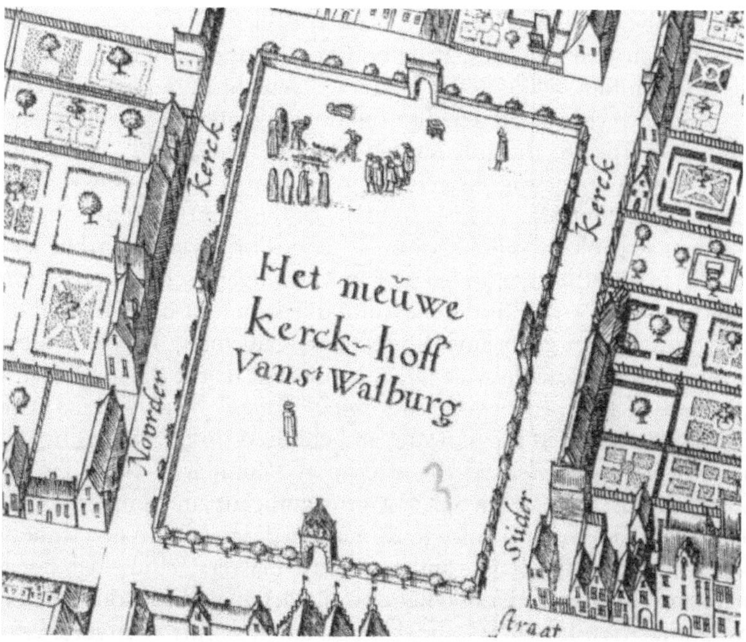

Figure 6.4 The Nieuwe Kerkhof of St. Walburg during the plague of 1623, Groningen

Source: Haubois, *Caerte.* Image taken from: https://commons.wikimedia.org/wiki/File:Grote_Haubois.jpg. Women are in hooded dresses to the left and men are to the right.

be linked to the potential for creating miasmatical conditions of concern. Thus, in Amsterdam during the plague of 1602, women were banned from funerals because their presence increased the danger of "contaminated air" rising from the graves.[88] These announcements were not uncommon. Women were banned in Amersfoort in 1599 on the grounds of the potential for abuses (*misbruiken*), but also during the "hot plague" (*peste van heete sieckte*) in 1603 in Leiden, the severe plague in 1636 in Haarlem, and during the plague period of 1664–6 in Rotterdam.[89] In Delft, the ban on women attending funerals and children from school (if their house was considered infected) in 1602 was later repeated publicly on 22 July 1624 during another epidemic outbreak along with the ringing of church bells.[90] Female spreading anxieties had long historical roots that often cut across cultural contexts. In the medieval imaginary, leprous blood was linked to menstruation, and said to be discharged by "impure" women, and this continued into the early modern period, as menstrual blood came to be seen through the moral lenses of decency and shame, and thus a form of pollution or corruption.[91] Medical theories derived from Galenism and the Hippocratic Corpus, as mentioned in Chapter 2, created the view that the female body was inferior and thus more susceptible to these dangerous miasma.[92]

Restrictions such as these cannot have been anything other than highly distressing for the women involved, if we consider, as mentioned already in Chapter 4, that communities, neighbourhoods, and families went to great lengths to maintain religious observance, even during epidemics, and significant importance was attached to the time-honoured customary duties of carrying the corpse to the consecrated burial site and being physically present to observe the passing.[93] Accordingly, it is also no surprise that women were at the forefront of resistance to many of these impositions—just as they were with the revolts against high bread prices or perceived arbitrary taxation.[94] The previously mentioned riot in Groningen (see Chapter 4) during the plague of 1623—one of the most notable standout cases of civil disobedience against urban government directives—had many female protesters.[95] A chronicle notes that this was likely connected to the place women traditionally had in this practice—adults (*oude doden*) being carried to burial sites by older women in the morning and children (*jonge doden*) by younger women or girls (*maagden*) in the afternoon.[96] Similarly, along the Rue du Curé in Brussels in 1668, women were significant and numerous in their opposition and acts of resistance to the enforced occupation of vacant houses by those infected by the plague and pest house masters.[97] In Leiden, the books of correction shine considerable light on the defiance that women often held against authorities. In 1483/4 and 1515, women simply refused to carry the obligatory white stick in public spaces that signalled infection or proximity to infection, and in 1538 one woman challenged the written regulation that corpses could not be kept domestically for more than 36 hours—disputing the precise diagnosis of her husband's death from *pest*.[98]

Many of these social controls were connected to wider moral concerns over women's sexual behaviour. One of the most valuable early references comes from the time of the Black Death, where it was noted in the financial accounts of Deventer that the aldermen had banned the women of the Overstrate (centre of the city), who were likely sex workers, on account of the *mortalitate*.[99] From the late fifteenth century, towns such as Abbeville in Picardy were restricting the freedoms of sex workers during epidemics—especially restricting collective resources and rights such as the ability to use public ovens and venture outside the city walls for firewood.[100] Such condemnation was specifically reserved for those "indecent" women who were working within certain trades. For example, some "bad" foods were seen to pose a threat to public health if sold by the hand of a corrupted woman.[101] These restrictions, moreover, not only continued but became stricter into the early modern period. Medics tended to moralise the connection between epidemic diseases and the sexual behaviour of women, where women were seen to entice men into the sex act, weaken men's bodies, and therefore make them more susceptible to afflictions such as the plague.[102] For the seventeenth-century medic Johan van Beverwijck, this was interpreted within the polarity of female behaviour—at one end the "learned chaste housewife" and at the other the "desires of the whore".[103] Hence, in a plague ordinance announced in 1605 in the town of Sluis, the ongoing infection within the community was explicitly linked to God's wrath at "loose women and whores" (*lichte vrouwen en hoeren*). As a result, sex workers were ordered to leave the city three days after publishing the ordinance, and further, were reported to authorities if they refused to move, and could not be harboured at any local inn or tavern.[104] Elsewhere, in Leiden in 1681, one 23-year-old woman who was said to be guilty of prostitution was initially meant to be taken into a house of correction (*tuchthuis*), but the feared link with epidemic disease was so great that, upon learning of her visible *pokken* (possibly syphilis), she was released by the authorities and simply banned from the Rijnland area.[105]

Not all problems were impositions from authorities from above, however. Indeed, local communities also created heightened levels of vigilance about women's actions during times of epidemics. Thus, on 23 March 1519 in the town of Kampen, one local witness testified in a legal proceeding of a one Peter Baeck against a maid, Wyllemken Claesdr., that she had continued to go to the house of Peter, spending the night with him on one occasion, despite the fact she was afflicted with *pest*.[106] And more simply and straightforwardly, it is clear that women faced several vulnerabilities from outside their own communities. Eruptions of military activity brought bands of soldiers, especially to rural settlements, creating risks of sexual violence. It is perhaps no coincidence, then, that in times of conflict we also see increased references to deaths through sexually transmitted diseases. In the Campine village of Lille which was overrun by *Croat* soldiers in 1625 and 1626, the term Croats Sickness (*crawatensieckte*) was frequently used in the burial registers, and one woman, Elisabeth Peeters, was recorded as dying *inden Crawatentijt vande pocxkens*—a very likely reference to syphilis.[107]

Representing women

It should be noted that women explicitly wrote about the epidemics that they were experiencing, even if that pool of information is rather restricted. A Norwegian sailor's wife made several comments about the outbreak of plague of 1664 that was occurring in Amsterdam, and during the same episode, a very detailed analysis was made into the precise number and scale of deaths seen and their impact upon the local community in one woman's extensive set of diaries.[108] One woman, Margaretha Jongh, is found in the burial registers during certain years of high mortality making poems about the redundant nature of wealth in great houses, land, and money (*hooge huijsen, lant en gelt*) when faced with the inevitable journey of death.[109] This conforms to the point developed by early modern medical treatises and religious tractates that regardless of whether someone is privileged or poor, true wealth lies ultimately in God's favour.[110] In one case, Elisabeth Strouven, the shoemaker's daughter who eventually founded a devout community for women in Maastricht, described the case of another woman, Lijsbeth Dries, who upon joining the institution, had been infected with the plague in 1633. In her autobiography, Elisabeth mentions that Lijsbeth, on her deathbed, was tempted by the devil—but fortunately resisted and scorned him.[111] Similar tropes were seen centuries earlier in a "sister book" compiled by women at the convent of St. Mary and St. Agnes in Diepenveen, Overijssel, in the fifteenth century, which uses the trauma of a plague outbreak in 1452 to warn of a communal tragedy that could serve as an instructive lesson to the unaffected virtuous.[112]

Nevertheless, historical sources are not necessarily neutral or straightforward reconstructions of female experiences of epidemics but instead subjective perceptions from outside—often elite, official, and male. Most sources we have on this subject are produced by men. Hence, we should also recognise that some of the material we have actually might be best seen as societal expectations of what women do and experience during epidemics, sometimes presented in moralising terms of how women should behave or act—a prescribed role, often connected to the physical body, as part of the male gaze.[113] In broader literature from cultural studies or media history, these depictions are often said to fall within broader tropes of an Outbreak Narrative connected to epidemics—the vulnerable woman, the burdened woman, the female saviour, and the female spreader—and perhaps do not capture either the nuances or the realities of female epidemic impacts.[114] Many of these tropes show parallels with the feminised representation said to characterise famine images and material culture of the past—at least, those seen from the nineteenth century onwards—often with deliberate intentions to foreground blame and victimhood.[115] To end this section, then, I more explicitly focus on female representation—and especially how women were visualised in epidemic contexts in the Low Countries. I also reflect on those few occasions in the sources where we have evidence of female interpretation of epidemic disease.

Overall, women are at the heart of interpreting medieval and early modern epidemic diseases such as plague in the Low Countries—likely in line with other parts of preindustrial and early industrialising Europe.[116] Much of the imagery and material culture we have connected to epidemics tends to see women as inherent sources of protection for communities, and yet, a source of danger—seeding infections, even—particularly framed in a narrative of female deviation from the prescribed norms of what their role should entail. This situation has even been entrenched within modern popular culture. For example, *Mariken van Nieumeghen* (Jos Stelling, 1974), the first Dutch film to be entered at Cannes Film Festival, was based on a play (*mirakelspel*) written in Middle Dutch in the late fifteenth or early sixteenth century, where a woman, Marieke, travels from Nijmegen to Antwerp, and is eventually blamed for a plague outbreak on the grounds that she had cohabited with the devil for seven years. This trope then shifts to one of burdens, as in recompense she embarks on a pilgrimage to the Pope in Rome and carries out a penance in a convent for the equivalent number of years.[117]

Regarding protection, processions to female figures urging deliverance and protection from epidemic disease can be found from well before the Black Death—during the 1272 outbreak, the people of Mechelen gathered in veneration of the image of Our Lady of Hanswijk.[118] Over time, although two saints often invoked were male, especially St. Rochus and St. Sebastian,[119] several female ones were invoked against plague and fevers in the Low Countries, and especially Agnes and Gertrudis of Nijvel—the last-mentioned name found on a c.1450 gravestone in Breda (pictured with black rodents) and on a part of the Lakenhal (cloth guild hall) in Leiden (pictured with a mouse climbing a staff).[120] Rosalia of Palermo, noted for being invoked during the 1624 plague processions in that part of Sicily, was a plague saint also explicitly introduced by the Jesuits into seventeenth-century Antwerp (Figure 6.5).[121] Jesuit rhetoric was frequently depicted in Antwerp paintings in the early seventeenth century seeking plague as a simile for heresy, and in the process creating a female allegory for the Catholic faith as a cure.[122] Dominican orders often propagated devotion to the protective function of Mary Magdalene, appeasing God's wrath, but this was not something entirely restricted to Catholicism in the Low Countries.[123] In a processional hymn of 1566 at the Leiden monastery of Mariënpoel, developed from a fifteenth-century antiphon against the plague, a "lady of powers" (*vrouwe der crachten*) was urged to deliver the community from the threat of the serpent leading to a hasty inconsiderate death (*haestighe onuersienige doot*).[124]

Nevertheless, women's epidemic powers also were seen as a vulnerability—not so much for themselves but for exposing the wider community at large. Early modern plague paintings in the Low Countries tended to foreground female distress, where a recurring moralising motif was employed depicting

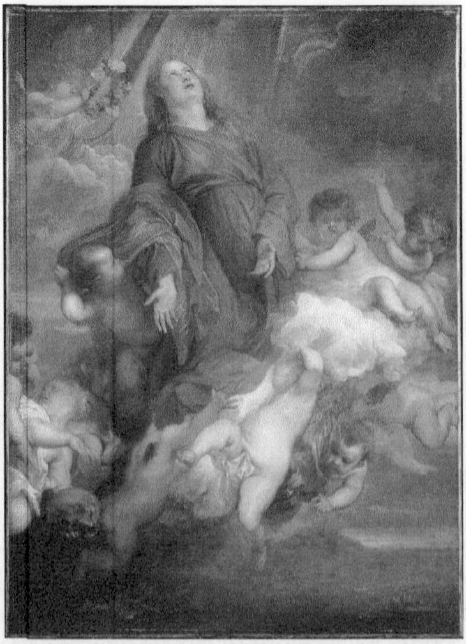

Figure 6.5 St. Rosalie Interceding for the Plague Victims of Palermo painting, Anthony Van Dyck (c.1625)

Source: Kemps, Heilige Rosalia.

cases of vulnerable children who had been made motherless through their experiences with disease.[125] Such a scene was depicted in Rombout Verhulst's sculpted stonework of the Leiden pest house, where a woman is pulling out her hair after "Fury", symbolising the plague, has taken her child (Figure 6.6). A variation on the theme was Gerard de Lairesse's *Niobe Punished for her Pride*, which depicted a plague outbreak because of a woman's "pride leading to a fall", where she had boasted about the number of children she had (Figure 6.7).[126]

Conclusion

Female experiences of epidemic disease were often harsh, burdensome, and traumatic, and could combine a variety of imposed restrictions or losses of fortune—some of which were of course shared with men, but some were accentuated or distinctive. Although women could adapt to conditions of spiked mortality, it is unclear whether new roles or the opening of access to new resources truly benefitted women, or rather, women were able to secure and keep hold of this wealth or status. Interestingly, however, and mirroring more general observations about social resistance in Chapter 4, women in the preindustrial Low Countries often used epidemic disease as a vehicle for

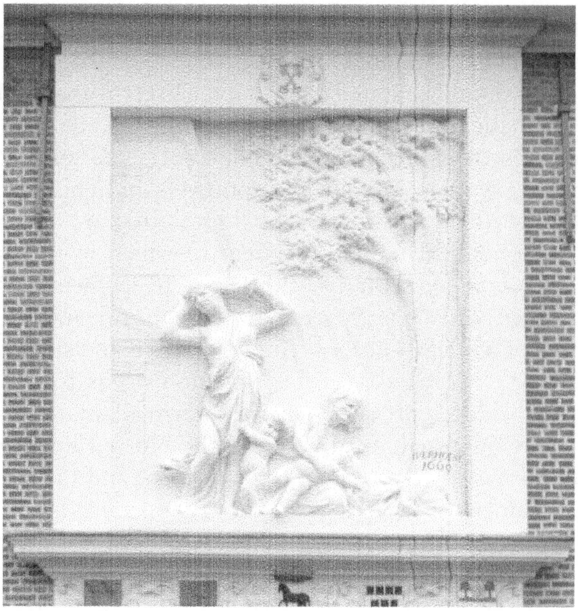

Figure 6.6 Allegory of the Plague stonework, Rombout Verhulst (Leiden pest house, 1660)

Source: Van Asperen, Nothing Else than Decay, 7.

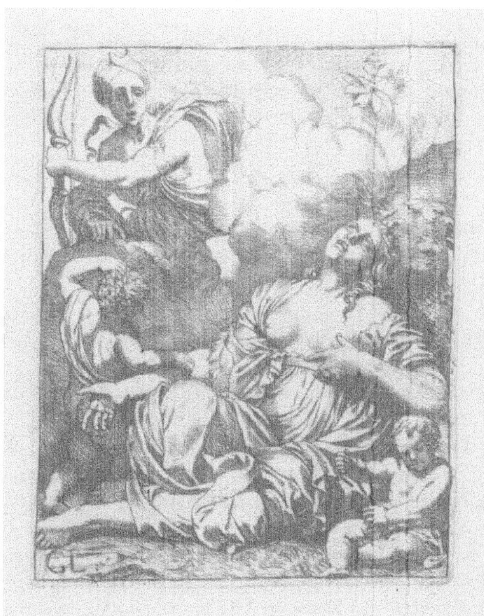

Figure 6.7 Niobe Punished for Her Pride painting, Gerard de Lairesse (Amsterdam, 1668)

Source: Van Asperen, Nothing Else than Decay, 10.

pushing back against perceived restrictions—and were at the forefront of some significant epidemic-related protests.

Nevertheless, it should be stated that Chapter 6 serves as a foundation point for a more systematic and focused future research agenda that foregrounds female experiences of epidemics (including representation of women and representations by women in epidemic contexts) and epidemic impacts on women.[127] Now, we have identified several areas that are deserving of more fundamental treatment including the extent to which women's experiences were qualitatively and quantitatively different from men's, how women's experiences differed across contexts, and by the same token, how they differed across the status of women—old and young, married and single, wealthy and poor, and so on.[128] Moreover, further attention needs to be addressed to temporality and the differences between short-term adaptations and long-run structural impacts on female fortunes, and the blurred lines between what were likely moral narratives, often created by men, and the actual epidemic experiences of women themselves.

Notes

1 Neumayer and Plümper, The Gendered Nature; Rivers, Women.
2 Smith, Overcoming; Harman, Ebola; Davies and Bennett, A Gendered Human Rights Analysis; Wenham et al., COVID-19; Wenham et al., Women. More broadly on the lack of gender- and sex-disaggregated data collection and analysis, including specific reference to epidemics: Criado Perez, *Invisible Women*, 298–300.
3 Belich, *The World the Plague Made*, 98. In a study of the impact of the Black Death on women's participation in the brewing industries in England, it was noted that it was not "a story of transformation in women's lives but instead as a story of remarkable stability for women despite considerable socioeconomic change": Bennett, *Ale*, 7.
4 Ogilvie, The Lion's Share.
5 Scheidel, *The Great Leveler*.
6 A disproportionate amount of evidence on this topic has been derived from England. On the dimensions of an earlier debate on women's welfare and the Black Death: Rigby, Gendering.
7 Horrell et al., Malthus's Missing Women; Humphries and Weisdorf, The Wages.
8 De Pleijt and van Zanden, Two Worlds; Drelichman and Agudo, The Gender Wage Gap.
9 A long and ongoing discussion: Hatcher and Stephenson, eds., *Seven Centuries*.
10 Whittle, A Critique.
11 Griffin, *Bread Winner*; Van Nederveen Meerkerk, Market Wage; Dennison and Ogilvie, Does the European Marriage Pattern?; Molinder and Pihl, Women's Work. The original relevant work on this issue: Howell, *Women*.
12 Curtis, The Female Experience.
13 Massong, The Mobile Woman; Munkhoff, Searchers; Winer, The Enslaved Wet Nurse; Cohn, Last Wills; Carmichael, The Last Past Plague; Feci, Trame.
14 Van Zanden et al., *Capital Women*; Van den Heuvel, *Women*; Schmidt and van der Heijden, Women; De Moor and van Zanden, Girl Power.

15 Boter and Woltjer, The Impact; Schmidt and van Nederveen Meerkerk, Reconsidering; Schulz et al., When Women Disappear. For an insightful statement on the concept for England: Griffin, *Bread Winner*.
16 Van den Heuvel, Gender; Roelens, Visible Women, 17–22; Hutton, Women. Of course, this contrasts with other places in Europe such as southern Italy, where women's visibility within the fields or in other people's houses as domestic servants was entirely limited, even if the explanations for this are still subject to debate: Curtis, An Agro-Town Bias?
17 De Moor and van Zanden, "Every Woman Counts", 207; and the recent essays in Moran and Pipkin, eds., *Women*.
18 Schmidt, Generous Provisions; Zuijderduijn, Grave Concerns; De Haan and Hoppenbrouwers, Intergenerational Transfer, 345.
19 For the Low Countries; Howell, The Problem; and the broader critical remarks on the enduring concept of agency for women in the past: Thomas, Historicising Agency. I have criticised the use of the above-mentioned demographic markers as evidence for female agency, noting that they only have relevance when embedded within specific economic and cultural contexts: Curtis, An Agro-Town Bias? Indeed, wide age gaps between spouses in southern Europe, for example, gave younger women less autonomy but potentially more in later life: Ogilvie, *Controlling Contagion*, 392. The notion of historically few single women in the Mediterranean has also been skewed by lack of receptiveness to strong regional divergences and the persistence of modernist biases, as critiqued in: Armstrong-Partida and McDonough, Singlewomen; Curtis, An Agro-Town Bias?
20 A summary of the literature on women's social and economic status in the northern Low Countries has recently appeared although it does not mention once any potential impact of epidemic disease: Schmidt, Women.
21 Curtis, Was Plague an Exclusively Urban Phenomenon? 152; Curtis and Roosen, The Sex-Selective Impact, 252, 255–6. And this is something that we can also see anecdotally in the sources—occasions where an adult might lose their partner and three, four, or even five children in a short space of time.
22 On the importance of female medical care within medieval and early modern households: Green, Women's Medical Practice; Rawcliffe, *Medicine*, 182–3; Cabré, Women; Pelling, *The Common Lot*, 155–202.
23 Ogilvie, *Controlling Contagion*, 395.
24 HUA, Notarissen in de stad Utrecht 1560–1905, no. 4 [10/9/1604] [AO].
25 Alink, ed., Getuigenissen, no. 890, fo. 224v.
26 SD, Groote (vroeger Heilige Geesten-) en Voorster gasthuis te Deventer, 0767, no. 1304 [AO].
27 Heyning, *Turbulente tijden*, 47. Something also seen in northern France during dysentery outbreaks: Broomhall, *Women's Medical Work*, 157–8.
28 Hachez, Les fondations charitables, 189.
29 SNV, Stadsbestuur Harderwijk, (1190) 1231–1813, 5001, no. 607 [30/10/1525] [AO].
30 SNV, Stadsbestuur Harderwijk, (1190) 1231–1813, 5001, no. 861 [28/9/1547] [AO].
31 Ufkes, De verzorging, 30.
32 In various contexts: Jacquet-Ladrier, Les épidémies, 131; Vis, *Het weeshuis*, 150–1; SB, Stadsbestuur Breda (oud administratief archief) 1280–1810, Stadsrekeningen, no. 617, fo. 100v.
33 Moquette, Pestepidemieën, 12.
34 Kappelhof, ed., Kroniek, 56.
35 Jacquet-Ladrier, Les épidémies, 134.

36 Simons, *Cities*, 76–9.
37 Wiersma, Observaties, 2620.
38 See, also, the reference above to early modern women receiving structural aid such as poor relief more readily than men. Similarly, during nineteenth-century cholera outbreaks, citizens' committees in Utrecht disproportionately supported struggling widows: Tanis, *An Epidemic*, 65.
39 Ladan, *Gezondheidszorg*, 102–3. However, as noted in Chapter 3, the notion that Leiden had substantially more women than men by the seventeenth century is perhaps not as strong as one might presume.
40 Van de Pol and Kuijpers, Poor Women's Migration.
41 Own database of patients calculated from ZAM, Godshuizen Middelburg 1343–1812, 'Lootjesboeken', register van personen, die voor rekening van het gesticht ter verpleging zijn opgenomen, voornamelijk vreemdelingen en arme ingezetenen, 1584–1812, no. 22, fo. 1–20r [AO].
42 Bruneel, L'assistance, 239. We also see transfers of patients. For example, at Leiden during the last phases of the epidemic in 1636, the St. Catharina hospital decided to send 18 of their sick to the new wooden pest house that had been built outside the Morschpoort on the city periphery, and claimed for all the costs down to the exact number of days they had stayed at the *gasthuis*. Many apparently did not have plague, or had recovered, since they had spent as much as half a year at the institution: ELO, Archieven van de Gasthuizen, 1311–1873, 0504, no. 1696.
43 WBA, Archief van de stad Bergen op Zoom, 1397–1810, 0005, no. 6, fo. 252r–4v; Van Zuijlen, ed., *Inventaris*, II, no. 1167.
44 Ladan, *Gezondheidszorg*, 102–3.
45 Moquette, Pestepidemieën, 25.
46 SDEL, Archieven van het stadsbestuur van Delft 1246–1813, Register van vonnissen in strafzaken, no. 2387, fo. 122v [6/4/1665] [AO]. Thanks to Eveline Kaiser, Stadsarchief Delft, for directing me to this document [14/4/2020].
47 Weeda, Doing the Dirty Work.
48 Curtis, The Female Experience, 5. More systematic work on who these people were is needed. The relative likelihood of women or men doing the job likely deviated across region, as in some contexts we see certain categories of men more likely to do the job, sometimes of considerable influence, and in others certain categories of women more frequently appearing as plague cleaners, who were sometimes the poorest and most marginalised: Johnson, The Johnes; Craig, "Villanies"; Harkness, A View; Newman, Shutt Up. In a recent statement for plague nurses in seventeenth-century London, it was argued that "by an overwhelming majority, these nurses tended to be female" and "these women in fact came from diverse backgrounds": Thorpe, "In Middest of Death", 18, 224.
49 The pioneering work remains Munkhoff, Searchers; with important additions for the eighteenth century: Siena, Searchers. However, in early modern England, searchers (public codifiers of corpses) were apparently separate from household plague nurses, while in the Low Countries both tasks can be found falling under the remit of the domestic *schrobster*.
50 BHIC, Schepenprotocol Dinther, 7603, no. 4, fo. 39 [AO].
51 Gooskens, Pestepidemieën, 52.
52 BHIC, Schepenprotocol Dinther, 7603, no. 11, fo. 217v [AO].
53 BHIC, Schepenprotocol Schijndel, 5122, no. 86, fo. 52 [26/9/1605] [AO].
54 For the older female searchers profile: Munkhoff, Searchers, 1–2.
55 BHIC, Schepenprotocol Dinther, 7603, no. 12, fo. 33r, 35r [AO]. Meanwhile, another woman, Lijsken Peters, in the same household of Stoffel Lamberts at the same time earned less for seven weeks' work—50 guilders. Where two plague

cleaners worked in the same house simultaneously brings up the question of whether it was work for two people, or whether each *schrobster* was in charge of different infected people or different tasks.

56 One plague tractate from Antwerp cleric, Jan vander Linden, gave a personal account of how he was, as an infant, found next to his mother who had died of the *haestighe sieckte* in 1577 under the constant supervision of a *schrobster*: Vander Linden, *Cort verhael*, 25.

57 Beijers, ed., Meierijse schoutsrekeningen, no. 12996, fo. 229, 233, 241–2, 258. Again, a demonstration of the early presence of some contagionist principles, as mentioned in Chapter 3.

58 De Waardt, *Toverij*, 94.

59 De Waardt, *Toverij*, 94.

60 Monballyu, ed., "Geexecuteert metten viere", no. 17, 21.

61 De Brouwer, Erfenisperikelen, 75.

62 Beijers, ed., Meierijse schoutsrekeningen, no. 12995, fo. 12.

63 Doedeijns, ed., Uitreksels, 197 [28/1/1631].

64 Kuijpers, *Migrantenstad*, 315–16. Church meetings were often disrupted. In Leiden, the Walloon Church members had to conduct meetings elsewhere on account of plague mortality in 1655: ELO, Archieven van de Waalse gemeente te Leiden, 1584–1983, 0535, no. 72.4.

65 In other places such as Roosendaal and Oudenbosch in west Brabant, we have explicit references to long periods where no lessons were given at school as a result of the epidemic of 1625: Goyarts, De pest, 34.

66 This whole episode is usefully recorded in some detail in Polak-de-Booy, Dansen.

67 AEA, Stadsbestuur Amersfoort, 1300–1810, 0001, no. 18, fo. 52v [26/11/1599] [AO]. In other documents, Gerrit van de Dashorst is referred to as both a master in the hospital and a painter: AEA, Stadsbestuur Amersfoort, no. 19, fo. 524, 537v, 610v [AO].

68 HUA, Notarissen in de stad Utrecht 1560–1905, no. 157 [8/9/1636] [AO].

69 SB, Schepenbank Breda 1499–1811, Vestbrieven 1521, no. 428, fo. 259r–60v [22/10/1521].

70 HUA, Notarissen in de stad Utrecht 1560–1905, no. 139 [11/8/1637] [AO].

71 BHIC, Schepenprotocol Berlicum, 5120, no. 55, fo. 28v–9v [1/1/1630] [AO].

72 Dröge, De bouwgeschiedenis, 76.

73 Erickson, Afterword, 267.

74 A continuity in situation both before the Black Death: Bennett, Women; and after: Whittle, Inheritance; Bardsley, Peasant Women. Corroborating the story of (younger or unmarried) women's minimal "Black Death bonuses" compared to male wages: Humphries and Weisdorf, The Wages. Recently, it was stated that "[post Black Death in England] young women did not increase their participation in the land market in order to construct a marriage fund": Bailey, The Black Death, 493. Older literature pointed to pre- and post-Black Death differences, suggesting that women before the mid-fourteenth century tended to operate full sized holdings independently: Franklin, Peasant Widows' "Liberation".

75 Vervaet, Women; Vervaet, The Economic Opportunities.

76 Curtis, *Coping*, 23–62.

77 Curtis, In One Hand and Out the Other?

78 Hilkens, *Living*.

79 There was, in this area, a locally significant epidemic around 1617/18 that can account for the earlier spike in women's landownership already by 1620, which persisted to 1628.

80 Arnold, *Colonizing the Body*. The same process has been shown outside of colonial contexts though. For example, during the quarantine of Chinatown

during the plague outbreak in Honolulu in 1899/1900, sanitary commissions at mandatory disinfecting stations forced Japanese women and men to be naked during collective fumigations: Mohr, *Plague*, 116–18.

81 Sellers-García, A Hidden Plague; Carmichael, The Last Past Plague, 145; Rose, Plague, 1006.

82 Curtis, The Female Experience; Cohn, *Epidemics*, 211, 213, 217–18, 287–8; Burrell and Gill, The Liverpool Cholera Epidemic, 485.

83 Byfield, Taxation; Bohstedt, Gender; and seen especially in the context of late-medieval political revolts and early modern food, tax, and other riots related to perceived injustices in different parts of the Low Countries: Demets, Spies; Dekker, *Holland*, 51–9.

84 Massong, The Mobile Woman.

85 An argument derived more generally from Dekker, Women, 350.

86 Kerkhoff, *Per imperatief plakkaat*, 38–9.

87 Seen in other parts of Europe: Cohn, *Cultures*, 246.

88 Noordegraaf and Valk, *De gave Gods*, 80; Steendijk-Kuypers, *Volksgezondheidszorg*, 176–7.

89 AEA, Stadsbestuur Amersfoort, 1300–1810, 0001, no. 18, fo. 17 [7/8/1599] [AO]; Van Hout, *Ordonnantie*, 165 [no. 4]; Anon., ed., Ordonnantie Haarlem, no. 15; Moquette, Pestepidemieën, 51.

90 Van der Wiel and Ekamper, Kromme sikkel, 84–5.

91 Zimmerman, Leprosy; Read, "Thy Righteousness is but a Menstrual Clout", 19.

92 Whaley, *Women*, 48–9.

93 Huisman, *Stadsbelang*, 157; Bogaers, Geleund, 350; Rommes, Op het spoor, 114; Curtis, Preserving, 285–7. On the precise phases of preparation of the corpse, procession preparation, procession to the church, church service, procession to the grave, the burial, return to the church, and uses of liturgy and music, and the importance that specifically women attributed to all these phases: Wendling, Death.

94 Dekker, *Holland*, 51–9; Dekker, Women.

95 Lonsain, Een oproer, 57.

96 Reilingh, *Geschiedkundig-geneeskundige beschouwing*, 28.

97 Van Honacker, Résistance locale, 46–7.

98 Ladan, *Gezondheidszorg*, 63; Tamis, Ook zij slaat wel eens terug, 89.

99 Coomans, *Community*, 221.

100 Murphy, Plague Ordinances, 152. On related issues: Coomans and Geltner, On the Street, 71.

101 Coomans, Policing, 108.

102 Noordegraaf and Valk, *De gave Gods*, 134.

103 Van Gemert, The Power, 49.

104 ZAM, Vrije van Sluis 1584–1796, 7, Stukken betreffende maatregelen tegen besmetting met pest, 1605, 1770–1771, no. 363, fo. 3r [AO].

105 Van den Heuvel, ed., Crimineel klachtboek, 689 [7/1/1681].

106 Alink, ed., Getuigenissen, no. 633, fo. 165v [21/3/1519].

107 Janssens and Van den Branden, De pest, 81–2. *Croat* was a generic term for light cavalry operating on the side of the Catholic League during the Thirty Years' War rather than a specific ethnic designation.

108 Sogner and van Lottum, An Immigrant Community? 165; Van Wijngaarden and van der Hoeven, eds., De familienotities, 22.

109 SA, Archief van de Burgerlijke Stand: Doop-, trouw- en begraafboeken van Amsterdam, 5001, no. 1092, fo. 108v [AO].

110 Van Asperen, Nothing Else than Decay, 15–16.

111 Strouven, *La vie*, 205–7.

112 Perk, Adapting Saints, 208–9.
113 Although clearly women did not always conform to these imposed rules and institutional norms during epidemics: Singer, *Erotic Welfare*.
114 Han and Curtis, The Female Burden; Han and Curtis, Cinematic Representation; Han and Curtis, *Infectious Inequalities*, 85–106; Wald, *Contagious*, 68–113; Ostherr, *Cinematic Prophylaxis*, 5–11.
115 Kelleher, *The Feminization*; with some pushback against this emphasis on victimhood in popular famine representation and memory: Steiner, Heroines. Clearly, it is difficult to separate tropes of suffering and survival strategies: Edgerton-Tarpley, Family; Kis, Defying Death. For feminised famine imagery used in Dutch contexts of the 1845–50 potato harvest failure: Corporaal and Jensen, Famine, 1370.
116 For the cult of the Virgin Mary and plague survival: Lopez, *Queen of Sorrows*.
117 Han and Curtis, Cinematic Representation, 128–9. The sixteenth-century play was widely reproduced in several languages including Arabic and Latin. On the role of the plague in the text, and in German versions of the story: Peeters, Mariken van Nieumeghen, 85–6.
118 Delafaille, *Hongersnooden*, 16–17.
119 Especially St. Sebastian worked into Caravaggisti paintings of the 1620s. From Utrecht: De Meyere, Sint Sebastiaan.
120 Dippel, Kanttekening, 255.
121 Kemps, Patronesse.
122 As seen in Peter Paul Rubens' painting from 1617, *The Miracles of St. Francis Xavier*: Boeckl, *Images*, 127–9.
123 Timmers, *Symboliek*, 495–7. On this phenomenon more broadly: Delumeau, *La peur*, 185.
124 Vanden Bossche, Een pest-antifoon, 12.
125 Van Asperen, Nothing Else than Decay, 7.
126 Van Asperen, Nothing Else than Decay, 10–11.
127 Curtis, The Female Experience.
128 To be developed in the forthcoming: Curtis, *The Impact*.

7 Conclusion

Accommodating epidemics

Historical research into epidemic diseases is back in fashion. COVID-19 played some role, of course, but this trend was something already in motion well before the global pandemic and stimulated by interdisciplinary and within-discipline developments.[1] Research into epidemics has been ignited in the past 15 or 20 years through a laboratory revolution that has enhanced the quality and quantity of relevant findings connected to sequencing ancient DNA in genetics and the excavations of skeletons in the palaeo sciences. In tandem, this has stimulated a desire to widen the geographical scale of our epidemic disease stories and analyses—particularly for medieval plagues—introducing new kinds of evidence for places where documents are scarce or missing.[2] And all this fits very neatly with the increasing desire in the historical discipline to "go bigger"—even if there are ongoing debates about what the global exactly means when we are talking about society-disease interaction and the difficulties of aligning the scales and temporality at which independent and dependent variables play out.[3]

In recent years, much of the focus on epidemic diseases in the past has been on their capacity to invoke substantial changes within societies. Substantial books have been written on the impact of epidemics to shape the fortunes of political entities—be that the decline or reshaping of feudal institutions, the centralisation of "disaster response", the role played in the formalisation of states and their boundaries, or conversely their contribution to helping destabilise large empires.[4] This work, especially on the decline of large polities or empires, has been given further credence by the growing awareness of historical climate information and the movement of climate-induced "explanations" away from environmental determinism (previously seen as bad by historians) to something much more trendy. Elsewhere, on the subject of economic impact, scholars have pointed to epidemics and their role in creating transitions, divergences, or paths of redistribution at different scales.[5] Likewise, socio-cultural forms of change have also been foregrounded—from the long-established (and contended) idea that the Black Death ushered in mentality effects on the way people thought and felt about life, death, health, and sickness, to European-colonial era epidemics connecting the subject of race and disease resistance and how these associations were used by those with wealth and power to justify unequal and coercive institutions such as

DOI: 10.4324/9781003694908-7

plantation slavery.[6] Building on older work, scholars are integrating new evidence to make grandiose claims about epidemic diseases shaping the whole course of human history and seen in titles such as "The World the Plague Made" or "The Spanish Flu of 1918 and How it Changed the World".[7]

The findings of my book, taken together, are something of a departure from much of the recent literature, and perhaps also a departure from what is trending within historical research into epidemics now. Global scales of analysis are welcome when our evidence bases are non-documentary and we are incorporating data from samples of *Yersinia pestis* DNA, for example. But this kind of evidence inevitably leads itself to certain kinds of questions—questions that revolve around why diseases emerge in a particular time or place, why they spread in a particular direction, and their recurring or different characteristics. These questions are not unimportant, but as a historian, they strike me as descriptive questions with clear limits. At best, they are necessary preliminary foundations to more analytical questions. Global scales might also be an important vehicle behind understanding temporal and spatial dimensions of stories and discourses surrounding epidemic disease and who controls these narratives—but this would require a systematic cultural history approach integrating other disciplines that has yet to be attempted.[8] Impact questions, however—those revolving around society-epidemic interaction—in my view can still only be solved at a more restricted scale using historical documents at the core (at least for the past 1,000 years) and supplemented with other kinds of palaeo or material evidence, even if it is unfashionable to say so.

Indeed, broad temporal lines might be more important than broad spatial scales—especially when we aim to understand supposed changes wrought by epidemic diseases of the past—or perhaps alternatively, high-resolution evidence of impact that can be tightly placed against markers of epidemic activity. In my view, when we reduce the scale of analysis down to the level at which people of the past thought about their own lives—households, neighbourhoods, associations, and communities—most of the interesting components of epidemic-society interaction are connected to their recurring nature, the adaptation to this recurring nature, and the attempts to prevent change or dampen down the pressure points that epidemics create. To be sure, I am not disputing the findings of the literature I have mentioned above but simply showing an alternative narrative exists and is driven by which scale we decide to work at. Both (and more) narratives deserve to be told.

In one of the most well-known passages from the famous novel penned just after the Second World War by Albert Camus, *La Peste*, it is remarked that "Everybody knows that pestilences have a way of recurring in the world; yet somehow, we find it hard to believe in ones that crash down on our heads from a blue sky. There have been as many plagues as wars in our history; yet always plagues and wars take people equally by surprise".[9] Such a view has tended to inform much of the historical literature about epidemic-society interaction, with a temptation to see these epidemic outbreaks as clear "shocks" that push society from a state of normality to the exceptional, the atypical, or the sub-normal.[10] The adherence to the shock concept can be seen especially within the disciplines of economics and economic history—probably driven by the desire to draw much tighter correlating or causal links between two or more clearly discernible processes, developments, or conditions. In my view, based on what I have shown from the long-run history of epidemics occurring in the Low Countries, little support can be given to that contention. Recurring epidemics seem to be entirely anticipated, and most of the reactions, responses, and changes seen are the product of frequent and incremental adaptations. Where epidemics are concerned, the lines between the normal and the sub-normal are blurry, and the idea of "managing" epidemics as a kind of deviation from the norm becomes rather modernist and anachronistic.[11] Accommodating epidemic outbreaks meant living alongside them, incorporating them into the rhythms of everyday life, and which included incremental adaptations to practices and institutions made outside of epidemic periods. Of course, this complicates incessant calls for "learning" from past epidemics—an aspect I address below.

Where I have tried to intervene most strongly in the historical discussion on epidemic impacts on society is on the subject of structural change, and in the process calling for more clarity in what I perceive to be again a rather blurry dividing line between reactions and responses to epidemics and their capacity to affect communities and societies structurally.[12] The two things are quite different. Thus, to use just one prominent example, in recent historical debates on the Plague of Justinian (the first episode of the First Plague Pandemic beginning in the 540s), the impact of this outbreak is seen to be either exaggerated or not made prominent enough as a historical agent, and yet it is not entirely clear whether the scholars involved in the discussion are addressing the same outcome variables.[13] Many of the reactions and responses in the Low Countries in the short run did not conform to our expectations. Rather than oppression and social control from authorities and elites, or panicked and fearful communities, we saw communities push back against these authorities and elites to maintain continuities in practices under pressure. Many of the impositions remained theoretical rather than what occurred in practice—an idealised form of a Foucauldian framework but with little tangible empirical support.[14] But, perhaps even more importantly, this book has made the point that even in those domains where epidemic-induced changes could be quantifiably measured, many were not meaningful to ordinary people's lives (see the seventeenth-century Leiden housing market case and the statuses of "new" homeowners that emerged from the mass turnover) or not long lasting. Land markets tended to work to restore pre-existing distributions seen before an outbreak; collectively pooled resources such as commons offered interventions that saw continuities in access to commoners with privileged rights; and women who managed to newly gain independent access to resources through the deaths of their husbands often found that within some years these resources were now in the hands of other men, even if we might concede that women sometimes used these resources to acquire other sources of wellbeing.

Overall, it was the intention of this book to escape some of the preconceptions that have tended to go hand in hand with studying topics such as plague and epidemic disease and their societal impacts. In my view, our line of attention should not be how and why these outbreaks helped substantially change societies, but why, given oftentimes significant levels of mortality (or the threat of), was change so modest? How did societies achieve this with the tools and ideas at their disposal? And around the world in those cases where strong cultural or institutional change was seen down specific measurable dimensions, what were the variables or conditions that allowed these apparently rare developments to happen?

I also hope that this book is an intervention in what is an unhelpful recent field-related tendency, often driven by a variety of university, funder, and public stakeholder desire for achieving a contrived form of "societal impact" (a concept still very poorly elaborated) in our work, as opposed to good science on its own terms and the intrinsic value that high-quality analytical research offers for society. Indeed, relevance is often a code word for actionable findings, but policy can be a straightjacket.[15] We need to make sure that we are not just creating checklists or templates from which "lessons from the past" can be drawn in how to succeed in the present, a kind of "generic moral guidebook", and to escape the myopic modernist view of epidemic diseases as conditions that have always needed to be "managed" or "dealt with".[16]

Frequently, when we look to the specific subject of epidemics and society interaction, we see claims for "useful knowledge" from the past "that can help us to better understand the present", and yet few theoretical or tangible methodological insights into how this is achieved.[17] Scholarship continues to identify standout tendencies during COVID-19 such as "misinformation", with the message that "these things happened in the past" or "happened in the past but slightly differently"—similarities between past and present, effectively—and yet, the analytical value of these kinds of approaches remains unclear.[18] Indeed, and as observed in the *American Historical Review* special issue on "The Pandemic and History", in the wake of COVID-19, some historians have assumed the positionality against which many of us were sternly warned in our training as students.[19] A good start might be to stop essentialising and "maximalising" epidemic diseases of the past—treating them as special—and instead considering them as fundamental and unexceptional components undetachable from the everyday life that historians of society, economy, culture, environment, and population hope to reconstruct and analyse.[20] Just as we have learned to move beyond the cliché literary corpus of Boccaccio and Pepys, perpetuating tropes of upheaval and disintegration, we should also be aware that a dichotomy between normalcy and vaguely elaborated notions of crisis will no longer do.[21] Perhaps we as historians might do well to remember that our command over dimensions of time need not only serve analytical insights into change but how things stay the same, even when continuity, on the surface at least, does not seem to be an obvious outcome.

Notes

1 COVID-19 stimulated a whole plethora of work from scholars who, to my knowledge, had never shown any direct expertise in epidemic diseases of the past. See, for example, Schama, *Foreign Bodies*. Interestingly, as COVID-19 recedes from our collective daily consciousness, the spike in "new" scholarship has disappeared from journals that in 2020–2 produced numerous review articles on subjects such as "pandemics and development", "pandemics and recovery", or "learning from pandemics".

2 Numerous summaries of these kinds of positions; perhaps the most prominent: Green, The Four Black Deaths; Harper, *Plagues*.

3 Although unification of the globe via disease is an idea already now more than 50 years old: Le Roy Ladurie, Un concept. For skeptical remarks about the global scope of disaster studies more broadly conceived, and the place of epidemic-society analysis within it: Curtis, Disasters.

4 Bailey, *After the Black Death*; Ermus, *The Great Plague Scare*; Varlik, *Plague*; Harper, *The Fate of Rome*.

5 Campbell, *The Great Transition*; Alfani, *Calamities*; Scheidel, *The Great Leveler*.

6 For the Black Death: Cohn, *Cultures*; Herlihy, *The Black Death*; for race, narratives of resistance, and yellow fever or malaria outbreaks: McNeill, *Mosquito Empires*; Seth, *Difference*; Olivarius, *Necropolis*.

7 Harper, *Plagues*; Belich, *The World the Plague Made*; Spinney, *Pale Rider*. For the older work, especially focused on linking disease and imperial power across large distances: McNeill, *Plagues*; Watts, *Epidemics*; Crosby, *The Columbian Exchange*.

8 The most important work remains the Outbreak Narrative of Wald, *Contagious*; although other significant frameworks have recently been developed: Lynteris, *Visual Plague*. The empirical dimensions of the Outbreak Narrative have yet to be coherently established in a systematic way across time and space. For a call for new systematic work on the spread and direction of disease and other environmental hazard stories: Curtis, Where's the Disaster in Disaster Studies?

9 Camus, *The Plague*, 37.

10 An unpredictability accepted and defended in Harper, Germs, 361.

11 In that sense, I concur with the views of Coomans, *Community*; Geltner, *Roads to Health*.

12 This is a point made at greater length in Curtis, Disasters; Curtis, Where's the Disaster in Disaster Studies?

13 For the "minimalist" view: Mordechai and Eisenberg, Rejecting Catastrophe; Mordechai et al., The Justinianic Plague. Which provoked a reassertion of strong plague impact: Sarris, New Approaches; Meier, The "Justinianic Plague". However, a very sharp elaboration on what is at stake in this debate has recently appeared: Kay et al., Burial Archaeology. My view on this subject, as an outsider, is that Mordechai and Eisenberg brought up highly relevant issues for the practice of comparative history which merited consideration.

14 A similar conclusion was made some time ago in: Slack, Responses, 417.

15 Haldon et al., Past Answers, 8.

16 For this growing tendency, see the conclusions on the role of applied history drawn in De Graaf et al., Aan de slag!; and the list of adaptive strategies seen during historical epidemics that are purportedly able to be applied today: De Graaf et al., Dancing; Jensen et al., Dear Government. The generic moral guidebook is used

appropriately as a criticism of the trend rather than endorsement in Kaal and van Lottum, Applied History, 139.

17 Doran, What Can We Learn from Historical Pandemics?

18 Greve and Roosen, Complottheorieën; Curtis, The Erasmian Way? 80.

19 Gómez, COVID-19, 1352.

20 On the maximalist narrative and its problems: Mordechai and Eisenberg, Rejecting Catastrophe. Relatedly, I agree with the recent cautionary statements about the prevalence of premature publication of overly "grand narratives" of epidemic disease origins, spread, and impact: Stathakopoulos et al., The First Plague Pandemic, 16.

21 Roitman, *Anti-Crisis*; Lachenal and Thomas, Epidemics, 684.

Bibliography

Archives

Archief Eemland, Amersfoort (AEA)

Sint Elisabeth Gast- of Ziekenhuis te Amersfoort, 1500–1970, 0102, no. 445 [AO].
Stadsbestuur Amersfoort, 1300–1810, 0001, nos. 18–21 [AO].
Stadsgerecht Amersfoort, 1435–1811, 0012, no. 436-02 [AO].
Stichting Armen de Poth te Amersfoort, 1342–1999, 0100, no. 571 [AO].

Archives de l'État à Liège (AEL)

Archives de la cité de Liège, 1434–1829, Registre aux enquêtes générales. 1634–1636, no. 10 [AO].

Archives de l'État à Mons (AEM)

Archives de la ville de Mons. Section ancienne, 1200–1836, Registres annuels de perception. 1496–1632, no. 1359 [AO].

Brabants Historisch Informatie Centrum, Den Bosch (BHIC)

Dorpsbestuur Schijndel, 1312–1811, 5016, no. 32 [AO].
Dorpsbestuur Veghel, 1310–1810 (1814), 7697, no. 65 [AO].
Illustre lieve vrouwe broederschap in 's-Hertogenbosch, (1291) 1318–2005, 1232, nos. 116–19 [AO].
Mechelse aanwinsten van het bisdom Den Bosch, 1330–1719, 2006, "regesten", no. 82 [AO].
Notarieel protocol Den Dungen, 5115, no. 3 [AO].
Raad en Rentmeester-Generaal Domeinen, 9, no. 18 [AO].
Resoluties Raad van State, 178, no. 186, 198–9, 202 [AO].
Schepenprotocol Berlicum, 5120, no. 55 [AO].
Schepenprotocol Dinther, 7603, no. 4, 11–12 [AO].
Schepenprotocol Lith, 7323, no. 41 [AO].
Schepenprotocol Oss, 7365, no. 65 [AO].
Schepenenprotocol Sint-Michielsgestel, 5121, no. 43, 47 [AO].
Schepenprotocol Schijndel, 5122, no. 86 [AO].
Schepenprotocol Veghel, 7700, no. 41 [AO].

Drents Archief, Assen (DAA)

Huisarchief Batinge, 0617, Recepten tegen de pest, het koliek en het maagkoliek, no. 340 [AO].

Erfgoedcentrum Achterhoek en Liemers, Doetinchem (EAL)

Huis Bergh, 1227–1842, 0214, no. 358, 445, 1128, 1676, 2734, 3268, 7268, 7282 [AO].
Stadsbestuur Groenlo, 1273–1811 (1852), 0138, no. 658 [AO].

Erfgoed Leiden en Omstreken (ELO)

Archieven van de Gasthuizen, 1311–1873, 0504, no. 1615A, 1696, 1711.
Archieven van de Waalse gemeente te Leiden, 1584–1983, 0535, no. 72.4.
Rekening van de gasthuismeesters van het Sint Catharinagasthuis, 334, no. 31.
Stadsarchief van Leiden, (1253) 1574–1816 (1897), 0501A, no. 49, 55, 79, 249, 1319, 3529–34.

Frysk Histoarysk en Letterkundich Sintrum, Leeuwarden (TRESOAR)

Familie Van Sminia, 327, Afschrift van een brief van Assuerus van Vierssen d.d. 1656 gericht aan zijn kinderen onder de indruk van de te Leeuwarden heersende pest, no. 596 [AO].

Gemeentearchief Steenwijk (GS)

Stad Steenwijk tot ca. 1811, 14, no. 151 [AO].

Groninger Archieven (GA)

Doop-, trouw- en begraafboeken enz. in de provincie Groningen, Kerkelijke gemeente Midwolda, Kerkeboek 1596–1811, 124, no. 294.
Hoge Justitiekamer en andere gewestelijke rechterlijke instellingen, 1444–1811, 136, no. 854.
Kerkeboek 1621–1743, Weiwerd, 124, DTB Groningen, no. 512.
Rechterlijke Archieven III, a9 [22/6/1604].
Register Feith, 1291–1815, 2041, Ordonnantiën op het begraven van de aan de pest gestorven, no. 878.
Stadsbestuur van Groningen (2), 1594–1815, 1605, no. 805, 1143.

Gelders Archief, Arnhem (GAA)

Brieven van en aan het Kwartier van Zutphen, 0124, no. 918 [AO].
Burgerweeshuis te Arnhem, 2090, no. 490 [AO].
Graven en hertogen van Gelre, graven van Zutphen, 0001, Rekeningen van de overste rentmeester Arnold van Ghoor, 1438–1450, no. 2997 [AO].
Hertogelijk Archief, Financieel beheer Rekeningen C1492–1543, no. 1332.209 [AO].
Huizen Nettelhorst en De Heest, 0418, no. 312 [AO].
ORA Arnhem, 2003, no. 399, 411–12 [AO].

Het Utrechts Archief (HUA)

Bisschoppen van Utrecht, 218-1, no. 170 [AO].
Notarissen in de stad Utrecht 1560–1905, no. 4, 139, 157, 181 [AO].
Stadsbestuur van Utrecht 1122–1577, 701, Buurspraakboek of Luiboek, 1385–1391, 1396–1536, 1542–1555, 1560–1579, no. 16.17 [1490–9] [AO].

Historisch Centrum Limburg, Maastricht (HCL)

Landen van Overmars, 01.075, no. 8677 [AO].

Noord Hollands Archief, Haarlem (NHAH)

Kloosters te Haarlem, 2123, Fundatieboek. Register van de te houden memories, met aantekeningen over bezittingen, bestuur en geschiedenis van het Begijnhof, periode 1272–1630, no. 419.

Regionaal Archief Alkmaar (RAA)

Collectie Wollebrand Gelijnsz de Jonghe, no. 53, brief 17 [AO].

Regionaal Archief Nijmegen (RAN)

Brouwersgilde Nijmegen, 1562–1770, 300, Publikatie van de magistraat over de afgelasting van de kermis in verband met de pest en het verbod bier aan klanten van buiten de stad te leveren, no. 49 [AO].

Regionaal Archief Rivierenland, Tiel (RAR)

Archief van het stadsbestuur van Culemborg, 1318–1813, 0826, no. 1596 [AO].

Regionaal Archief Zuid-Utrecht, Wijk-bij-Duurstede (RAZU)

Stadsbestuur Rhenen, 152, no. 843 [AO].
Stadsgerecht Rhenen, 066, no. 18, 619 [AO].

Regionaal Archief Zutphen (RAZ)

Archief van de Kerkmeesters van de Hervormde Gemeente te Zutphen. Rekening van kerkmeester Derrick van Thyll (buiten), 1576, no. 292 [AO].
Inventaris van de collectie Johannes Gimberg (1850–1930), 0142, no. 68 [AO].
Inventaris van de collectie K.O. Meinsma (1865–1929), 0138, no. 246 [AO].
Oud archief van de stad Zutphen (1206–1815), 0001, Rekeningen van Johan Ruter, 1598–1599, no. 1159 [AO].

Regionaal Historisch Centrum Eindhoven (RHCE)

Gemeentebestuur Gestel, 1620–1810, no. 336 [AO].

Rijksarchief te Leuven (RtL)

Archief van de Onze-Lieve-Vrouwparochie van Hamme, 880/47, no. 34296 [AO].
Archief van de schepenbank van Asse, 94, no. 842 [AO].

Stadsarchief Amsterdam (SA)

Archief van Burgemeesters: Stadsrekeningen, 5014, no. 125 [AO].
Archief van de Burgerlijke Stand: Doop-, trouw- en begraafboeken van Amsterdam, 5001, no. 1092 [AO].
Archief van de Notarissen ter Standplaats Amsterdam, 1578–1915, 5075, no. 3607 [AO].
Archief van de Notarissen ter Standplaats Amsterdam, 5075, Afschriften van notariele acten in banden, 1612–1644, no. 96560 [AO].

Stadsarchief Breda (SB)

Dekenaten Bergen op Zoom en Breda behorend tot Bisdom Antwerpen (1420) 1561–1802, ARC0007.3, no. 361.
Schepenbank Breda 1499–1811, Vestbrieven, no. 428, 765.
Stadsbestuur Breda (oud administratief archief) 1280–1810, Stadsrekeningen, no. 554, 615–19.

Stadsarchief Delft (SDEL)

Archieven van het stadsbestuur van Delft 1246–1813, Register van vonnissen in strafzaken, no. 2387 [AO].

Stadsarchief Deventer (SD)

Groote (vroeger Heilige Geesten-) en Voorster gasthuis te Deventer, 0767, no. 1304 [AO].

Sint Geertruiden Gasthuis, 0794, no. 23 [AO].

Stadsarchief Rotterdam (SR)

Archieven van de Notarissen te Rotterdam en daarin opgegane gemeenten, 18, no. 4, 42, 452, 588, 669.

State Archives of Belgium, Brussels (SAB)

Parochieregisters (various), accessed via https://agatha.arch.be/.

Streekarchivariaat Noordwest-Veluwe, Elburg (SNV)

Stadsbestuur Harderwijk, (1190) 1231–1813, 5001, no. 607, 861 [AO].

Streekarchief Voorne-Putten, Brielle (SVP)

Rekeningen Heilige Geest, no. 750 (Geervliet uitgaven; Abbenbroek uitgaven) [AO].

West Brabants Archief, Bergen op Zoom (WBA)

Archief van de stad Bergen op Zoom, 1397–1810, 0005, no. 6, 3112.

Doop-, trouw- en begraafboeken Oudenbosch, 1609–1811, 0302, no. 1, 3.

Dorpsbestuur Oudenbosch, 0300, nos. 0918–29, 0960–8.

Notaris Wouter de Witte, Minuutakten van andere akten, 1625–7, 0050, no. 64.

Zeeuws Archief, Middelburg (ZAB)

Godshuizen Middelburg, 1343–1812, 24.1, no. 19, 22 [AO].

Vrije van Sluis 1584–1796, 7, Stukken betreffende maatregelen tegen besmetting met pest, 1605, 1770–1771, no. 363 [AO].

Primary Literature

Amelang, James S., ed., *A Journal of the Plague Year: The Diary of the Barcelona Tanner, Miquel Parets, 1651*. Oxford: Oxford University Press, 1991.

Anon., ed., *Annales de la société médico-chirurgicale de Bruges*, XIII. Bruges: Vanhee-Wante, 1852.

Anon., ed., Gebed tegen de cholera. *Volkskunde: Nederlandsch Tijdschrift voor Volkskunde* 35, 1 (1930), 65–6.

Anon., ed., *Gheboden ende uutgheroepen. Al eest soo dat is verboden dat niemandt van sinte Claes (midts de groote infectie vande peste die aldaer is grasserende) binnen der stadt moghen logeren*. Antwerp: Jan I. Moretus, 1599.

Anon., ed., *Ordonnantie by de magistraet der stad Leeuwarden gemaeckt: tegens verscheydene Ongeregeltheden ende Misbruycken, soo in 't bekleden, op-draghen der Dooden…Met seeckere Tauxen op 't maecken van de dood-kisten. Ende een ordre voor de dood-gravers*. Leeuwarden: Claude Fonteyne, 1636.

Bavel, H. van, A.C.M. Kappelhof, G.M. van der Velden, and G. Verbeek, eds., *De kroniek van het St. Geertruiklooster te 's-Hertogenbosch: Die chronijcke der Stadt ende Meijerije van 's-Hertogenbosch*. Den Bosch: Stadsarchief 's-Hertogenbosch, 2001.

Beck, David. *Spiegel van mijn leven. Haags dagboek 1624*, ed. S.E. Veldhuijzen. Hilversum: Verloren, 1993.

Berger, Roger, ed., *Le nécrologe de la confrérie des jongleurs et des bourgeois d'Arras (1194–1361)*, II. Arras: Mémoires de la Commission Départementale des Monuments Historiques du Pas-de-Calais, 1970.

Bergsma, Wiebe, ed., *De wereld volgens Abel Eppens. Een Ommelander boer in de zestiende eeuw*. Groningen: Wolters-Noordhoff/Forsten, 1988.

Beurden, A.F. van, ed., *De handelingen van den magistraat der stad Roermond van het jaar 1596 tot en met het jaar 1696*. Roermond: M. Waterreus, 1903.

Billen, Claire, and Marc Boone, eds., *Bans et édits pour la ville de Tournai en temps de peste (1349–1351): Les transcriptions retrouvées de Frédéric Hennebert*. Brussels: Palais des Académies, 2021.

Blok, P.J., J.A. Feith, S. Gratama, J. Reitsma, and C.P.L. Rutgers, eds., *Oorkondenboek van Groningen en Drenthe*, I–II. Groningen: J.B. Wolters, 1896–9.

Brinkerink, Dirk A., ed., Biographieën van beroemde mannen uit den Deventer-kring. *Archief voor de Geschiedenis van het Aartsbisdom Utrecht* 27 (1901), 400–23.

Creemers, C., ed., Kronijk uit het klooster Maria Wijngaard te Weert 1442–1587: Opgesteld door suster Maria Luyten. *Publications de la société historique et archéologique dans le duché de Limbourg* 12 (1875), 145–248.

De Ketham, Joannes. Een tractaet van die pestelencie. In: *Fasciculus medicine houdende in hem dese nauolghende tractaten die allen cyrurginen ende andere menschen te wetene seer profitelijc ende nootsakelijc zijn*, trans. Petrus Antonianus. Antwerp: Claes die Graue, 1512.

Deusing, Anton. *Twee Diepzinnige en heilzame onderzoekingen Nopende de Pest ook besmettelijk zy?...* Amsterdam: Abraham Witteling, 1664.

De Vos, A., ed., Sprokkeling. Remedie tegen de pest. *Appeltjes van het Meetjesland: Jaarboek van het Heemkundig Genootschap van het Meetjesland* 2 (1950), 62.

Dijstelberge, Paul, and Leo Noordegraaf, eds., *Plague and Print in the Netherlands: A Short-Title Catalogue of Publications in the University Library of Amsterdam*. Rotterdam: Erasmus Publishing, 1997.

Dooren, Berend van, ed., Thuisisolatie in 1533. *Ons Voorgeslacht* 75 (2020), 400.

Doorninck, Pieter N. van, ed., *Acten betreffende Gelre en Zutphen 1400–1404 uit het staatsarchief te Dusseldorp, Register B No. 25*. Haarlem: Gebrs. van Brederode, 1901.

Drost, Aernout. *De pestilentie te Katwijk (1625)*. Amsterdam: G.J.A. Beijerinck, 1835.

Eeghen, Isabella H. van, ed., *Dagboek van broeder Wouter Jacobsz. (Gualtherus Jacobi Masius) Prior van Stein. Amsterdam 1572–1578 en Montfoort 1578–1579*, I. Groningen: J.B. Wolters, 1959.

Even, Edward van, ed., Reglement over de pest, afgekondigd door het stedelyk bestuer van Leuven, anno 1473. *Vaderlandsch Museum voor Nederduitsche Letterkunde, Oudkunde en Geschiedenis* 2 (1858), 132–5.

Formsma, W.J., and R. van Roijen, eds., *Diarium van Egbert Alting 1553–1594*. The Hague: Nijhoff, 1964.

Franquinet, G.D., ed., Eene verordening der stad Venlo in tijd van pest (1615 en 1623). *De Maasgouw: Orgaan voor Limburgsche Geschiedenis, Taal- en Letterkunde* 13 (1891), 142.

Fruin, Robert, ed., *Informacie up den staet faculteyt ende gelegentheyt van de steden ende dorpen van Hollant ende Vrieslant: Om daernae te reguleren de nieuwe schiltaele, gedaen in den jaere MDXIV*. Leiden: A.W. Sijthoff, 1886.

Haecht, Godevaert Van. *Kroniek over de troebelen van 1565 tot 1574 te Antwerpen en elders*, II, ed. R. van Roosbroeck. Antwerp: De Sikkel, 1930.

Hamaker, Hendrik Gerard, ed., Historische aanteekeningen in het Memoriale Fautorum Capituli Sti Pancratii te Leiden, 1367–1408. *Bijdragen voor Vaderlandsche Geschiedenis en Oudheidkunde* 6 (1870), 126–43.

Haubois, Egbert. *Caerte van de vermaerde ende antique stad Groeningen (Grote Haubois)*. Groningen: Jan Lubberts Langeweerd, 1665 [1634].

Hendrik Hering, Johan. *Bespiegeling over Neêrlandsch watersnood, tusschen den 14den en 15den Nov. MDCCLXXV*, I. Amsterdam: Wed. Loveringh en Allart, 1776.

Horrox, Rosemary, ed., *The Black Death*. Manchester: Manchester University Press, 1994.

Hout, Jan van. *Ordonnantie Ende Ghebot Nopende De Heete Ziecte, Ofte Peste*. Leiden: Raedthuys, 1603.

Joosting, J.G., ed., Cornelis Block's kroniek van het regulierenklooster te Utrecht. *Bijdragen en Mededelingen van het Historisch Genootschap* 16 (1895), 1–93.

Kaisin, J., ed., *Annales historiques de la commune de Farciennes*, I. Tamines: C. Duculot-Roulin, 1889.

Linden, Jan vander. *Cort verhael oft Tractaet, Vande Contagieuse Sieckte, de Peste*. Antwerp: Godtgaf Verhulst, 1634.

Matthieu, E.M., ed., Mesures réglementaires contre la peste à Braine-le-Comte en 1575. *Annales du cercle archéologique d'Enghien* 2 (1883), 245–6.

Oomius, Simon. *Des Heeren verderflicke pyl: ofte Twee boeken van de pest...* Amsterdam: Willem van Beaumont, 1665.

Oosterbaan, D.P., ed., Kroniek van de Nieuwe Kerk te Delft. *Haarlemsche Bijdragen: Bouwstoffen voor de Geschiedenis van het Bisdom Haarlem* 65 (1958), 2–336.

Oudenhoven, Jacob van. *Antiquitates Cimbricae renovatae, dat is, vernieude oudtheden der Cimbren of een raer verhael van de Cimbren ende Cimberische vloet ende van 't hoogh water 1681 en hoogen vloet van den 26 January, 1682*. Haarlem: Symon Swart, 1682.

Reygersbergh, Jan. *Dye cronijcke van Zeelandt*. Antwerp: Heyndrick Peetersen van Middelburch, 1551.

Romen, J.J., ed., Kronijk tot 1620. *Publications de la société historique et archéologique dans le duché de Limbourg* 10 (1873), 98–343.

Schevensteen, A.F.C. Van, ed., *Documents pour servir à l'étude des maladies pestilentielles dans le marquisat d'Anvers jusqu'à la chute de l'Ancien Régime*, I. Brussels: Lamertin, 1931.

Scholtens, Hendrik Jan Joseph, ed., Necrologie van de Utrechtse Kartuizers. *Archief voor de Geschiedenis van het Aartsbisdom Utrecht* 71 (1952), 97–150.

Strouven, Elisabeth. *La vie de la vénérable mère Elizabeth Strouven, fondatrice et première supérieure du monastère nommé le Mont Calvaire à Maestricht*. Liège: Jean-Philippe Gramme, 1722.

Teding van Berkhout Jr., P.J., ed., *Register op het oud-archief van Hasselt*. Zwolle: De Erven J.J. Tijl, 1883.

Teellinck, Willem. *Wraeck-sweert, Bepleytende Het recht van Gods Verbondt door Bloedighe Oorloghe, Diere tijdt, Bleecke pestilentie...* Middelburg: Marten Jansz. Brandt, 1624.

Thelwall, Algernon Sydney. *Keert U tot Hem die Slaat: Eene christelijke opwekking aan de Nederlanders; bij gelegenheid van de tegenwoordige overstroomingen*, 2nd ed. Amsterdam: P. den Hengst en Zoon, 1825.

Wassenbergh, A., ed., Reisindrukken van den Franschen gezantschapssecretaris Charles Ogier uit Friesland en Groningen in het jaar 1636. *De Vrije Fries* 37 (1943), 162–71.

Weiler, A., ed., *Necrologie, kroniek en cartularium c.a. van het Fraterhuis te Doesburg (1432–1559)*. Leiden: Brill, 1974.
Wijngaarden, C.H. van, and L.M. van der Hoeven, eds., De familienotities van Elisabeth Willemsdr. Cortenhoff. *Ons Voorgeslacht* 73 (2018), 1–25.
Zuijlen, R.A. van, ed., *Inventaris der Archieven de Stad 's-Hertogenbosch, 1568–1700*, I–II. Den Bosch: W.C. van Heusden, 1863–6.

Films

Stelling, Jos. *Mariken van Nieumeghen*. Jos Stelling Producties, 1974.

Websites

Adriaensen, Erik, ed., Turnhout in het verleden. https://adoc.pub/erik-adriaensen-turnhout-in-het-verleden-2006.html (2006).
Alink, Annink M., ed., Getuigenissen en gichten. https://kampen-notarieel.nl/images/GGpdfs/akten9.pdf (2017).
Anon., ed., Arch. Klerken- en fraterhuis, inv.nr. 0278, reg. 341. http://www.cartago.nl/nl/oorkonde/kfh341.xml (2020).
Anon., ed., Beek RK overlijdens, 1650–1654. https://www.genbronnen.nl/bronnen/limburg/beek/overlijdens/1650-1654.html (2006).
Anon., ed., Criminele sententies (vonnissen). https://hetutrechtsarchief.nl/hulp-bij-onderzoek/online-bronnen/criminele-sententies-vonnissen.
Anon., ed., Dataschurk. https://www.erfgoedshertogenbosch.nl/onderzoek/hulp-bij-onderzoek/dataschurk.
Anon., ed., Een geplunderde woning in Hasselt. https://watstaatdaer.nl/oefenen/complete-teksten/een-geplunderde-woning-hasselt.
Anon., ed., Klooster Ter Apel, inv.nr. 0001, fol. 021r, reg. 61. http://www.cartago.nl/nl/oorkonde/kta061a.xml (2020).
Anon., ed., Lottum overlijdens, 1690–1694. https://www.genbronnen.nl/bronnen/limburg/lottum/overlijdens/1690-1694.html (2006).
Anon., ed., Naarden, Begraven 1644–1667. https://www.familysearch.org/ark:/61903/3:1:3QSQ-G9QK-MFY2?cc=2037985 (2014).
Anon., ed., Ordonnantie Haarlem 1636. http://www.cranendonk.demon.nl/Figuren/Ordonnanties/Haarlem-1636.html (2017).
Anon., ed., Ordonnantie Haarlem 1655. http://www.cranendonk.demon.nl/Figuren/Ordonnanties/Haarlem-1655.html (2017).
Anon., ed., Ordonnantie Leiden 1655. http://www.cranendonk.demon.nl/Figuren/Ordonnanties/Leiden-1655.html (2017).
Anon., ed., Ordonnantie Roermond 1598. http://www.cranendonk.demon.nl/Figuren/Ordonnanties/Roermond-1598.html (2017).
Anon., ed., https://en.wikipedia.org/wiki/Xenophobia_and_racism_related_to_the_COVID-19_pandemic (2024).
Asseldonk, Martien van, ed., Regesten van resoluties van het dorpsbestuur van Veghel 1807–1809. http://www.oudzijtaart.nl/Reconstructie%20van%20Veghel/Downloads/Resoluties%20dorpsbestuur%201807-1809.docx (2014).
Auwerda-Berghout, S.M., ed., Voorne en Putten in de exploiten uit de grafelijkheidsrekenkamer 1480-1631. https://www.onsvoorgeslacht.nl/genealogische-databank/bronbewerkingen/grafelijkheidsrekenkamer-van-holland-voorne-en-putten-1480-1631/3/ (2011).
Beijers, Henk, ed., Meierijse schoutsrekeningen 1368–1638. http://www.henkbeijersarchiefcollectie.nl/historisch_onderzoek/schoutsrekeningen.htm (2005).

Boterbergh, Tom. Burgers, boeren en soldaten. Militaire lasten in de twee steden en het Land van Aalst, 1621–1648. Licentiaat in de Geschiedenis, University of Ghent, http://www.ethesis.net/boeren_burgers/bbs_inhoud.htm (2000).

Braber, Hans den, ed., Overlijdensregister RK Parochie Oudenbosch 1704 t/m 1721. Overlijdens RK Oudenbosch 1704–1721. https://web.archive.org/web/20210509140101/http://www.den-braber.nl/genealogie/bronnen/oudenbosch/odb_ov17041721.html (2002).

Brand, Rien van den, ed., Maashees testament 1636. http://home.kpn.nl/rien.vandenbrand/docs/Maasheestestament1636.doc.

Curtis, Daniel R., ed., Database of those Recorded as Deceased in the Haarlem "Bells and Graves" Register, 1412–1547. https://doi.org/10.34894/LYSYEV (2023).

Curtis, Daniel R., ed., Original Burials Data for the Book: Epidemic Disease and Society in the Premodern Low Countries: Inequality and Community (Abingdon: Routledge, 2026). DataverseNL. https://doi.org/10.34894/LRAMMV (2025).

Curtis, Daniel R., and Bram van Besouw. Not Learning from History. Learning from COVID-19. *Wiley: COVID-19 Resources for the Research Community*. https://www.wiley.com/en-us/network/publishing/research-publishing/trending-stories/not-learning-from-history-learning-from-covid-19 (2020).

De Keijzer, B., ed., Nieuwpoort, DTB inv.nr. 8 (aantekenboek 1) 1598–1602. https://www.hogenda.nl/hogenda-bronnen/?id=10799 (2016).

De Veer, E.J.C. De pest in Leerdam. https://www.historischeverenigingleerdam.nl/historische-artikelen/de-pest-in-leerdam/ (2015).

De Vos, Pieter-Jan. #VVDW: Het eerste pesthuis van Leiden. https://www.erfgoedleiden.nl/nieuws/vondst-van-de-week/1132-vvdw-het-eerste-pesthuis-van-leiden (2020).

Doedeijns, C., ed., Uittreksels uit de criminele vonnisboeken van Gouda over de periode 1447–1810. https://www.archiefhond.nl/nt/Gda/Gda_crimvonn.pdf (2001–3)

Cailleau, Hubert. Peste à Valenciennes en 1515. In: Louis de la Fontaine, ed., *Recueil des antiquités de Valenciennes*, III. Valenciennes, 1551–4, fo. 33r. http://initiale.irht.cnrs.fr/decor/56276 (2001).

Graaf, Beatrice de, Lotte Jensen, Rina Knoeff, and Catrien Santing. Aan de slag! Een manifest voor "Applied History". https://www.historici.nl/aan-de-slag-een-manifest-voor-applied-history/ (2020).

Green, Monica H. Climate and Disease in Medieval Eurasia. *Oxford Research Encyclopedia of Asian History*, https://oxfordre.com/asianhistory/view/10.1093/acrefore/9780190277727.001.0001/acrefore-9780190277727-e-6 (2018).

Green, Monica H. Hidden Plagues: Rediscovering the History of Plague during Times of Famine, https://www.academia.edu/115046429/Hidden_Plagues_Rediscovering_the_History_of_Plague_During_Times_of_Famine (2024).

Green, Monica H., and André Filipe Oliveira da Silva. Shifting Paradigms in Black Death Chronologies. *Religion and Urbanity: Reciprocal Formations*. https://urbrel.hypotheses.org/5550 (2023).

Harmeling, Florien. Het heksenproces tegen Lyssen Thys. https://www.erfgoedshertogenbosch.nl/verhalen/het-heksenproces-tegen-lyssen-thys (2023).

Heijmans, P., ed., Nadere toegang op inv.nr 51A-B uit het archief van het Stadsbestuur Wijk bij Duurstede, 1300–1810 (1). https://www.ewab-applications.nl/RHCZOU/PDF/NT00001_51A_B.pdf.

Helms van Eis, L., ed., Landpachters in het Oudeland van Strijen en het Oostzomerland voor Heinenoord anno 1657 voor notaris Adriaen de Haen. https://www.onsvoorgeslacht.nl/genealogische-databank/bronbewerkingen/landpachters-in-het-oudeland-van-strijen-en-het-oostzomerland-voor-heinenoord-anno-1657-voor-notaris-adriaen-de-haen/1121/ (2016).

Heuvel, Hans M. van den, ed., Crimineel klachtboek, 1533–1811. https://www.erfgoedleiden.nl/collecties/uw-verhalen/uw-verhalen/verhaal/id/270 (2013).

Holtman, Ritzo, ed., De oude Nederlandse maten en gewichten. https://mgw.meertens.knaw.nl/ (2023).

Jensen, Lotte, Beatrice de Graaf, Rina Knoeff, and Catrien Santing. Dear Government, Please Make Use of Historical Knowledge to Defeat the Pandemic. https://www.the-low-countries.com/article/dear-government-please-make-use-of-historical-knowledge-to-defeat-the-pandemic (2021).

Kappelhof, Ton, ed., Kroniek Breda en Baronie, 150–1829. https://www.academia.edu/121141609/Kroniek_Breda_en_Baronie_150_1829 (2024).

Kemps, Lotte. Heilige Rosalia bemiddelt voor de door de pest geteisterde inwoners van Palermo, Anthony Van Dyck, ca. 1625. https://expo-rg.flw.uantwerpen.be/exhibits/show/intro-heiligen-rosalia/item/153 (2023).

Kemps, Lotte. Patronesse van de peste – Rosalia van Palermo. https://expo-rg.flw.uantwerpen.be/exhibits/show/intro-heiligen-rosalia/rosalia-pest (2023).

Monballyu, Jos, ed., "Geexecuteert Metten Viere": Omwille Van Hekserij in Het Graafschap Vlaanderen, 1600–1624. https://kulak.kuleuven.be/facult/rechten/Monballyu/Rechtlagelanden/Heksenvlaanderen/Vonnissenhekserij/Vonnissenhekserijtekst1600-1624.htm (2001).

Ogilvie, Sheilagh. The Lion's Share: A Discussion on Alfani and Di Tullio's Book on Inequality in Preindustrial Europe #1. https://inequalityandhistory.blogspot.com/2020/03/the-lions-share-discussion-on-alfani.html (2020).

Stapel, Rombert, Isabel Flens, Daria Vaccari, and Rosalie Versmissen, eds., "(Re)counting the Uncounted": Repository of Digitised Premodern Censuses in the Low Countries. IISH Data Collection, V11, https://hdl.handle.net/10622/E5BC1Y [file number: census_NED1849a.tab] (2023).

Tielhof, Milja van. Droogte, drinkwater en sterfte. De Groninger ziekte van 1826. https://copingwithdrought.com/2022/08/30/droogte-drinkwater-en-sterfte-de-groninger-ziekte-van-1826/ (2022).

Walle, Kees, ed., West Vreugdenrijk. https://www.oudleiden.nl/werkgroepen/jan-van-hout-archiefonderzoek/buurthouden-1400-1795/buurtindeling-1600-1795-210-gebuurten-a-z/west-vreugdenrijk-015 (2006).

Secondary Literature

Aberth, John. *From the Brink of the Apocalypse: Confronting Famine, War, Plague, and Death in the Later Middle Ages*. Routledge: New York, 2001.

Adriaenssen, Leo, and Marjolein 't Hart. *Farming Communities at Risk. War and Economic Structures in the Netherlands; Some Evidence from the Meierij and Westerwolde, c. 1550–1700*. Unpublished Paper: University of Amsterdam, 2005.

Adriaenssen, Leo. *Staatsvormend geweld: Overleven aan de frontlinies in de Meierij van Den Bosch, 1572–1629*. Tilburg: Stichting Zuidelijk Historisch Contact, 2007.

Adrichem, Donatus van. Een pest-instructie van 1644 voor de Minderbroeders te Weert. *De Maasgouw: Orgaan voor Limburgsche Geschiedenis, Taal- en Letterkunde* 37 (1915), 49–50.

Agresta, Abigail. From Purification to Protection: Plague Response in Late Medieval Valencia. *Speculum* 95, 2 (2020), 371–95.

Alexander, John. *Bubonic Plague in Early Modern Russia: Public Health and Urban Disaster*. Baltimore, MD: John Hopkins University Press, 1980.

Alfani, Guido. The Effects of Plague on the Distribution of Property: Ivrea, Northern Italy 1630. *Population Studies* 64, 1 (2010), 61–75.

Alfani, Guido. Plague in Seventeenth-Century Europe and the Decline of Italy: An Epidemiological Hypothesis. *European Review of Economic History* 17, 4 (2013), 408–30.

Alfani, Guido. *Calamities and the Economy in Renaissance Italy. The Grand Tour of the Horsemen of the Apocalypse*. Basingstoke: Palgrave Macmillan, 2013.

Alfani, Guido. Economic Inequality in Northwestern Italy: A Long-Term View (Fourteenth to Eighteenth Centuries). *Journal of Economic History* 75, 4 (2015), 1058–96.

Alfani, Guido. La popolazione dell'Italia settentrionale nel XV e XVI secolo: Scenari regionali e macro-regionali. In: Guido Alfani, Angelo Carbone, Beatrice Del Bo, and Riccardo Rao, eds., *La popolazione italiana del quattrocento e cinquecento*, 19–40. Udine: Forum, 2016.

Alfani, Guido. Economic Inequality in Preindustrial Times: Europe and Beyond. *Journal of Economic Literature* 59, 1 (2021), 3–44.

Alfani, Guido. Epidemics, Inequality, and Poverty in Preindustrial and Early Industrial Times. *Journal of Economic Literature* 60, 1 (2022), 3–40.

Alfani, Guido, *As Gods Among Men: A History of the Rich in the West*. Princeton, NJ: Princeton University Press, 2023.

Alfani, Guido, and Francesco Ammannati. Long-Term Trends in Economic Inequality: The Case of the Florentine State, c. 1300–1800. *Economic History Review* 70, 4 (2017), 1072–102.

Alfani, Guido, and Marco Bonetti. A Survival Analysis of the Last Great European Plagues: The Case of Nonantola (Northern Italy) in 1630. *Population Studies* 73, 1 (2019), 101–18.

Alfani, Guido, Marco Bonetti, and Mattia Fochesato. Pandemics and Socio-Economic Status. Evidence from the Plague of 1630 in Northern Italy. *Population Studies* 78, 1 (2024), 21–42.

Alfani, Guido, and Marco Percoco. Plague and Long-Term Development: The Lasting Effects of the 1629–30 Epidemic on the Italian Cities. *Economic History Review* 72, 4 (2019), 1175–201.

Alfani, Guido, and Matteo Di Tullio. *The Lion's Share. Inequality and the Rise of the Fiscal State in Preindustrial Europe*. Cambridge: Cambridge University Press, 2018.

Alfani, Guido, Matteo Di Tullio, and Mattia Fochesato. Wealth Inequality and Epidemics in the Republic of Venice (1400–1800). *Economic History Review* (2025) early view.

Alfani, Guido, and Tommy E. Murphy. Plague and Lethal Epidemics in the Pre-Industrial World. *Journal of Economic History* 77, 1 (2017), 314–43.

Alfani, Guido, Victoria Gierok, and Felix Schaff. Economic Inequality in Preindustrial Germany, ca. 1300–1850. *Journal of Economic History* 82, 1 (2022), 87–125.

Allan, Francis. *De stad Enkhuizen en hare geschiedenis*, I. Schagerbrug: Wed. J.C. Honigh, 1856.

Almenar Fernández, Luis. Wealth Inequality and Land Ownership Before and After the Black Death. A Quantitative Analysis of Peasant Probate Inventories from the Kingdom of Valencia (1283–1400). In: Davide Cristoferi, ed., *Socio-Economic Inequalities during the Conjuncture of the Fourteenth Century: Sources and Methods, Dynamics and Representations (Italy and Europe, c. 1270 –c. 1350)*, 177–99. Florence: Firenze University Press, 2025.

Alter, George. Plague and the Amsterdam Annuitant: A New Look at Life Annuities as a Source for Historical Demography. *Population Studies* 37, 1 (1983), 23–41.

Alter, George, and Ann Carmichael. Classifying the Dead: Toward a History of the Registration of Causes of Death. *Journal of the History of Medicine and Allied Sciences* 54, 2 (1999), 114–32.

Álvarez-Nogal, Carlos, and Leandro Prados de la Escosura. The Rise and Fall of Spain (1270–1850). *Economic History Review* 66, 1 (2013), 1–37.

Ammannati, Francesco. La Peste Nera e la distribuzione della proprietà nella Lucchesia del tardo medioevo. *Popolazione e Storia* 16, 2 (2015), 21–45.

Ammannati, Francesco. La disuguaglianza economica in area marchigiana: Uno studio di un lungo periodo (1400–1800). In: Giampiero Nigro, ed., *Disuguaglianza economica nelle società preindustriali: Cause ed effetti / Economic Inequality in Pre-Industrial Societies: Causes and Effects*, 37–63. Florence: Firenze University Press, 2020.

Andel, M.A. van. Pestepidemieën te Gorinchem. *Nederlandse Tijdschrift voor Geneeskunde* 57 (1913), 1844–62.

Andreski, Stanislav. The Syphilitic Shock: A New Explanation of the "Great Witch Craze" of the 16th and 17th Centuries in the Light of Medicine and Psychiatry. *Encounter* 58, 5 (1982), 7–26.

Anon., ed., *De pest in de Nederlanden. Medisch-historische beschouwingen 650 jaar na de Zwarte Dood.* Brussels: Koninklijke Academie voor Geneeskunde van België, 1999.

Anon., ed., *Épidémies et endémies à Ath et en Hainaut du Moyen Âge au XIXe siècle. Colloque de Chièvres, 1989.* Ath: Cercle royal d'histoire et d'archéologie d'Ath et de la région, 1998.

Anon., ed., *Villages désertés et histoire économique, XI–XVIIIe siècle.* Paris: S.E.V.P.E.N., 1965.

Antonio Luque de Haro, Víctor. Social Inequalities in Adult Mortality across Europe (XVIII–XXI Centuries): A Critical Analysis of Theories and Evidence. *Economics & Human Biology* 55 (2024), 101438.

Appleby, Andrew B. Famine, Mortality, and Epidemic Disease: A Comment. *Economic History Review* 30, 3 (1977), 508–12.

Archambeau, Nicole. Healing Options during the Plague: Survivor Stories from a Fourteenth-Century Canonization Inquest. *Bulletin of the History of Medicine* 85, 4 (2011), 531–59.

Arickx, Valere. De armendis te Pittem tussen 1486 en 1498. *Biekorf* 51 (1950), 169–79.

Armstrong-Partida, Michelle, and Susan McDonough, Singlewomen in the Late Medieval Mediterranean. *Past and Present* 259, 1 (2023), 3–42.

Arnold, David. *Colonizing the Body: State Medicine and Epidemic Disease in Nineteenth-Century India.* Berkeley, CA: University of California Press, 1993.

Arrizabalaga, Jon. Medical Causes of Death in Preindustrial Europe: Some Historiographical Considerations. *Journal of the History of Medicine and Allied Sciences* 54, 2 (1999), 241–60.

Arrizabalaga, Jon. Problematizing Retrospective Diagnosis in the History of Disease. *Asclepio* 54, 1 (2002), 51–70.

Arrizabalaga, Jon, John Henderson, and Roger French. *The Great Pox: The French Disease in Renaissance Europe.* New Haven, CT: Yale University Press, 1997.

Asperen, Hanneke van. Nothing Else than Decay: Theodoor van der Schuer's *Allegory of Human Deprivation* for Leiden's Plague Hospital. *Journal of Historians of Netherlandish Art* 12, 2 (2020), 1–28.

Asseldonk, Martien van. Recepten voor Veghelse medicijnen uit 1672. *Van Vehchele tot Veghel* 5 (1985), 68–73.

Asseldonk, Martien van. *Veghel; een goet ende vet Dorp. Het ontstaan van Veghel, de ontwikkeling van landschap en samenleving, 600–1810: Nieuwe instrumenten voor de historische geografie.* Woudrichem: Pictures Publishers, 2016.

Aubry, Martine. Les mortalités lilloises (1328–1369). *Revue du Nord* 65, 257 (1983), 327–42.

Audoin-Rouzeau, Stéphane. *Les chemins de la peste: Le rat, la puce et l'homme.* Rennes: Presses universitaires de Rennes, 2003.

Baer, William C. Landlords and Tenants in London, 1550–1700. *Urban History* 38, 2 (2011), 234–55.

Bailey, Mark. *After the Black Death: Economy, Society and the Law in Fourteenth-Century England.* Oxford: Oxford University Press, 2021.

Bailey, Mark. The Black Death, Girl Power, and the Emergence of the European Marriage Pattern in England. *Journal of Medieval and Early Modern Studies* 54, 3 (2024), 493–528.

Barbieri, Rémi, Michel Signoli, D. Chevé, C. Costedoat, Stefan Tzortzis, G. Aboudharam, et al. *Yersinia pestis*: The Natural History of Plague. *Clinical Microbiology Review* 34, 1 (2021), e00044-19.

Barbieri, Rémi, Michel Drancourt, and Didier Raoult. The Role of Louse-Transmitted Diseases in Historical Plague Pandemics. *The Lancet Infectious Diseases* 21, 2 (2021), e17–e25.

Bardsley, Sandy. Peasant Women and Inheritance of Land in Fourteenth-Century England. *Continuity and Change* 29, 3 (2014), 297–324.

Barker, Hannah. Laying the Corpses to Rest: Grain Embargoes and the Early Transmission of the Black Death in the Black Sea, 1346–1347. *Speculum* 96, 1 (2021), 97–126.

Barla, Nicolas. *Pour la necessitet du povre peuple: La gestion des crises alimentaires dans les Pays-Bas méridionaux en période d'affirmation des pouvoirs urbains et princiers (XIe–XVe siècle): Chronologie des crises, analyse historiographique, étude de cas (Lille et Mons au XVe siècle).* PhD Thesis: Université Libre de Bruxelles, 2019/20.

Barnes, Kent B. Social Vulnerability and Pneumonic Plague: Revisiting the 1994 Outbreak in Surat, India. *Environment Hazards* 13, 2 (2014), 161–80.

Barnes, Kent B. The Gendered Dimensions of London's Last Bubonic Plague Epidemic 1665–1666. *Environment Hazards* 22, 4 (2023), 309–33.

Baron, Wilhelmina. *"Het belang en de welvaart van alle ingezetenen". Gezondheidszorg in de stad Groningen 1800–1870.* PhD Thesis: University of Groningen, 2006.

Barzilay, Tzafrir. *Poisoned Wells: Accusations, Persecution, and Minorities in Medieval Europe, 1321–1422.* Philadelphia, PE: University of Pennsylvania Press, 2022.

Bashford, Alison. Epidemics and Governmentality: Smallpox in Sydney, 1881. *Critical Public Health* 9, 4 (1999), 198–220.

Bauch, Martin, and Christan Oertel. Late Medieval Plague Waves in Eastern Germany and Bohemia. Combining Narrative, Administrative, Epigraphic, and Pictorial Sources with Quantitative Approaches. *Historical Studies on Central Europe* 4, 1 (2024), 30–67.

Bauch, Martin, and Ulf Büntgen. Climate-Driven Changes in Mediterranean Grain Trade Mitigated Famine but Introduced the Black Death to Medieval Europe. *Communications Earth & Environment* 6, 1 (2025), 986.

Baumann, E.D. De dysenterie te Nijmegen in 1736. *Nederlandse Tijdschrift voor Geneeskunde* 69, 2 (1925), 605–19.

Baumann, E.D. Iets over de dysenterie in de zestiende en zeventiende eeuw. *Nederlandse Tijdschrift voor Geneeskunde* 70, 2 (1926), 41–59.

Baumann, E.D. Bijdrage tot de geschiedenis der dysenterie in de achttiende eeuw. *Nederlandse Tijdschrift voor Geneeskunde* 70, 2 (1926), 1520–34.

Bavel, Bas J.P. van. People and Land: Rural Population Developments and Property Structures in the Low Countries, c. 1300–c. 1600. *Continuity and Change* 17, 1 (2002), 9–37.

Bavel, Bas J.P. van. The Land Market in the North Sea Area in a Comparative Perspective, 13th–18th Centuries. In: Simonetta Cavaciocchi, ed., *Il mercato della terra. Secc. XIII–XVIII*, 119–46. Florence: Le Monnier, 2004.

Bavel, Bas J.P. van. The Medieval Origins of Capitalism in the Netherlands. *BMGN: Low Countries Historical Review* 125, 2/3 (2010), 45–79.

Bavel, Bas J.P. van. Rural Revolts and Structural Change in the Low Countries, Thirteenth – Early Fourteenth Centuries. In: Richard Goddard, John Langdon, and Miriam Müller, eds., *Survival and Discord in Medieval Society. Essays in Honour of Christopher Dyer*, 269–86. Turnhout: Brepols, 2010.

Bavel, Bas J.P. van. *Manors and Markets: Economy and Society in the Low Countries 500–1600*. Oxford: Oxford University Press, 2010.

Bavel, Bas J.P. van. *The Invisible Hand? How Market Economies Have Emerged and Declined Since AD 500*. Oxford: Oxford University Press, 2016.

Bavel, Bas J.P. van. Wealth Inequality in Pre-Industrial Europe: What Role Did Associational Organizations Have? *Economic History Review* 75, 3 (2022), 643–66.

Bavel, Bas J.P. van, and Auke Rijpma. How Important Were Formalized Charity and Social Spending Before the Rise of the Welfare State? A Long-Run Analysis of Selected Western European Cases, 1400–1850. *Economic History Review* 69, 1 (2016), 159–87.

Bavel, Bas J.P. van, and Maarten Scheffer. Historical Effects of Shocks on Inequality: The Great Leveller Revisited. *Humanities and Social Science Communications* 8 (2021), no. 76.

Bavel, Bas J.P. van, and Oscar Gelderblom. The Economic Origins of Cleanliness in the Dutch Golden Age. *Past and Present* 205, 1 (2009), 41–69.

Bavel, Bas J.P. van, Daniel R. Curtis, and Tim Soens. Economic Inequality and Institutional Adaptation in Response to Flood Hazards: A Historical Analysis. *Ecology and Society* 23, 4 (2018), no. 30.

Bavel, Bas J.P. van, Daniel R. Curtis, Matthew Hannaford, Michail Moatsos, Joris Roosen, and Tim Soens. Climate and Society in Long-Term Perspective: Opportunities and Pitfalls in the Use of Historical Datasets. *WIREs Climate Change* 10, 6 (2019), e611.

Becuwe, F. De bouw van het pesthuis der kapucijnen in Veurne (1610–1611). *Biekorf* 91 (1991), 121–7.

Beeckaert, Esther, and Eric Vanhaute. Whose Famine? Regional Differences in Vulnerability and Resilience during the 1840s Potato Famine in Belgium. In: Jessica Dijkman and Bas van Leeuwen, eds., *An Economic History of Famine Resilience*, 115–41. New York: Routledge, 2020.

Béghin, Mathieu. Entre le cœur de ville et les faubourgs. La place de l'animal en milieu urbain dans le nord de la France aux XIVe et XVe siècles. In: Fabrice Guizard and Corinne Beck, eds., *Les animaux sont dans la place: La longue histoire d'une cohabitation*, 21–44. Amiens: Encrage Éditions, 2019.

Belich, James. *The World the Plague Made: The Black Death and the Rise of Europe*. Princeton, NJ: Princeton University Press, 2022.

Benedictow, Ole J. *The Black Death, 1346–1353: The Complete History*. Woodbridge: The Boydell Press, 2004.

Benedictow, Ole J. New Perspectives in Medieval Demography: The Medieval Demographic System. In: Mark Bailey and Stephen Rigby, eds., *Town and Countryside in the Age of the Black Death: Essays in Honour of John Hatcher*, 3–42. Turnhout: Brepols, 2012.

Benedictow, Ole J. *The Black Death and Later Plague Epidemics in the Scandinavian Countries: Perspectives and Controversies*. Berlin: De Gruyter, 2016.

Benedictow, Ole J. Biraben's Lists of the Plague Epidemics of the Second Plague Pandemic, 1346–c. 1690: Problems, Basis, Uses. *Annales de démographie historique* 138, 2 (2019), 213–23.

Benedictow, Ole J. *The Complete History of the Black Death*. Woodbridge: The Boydell Press, 2021.

Benedictow, Ole J. *The Complete History of Plague in Norway, 1348–1654*. Newcastle-upon-Tyne: Cambridge Scholars Publishing, 2022.

Beneker, Owyn, Ludovica Molinaro, Meriam Guellil, Stefania Sasso, Helja Kabral, Biancamaria Bonucci, et al. Urbanization and Genetic Homogenization in the Medieval Low Countries Revealed Through a Ten-Century Paleogenomic Study of the City of Sint-Truiden. *Genome Biology* 26 (2025), no. 127.

Bengtsson, Erik, and Patrick Svensson. The Wealth of the Swedish Peasant Farmer Class (1750–1900): Composition and Distribution. *Rural History* 30, 2 (2019), 129–45.

Benito i Monclus. Pere, Albert Reixach Sala, Alberto Barber Blasco, Adrià Mas Craviotto, and Guillem Roca Cabau. Assessing Epidemic Outbreaks in Late Medieval Catalonia (1348–1530): From Communities to Family Units. *The History of the Family* 30, 3 (2025), 371–412.

Benito i Monclus. Pere, Sandro Carocci, and Laurent Feller, eds., *Économies de la pauvreté au Moyen Âge*. Rome: École française de Rome, 2023.

Bennett, Judith M. *Ale, Beer, and Brewsters in England: Women's Work in a Changing World, 1300–1600*. Oxford: Oxford University Press, 1996

Bennett, Judith M. Women and Poverty: Girls on their Own in England Before 1348. In: John Langdon, Maryanne Kowaleski, and Philipp Schofield, eds., *Peasants and Lords in the Medieval English Economy: Essays in Honour of Bruce M. S. Campbell*, 299–324. Turnhout: Brepols, 2015.

Bennett, Judith M. Married and Not: Weston's Grown Children in 1268–1269. *Continuity and Change* 34, 2 (2019), 151–82.

Bennett, Judith M. Wretched Girls, Wretched Boys and the European Marriage Pattern in England (c. 1250–1350). *Continuity and Change* 34, 3 (2019), 315–47.

Berge, Erling, and Margaret A. Mckean. On the Commons of Developed Industrialized Countries. *International Journal of the Commons* 9, 2 (2015), 469–85.

Bergman, M. The Potato Blight in the Netherlands and its Social Consequences, 1845–47. *International Review of Social History* 12, 3 (1967), 390–431.

Berkner, Lutz K., and Franklin F. Mendels. Inheritance Systems, Family Structure, and Demographic Patterns in Western Europe, 1700–1900. In: Charles Tilly, ed., *Historical Studies of Changing Fertility*, 209–24. Princeton, NJ: Princeton University Press, 1978.

Besouw, Bram van. *On the Economic Consequences of Warfare in Early Modern Northwest Europe*. PhD Thesis: Utrecht University, 2019.

Besouw, Bram van, and Daniel R. Curtis. Estimating Warfare-Related Civilian Mortality in the Early Modern Period: Evidence from the Low Countries, 1620–99. *Explorations in Economic History* 84 (2022), 101425.

Besouw, Bram van, Daniel R. Curtis, and Roos van Oosten. Epidemic Mortality and Redistribution of Housing Wealth in Leiden, 1630–68. *SSRN* (2025). https://dx.doi.org/10.2139/ssrn.5418065.

Bever, Edward. Witchcraft Fears and Psychosocial Factors in Disease. *Journal of Interdisciplinary History* 30, 4 (2000), 573–90.

Beyerman, J.J. De (tweede) pokkenepidemie in Oud-Beijerland, 1883/1884. *Holland: Regionaal-Historisch Tijdschrift* 3, 1 (1971), 1–12.

Bieleman, Jan. Rural Change in the Dutch Province of Drenthe in the Seventeenth and Eighteenth Centuries. *Agricultural History Review* 33, 2 (1985), 105–18.

Binneveld, Hans, and Rudolf Dekker, eds., *Curing and Insuring. Essays on Illness in Past Times: The Netherlands, Belgium, England and Italy, 16th–20th Centuries*. Hilversum: Verloren, 1993.

Biraben, Jean-Noël. *Les hommes et la peste en France et dans les pays européens et méditerranéens*, I–II. Paris: La Haye, 1975/6.

Blažina Tomić, Zlata, and Vesna Blažina. *Expelling the Plague: The Health Office and the Implementation of Quarantine in Dubrovnik, 1377–1533*. Montreal: McGill-Queen's Press, 2015.

Blockmans, Wim P. The Social and Economic Effects of Plague in the Low Countries: 1349–1500. *Revue belge de philologie et d'histoire* 58, 4 (1980), 833–63.

Blockmans, Wim P. *Metropolen aan de Noordzee. De geschiedenis van Nederland, 1100–1560*. Amsterdam: Bert Bakker, 2010.

Blockmans, Wim P., Gerard Pieters, Walter Prevenier, and Remi van Schaïk. Tussen crisis en welvaart: Sociale veranderingen 1300–1500 (abnormale mortaliteit). In: Dirk P. Blok, ed., *Algemene Geschiedenis der Nederlanden*, IV, 42–86. Haarlem: Fibula-Van Dishoeck, 1980.

Bocquet, André. *Recherches sur la population rurale de l'Artois et du Boulonnais pendant la période bourguignonne, 1384–1477*. Arras: Mémoires de la commission départementale des monuments historiques de Pas-de-Calais, 1969.

Boeckl, Christine M. *Images of Plague and Pestilence: Iconography and Iconology*. Kirksville, MO: Truman State University Press, 2000.

Boeren, P.C. Een cellebroeder in Princenhage 1661/2. *Jaarboek De Oranjeboom* 16 (1963), 33–8.

Bogaers, Llewellyn. Geleund over de onderdeur: Doorkijkjes in het Utrechtse buurtleven van de vroege Middeleeuwen tot in de zeventiende eeuw. *BMGN: Low Countries Historical Review* 112, 3 (1997), 336–63.

Bohstedt, John. Gender, Household and Community Politics: Women in English Riots 1790–1810. *Past and Present* 120, 1 (1988), 88–122.

Bois, Guy. *Crise du féodalisme*. Paris: Presses de la F.N.S.P., 1976.

Bonenkampová, Viera. Waren "rijke stinkerds" rijk? De sociale stratificatie van de Delftenaren en hun graven in de Oude Kerk. In: Peter Bitter, Viera Bonenkampová, and Koen Goudriaan, eds., *Graven spreken: Perspectieven op grafcultuur in de middeleeuwse en vroegmoderne Nederlanden*, 193–204. Hilversum: Verloren, 2013.

Boomen, Nynke J.M. van den. *Born Close to Death. Region, Roman Catholicism and Infant Mortality in the Netherlands, 1875–1899*. PhD Thesis: Radboud University Nijmegen, 2021.

Boomen, Nynke J.M. van den. The Imperfections in Statistics: Interpretations of Causes of Infant Death in the Netherlands, 1875–1899. *Social History of Medicine* 35, 4 (2022), 1064–87.

Boone, Marc. *Gent en de Bourgondische Hertogen ca. 1384–ca. 1453: Een sociaal-politieke studie van een staatsvormingsproces*. Brussels: Paleis der Academiën, 1990.

Boschma, C. "Een pest, die Vrieslands Steeden, en luchtgewest bedorf". De bestrijding van de pokken. *De Vrije Fries* 64 (1984), 68–78.

Boter, Corinne, and Pieter Woltjer. The Impact of Sectoral Shifts on Dutch Unmarried Women's Labor Force Participation, 1812–1929. *European Review of Economic History* 24, 4 (2020), 783–817.

Bouman, Annechien, Maas Jan Heineman, and Marijke M. Faas. Sex Hormones and the Immune Response in Humans. *Human Reproduction Update* 11 (2005), 411–23.

Bourdelais, Patrice. *Les épidémies terrassées: Une histoire de pays riches*. Paris: La Martinière, 2003.

Bourgois, Danielle. Les Provinces Unies, les mesures contre la peste et le commerce dans la région baltique, 1709–1715. In: W.G. Heeres, L.M.J.B. Hesp, Leo Noordegraaf, and R.C.W. van der Voort, eds., *From Dunkirk to Danzig: Shipping and Trade in the North Sea and the Baltic, 1350–1850: Essays in Honour of J.A. Faber on the Occasion of his Retirement as Professor of Economic and Social History at the University of Amsterdam*, 191–202. Hilversum: Verloren, 1988.

Bourguignon, Mélanie, Yoann Doignon, Thierry Eggerickx, and Jean-Paul Sanderson. Le choléra en milieu rural: La pandémie de 1866 dans les provinces de Namur et Luxembourg. Espace populations sociétés 1 (2024), 1–30.

Bourin, Monique, John Drendel, and François Menant, eds., *Les disettes dans la conjoncture de 1300 en Méditerranée occidentale*. Rome: École française de Rome, 2011.

Bowers, Kristy Wilson. *Plague and Public Health in Early Modern Seville*. Woodbridge: Boydell & Brewer, 2013.

Bowsky, William M. The Impact of the Black Death upon Sienese Government and Society. *Speculum* 39, 1 (1964), 1–34.

Bowsky, William M. The Medieval Commune and Internal Violence: Police Power and Public Safety in Siena, 1287–1355. *American Historical Review* 73, 1 (1967), 1–17.

Bradley, Leslie. The Most Famous of All English Plagues: A Detailed Analysis of the Plague at Eyam, 1665–6. In: Paul Slack, ed., *The Plague Reconsidered: A New Look at its Origins and Effects in 16th and 17th Century England*, 63–94. Cambridge: Cambridge University Press, 1977.

Brandon, Pepijn. *War, Capital, and the Dutch State (1588–1795)*. Leiden: Brill, 2015.

Braudel, Fernand. *La Méditerranée et le monde méditerranéen á l'époque de Philippe II*, I. Paris: Armand Colin, 1966 [1949].

Brea-Martínez, Gabriel, and Joanna-Maria Pujadas-Mora. Estimating Long-Term Socioeconomic Inequality in Southern Europe: The Barcelona Area, 1481–1880. *European Review of Economic History* 23, 4 (2019), 397–420.

Breemen-Kruyt, N.C.J. van. De gave Gods in de Mallemolen. *Jaarboek "Die Haghe"* (1948/9), 47–72.

Brenner, Robert. Agrarian Class Structure and Economic Development in Pre-Industrial Europe. *Past and Present* 70, 1 (1976), 30–75.

Brenner, Robert. The Low Countries in the Transition to Capitalism. *Journal of Agrarian Change* 1, 2 (2001), 169–241.

Breuer, H.L.M., and Clé M. Lesger, *Dood en verderf: Over Leiden, de pest, en de Gouden Eeuw*. Leiden: Self Published, 2007.

Briggs, Asa. Cholera and Society in the Nineteenth Century. *Past and Present* 19, 1 (1961), 76–96.

Brookes, Edward. Plague Markings: Doors and Disease. *Cultural History* 12, 2 (2023), 145–67.

Broomhall, Susan. *Women's Medical Work in Early Modern France*. Manchester: Manchester University Press, 2004.

Brouwer, D. *Enkhuizen: Aanteekeningen uit het verleden*, III. Enkhuizen: Enkhuizer Courant, 1949.

Brouwer, Henk. Malaria in Nederland in de achttiende en negentiende eeuw. *Tijdschrift voor Sociale Geschiedenis* 9 (1983), 140–59.

Bruneel, Claude. *La mortalité dans les campagnes: Le duché de Brabant aux XVIIe et XVIIIe siècles*, I–II. Louvain: Nauwelaerts, 1977.

Bruneel, Claude. L'épidémie de dysenterie de 1779 dans les Pays-Bas autrichiens. *Bulletin de la commission royale d'histoire* 145, 3/4 (1979), 191–395.

Bruneel, Claude. L'assistance et la santé. In: Paul Janssens, ed., *La Belgique espagnole et la principauté de Liège (1585–1715)*, I, 231–44. Brussels: Dexia Banque, 2006.

Bruneel, Claude, and Yannick Coutiez. La dysenterie en Hainaut au XVIIIe siècle. In: Anon., ed., *Épidémies et endémies à Ath et en Hainaut du Moyen Âge au XIXe siècle. Colloque de Chièvres, 1989*, 127–46. Ath: Cercle royal d'histoire et d'archéologie d'Ath et de la région, 1998.

Brunner, H.G.H. Pest-epidemieën van de 15e tot de 17e eeuw te Rotterdam. *Nederlandse Tijdschrift voor Geneeskunde* 90, 2 (1946), 620–4.

Bruyndonckx, Marie. *Een cultuurgeschiedenis van de cholera Antwerpen in 1866: Emoties, opvattingen en dagelijkse praktijken.* MA Thesis: KU Leuven, 2023.

Buisman, Jan. *Duizend jaar weer, wind en water in de Lage Landen, 1450–1575*, III, ed. A.F.V. van Engelen. Franeker: Uitgeverij Van Wijnen, 1998.

Buning, Marius. Stench and the City: Urban Odors and Technological Innovation in Early Modern Leiden and Batavia. In: Bert De Munck and Antonella Romano, eds., *Knowledge and the Early Modern City: A History of Entanglements*, 104–29. Abingdon: Routledge, 2019.

Büntgen, Ulf, Christian Ginzler, Jan Esper, Willy Tegel, and Anthony J. McMichael. Digitizing Historical Plague. *Clinical Infectious Diseases* 55, 11 (2012), 1586–8.

Burrell, Sean, and Geoffrey Gill. The Liverpool Cholera Epidemic of 1832 and Anatomical Dissection—Medical Mistrust and Civil Unrest. *Journal of the History of Medicine and Allied Sciences* 60, 4 (2005), 478–98.

Buursma, Albert. *"Dese bekommerlijke tijden". Armenzorg, armen en armoede in de stad Groningen 1594–1795*. Assen: Van Gorcum, 2009.

Buwalda, J.M., and E.O. Buwalda-Prey. Eenige gegevens over de pest te Gouda in de 17de eeuw. *Nederlandse Tijdschrift voor Geneeskunde* 83, 4 (1939), 5663–71.

Buwalda-Prey, E.O. Bijdrage tot de geschiedenis van de pest en haar bestrijding te Gouda. *Oudheidkundige Kring "Die Goude"* (1940), 80–100.

Buylaert, Frederik, Thijs Lambrecht, Klaas Van Gelder, and Kaat Cappelle. The Political Economy of Seigneurial Lordship in Flanders, c.1250–1570. *Past and Present* 267, 1 (2025), 3–47.

Buzasi, Katalin, and Tim Riswick. The Rhythm of Death. Seasonality of Mortality in Amsterdam, 1812–1931. *Historical Life Course Studies* 15 (2025), 220–9.

Byfield, Judith A. Taxation, Women, and the Colonial State: Egba Women's Tax Revolt. *Meridians* 3, 2 (2003), 250–77.

Cabré, Montserrat. Women or Healers? Household Practices and the Categories of Health Care in Late Medieval Iberia. *Bulletin of the History of Medicine* 82, 1 (2008), 18–51.

Caferro, William. Petrarch's War: Florentine Wages and the Black Death. *Speculum* 88, 1 (2013), 144–65.

Callewier, Hendrik. De hondenslager van Kortrijk tijdens de late Middeleeuwen. *De Leiegouw* 64, 1 (2022), 23–30.

Camenisch, Chantal, Rudolf Brázdil, Andrea Kiss, Christian Pfister, Oliver Wetter, Christian Rohr, et al. Extreme Heat and Drought in 1473 and their Impacts in Europe in the Context of the Early 1470s. *Regional Environmental Change* 20, 19 (2020), 1–15.

Campbell, Bruce M.S. *The Great Transition: Climate, Disease and Society in the Late-Medieval World.* Cambridge: Cambridge University Press, 2016.

Campbell, Bruce M.S. Global Climates, the 1257 Mega-Eruption of Samalas Volcano, Indonesia, and the English Food Crisis of 1258. *Transactions of the Royal Historical Society* 27 (2017), 87–121.

Campbell, Bruce M.S., and Francis Ludlow. Climate, Disease and Society in Late-Medieval Ireland. *Proceedings of the Royal Irish Academy* 120C (2020), 159–252.

Camphuijsen, Frans, and Janna Coomans. De middeleeuwse stad en zijn varkens. *Madoc* 28, 3 (2014), 140–8.

Camus, Albert. *The Plague*. New York: Knopf Doubleday Publishing Group, 1991 [1947].

Canbakal, Hülya, and Alpay Filiztekin. Wealth Inequality in Northwestern Anatolia under the Ottomans, 1460–1870. *European Review of Economic History* 29, 1 (2025), 88–129.

Cantor, Norman F. *In the Wake of the Plague: The Black Death and the World it Made*. New York: The Free Press, 2001.

Carmichael, Ann G. Infection, Hidden Hunger, and History. In: Robert Rotberg and Theodore Rabb, eds., *Hunger and History: The Impact of Changing Food Production and Consumption Patterns on Society*, 51–66. Cambridge: Cambridge University Press, 1985.

Carmichael, Ann G. *Plague and the Poor in Renaissance Florence*. Cambridge: Cambridge University Press, 1986.

Carmichael, Ann G. The Last Past Plague: The Uses of Memory in Renaissance Epidemics. *Journal of the History of Medicine and Allied Sciences* 53, 2 (1998), 132–60.

Carmichael, Ann G. Universal and Particular: The Language of Plague, 1348–1500. *Medical History* 52, S27 (2008), 17–52.

Carmichael, Ann G. The Forensic Tradition in Milan's Civic Mortality Registers. *Journal of Early Modern Studies* (2022), 1–23.

Carpentier, Elisabeth. Autour de la peste noire: Famines et épidémies dans l'histoire du XIVe siècle. *Annales. Economies, sociétés, civilisations* 17, 6 (1962), 1062–92.

Casari, Marco. Emergence of Endogenous Legal Institutions: Property Rights and Community Governance in the Italian Alps. *Journal of Economic History* 67, 1 (2007), 191–226.

Casna, Maia, Carla L. Burrell, Rachel Schats, Menno L.P. Hoogland, and Sarah A. Schrader. Urbanization and Respiratory Stress in the Northern Low Countries: A Comparative Study of Chronic Maxillary Sinusitis in Two Early Modern Sites from the Netherlands (AD 1626–1866). *International Journal of Osteoarchaeology* 31, 5 (2021), 891–901.

Casna, Maia, Rachel Schats, Menno L.P. Hoogland, and Sarah A. Schrader. A Distant City: Assessing the Impact of Dutch Socioeconomic Developments on Urban and Rural Health Using Respiratory Disease as a Proxy. *International Journal of Paleopathology* 42 (2023), 34–45.

Casteels, Isabel. *Looking for Justice: Execution Spectators and the Revolt in the Low Countries, ca. 1520–1585*. PhD Thesis: Leiden University, 2025.

Castex, Dominique. Identification and Interpretation of Historical Cemeteries Linked to Epidemics. In: Didier Raoult and M. Drancourt, eds., *Paleomicrobiology: Past Human Infections*, 23–48. Berlin: Springer-Verlag, 2008.

Cervellati, Matteo, Elena Esposito, and Uwe Sunde. Epidemic Shocks and Civil Violence: Evidence from Malaria Outbreaks in Africa. *Review of Economics and Statistics* 104, 4 (2022), 780–96.

Cessford, Craig, Christiana L. Scheib, Meriam Guellil, Marcel Keller, Craig Alexander, Sarah A. Inskip, et al. Beyond Plague Pits: Using Genetics to Identify Responses to Plague in Medieval Cambridgeshire. *European Journal of Archaeology* 24, 4 (2021), 496–518.

Champion, Matthew S. *The Fullness of Time: Temporalities of the Fifteenth-Century Low Countries*. Chicago, IL: University of Chicago Press, 2017.

Chandavarkar, Rajnarayan. Plague Panic and Epidemic Politics in India, 1896–1914. In: Terence Ranger and Paul Slack, eds., *Epidemics and Ideas: Essays on the Historical Perception of Pestilence*, 203–40. Cambridge: Cambridge University Press, 1992.

Charlier, Jacques. *La peste à Bruxelles de 1667 à 1669 et ses conséquences démographiques*. Brussels: Pro Civitate, 1969.

Chiffoleau, Jacques. La violence au quotidien. Avignon au XIVe siècle d'après les registres de la Cour temporelle. *Mélanges de l'école française de Rome* 92, 2 (1980), 325–71.

Christakos, George, Ricardo A. Olea, Marc L. Serre, Hwa-Lung Yu, and Lin-Lin Wang. *Interdisciplinary Public Health Reasoning and Epidemic Modelling: The Case of the Black Death*. Berlin: Springer, 2005.

Christiaens, W., and M. Evers. *Patriotse illusies in Amsterdam en Harderwijk: De patriottentijd in Amsterdam en Harderwijk, weerspiegeld in de brieven van Steven Jan en Jakob van Geuns, zonen van de Harderwijkse hoogleraar Matthias van Geuns, 1784–1788*. Hilversum: Verloren, 2002.

Cipolla, Carlo. *Cristofano and the Plague: A Study in the History of Public Health in the Age of Galileo*. Berkeley, CA: University of California Press, 1973.

Cipolla, Carlo. *Fighting the Plague in Seventeenth-Century Italy*. Madison, WI: University of Wisconsin Press, 1981.

Claridge, Jordan, Vincent Delabastita, and Spike Gibbs. (In-Kind) Wages and Labour Relations in the Middle Ages: It's Not (All) About the Money. *Explorations in Economic History* 94 (2024), 101626.

Clauzel, Denis. Les maladies dans le Nord de la France au XIVe siècle. *De Franse Nederlanden - Les Pays-Bas Français* 12 (1987), 144–57.

Cluse, C.M. De Jodenvervolgingen ten tijde van de pest (1349–50) in de zuidelijke Nederlanden. In: *De pest in de Nederlanden. Medisch-historische beschouwingen 650 jaar na de Zwarte Dood*, 135–73. Brussels: Koninklijke Academie voor Geneeskunde van België, 1999.

Cnops, P. Het Sint-Elisabethklooster te Brussel tijdens de dysenterie van 1780. *Eigen Schoon en de Brabander* 51, 5/6 (1968), 265–8.

Coccoli, Lorenzo. The Moral Economy of Epidemics: Emergency, Charitable Institutions and Poor Relief in Early Modern Italian Plague Regulations. In: Tanja Skambraks and Martin Lutz, eds., *Reassessing the Moral Economy: Religion and Economic Ethics from Ancient Greece to the 20th Century*, 137–54. Cham: Palgrave Macmillan, 2023.

Coenen, Jean. *Baanderheren boeren & burgers. Een overzicht van de geschiedenis van Boxtel, Liempde en Gemonde*. Boxtel: Uitgeverij Æneas BV, 2004.

Cohn, Samuel K. Last Wills: Family, Women and the Black Death in Central Italy. In: Samuel K. Cohn, ed., *Women in the Streets: Essays on Sex and Power in Renaissance Italy*, 39–56. Baltimore, MD: John Hopkins University Press, 1996.

Cohn, Samuel K. *The Black Death Transformed: Disease and Culture in Early Renaissance Europe*. London: Arnold, 2001.

Cohn, Samuel K. *Popular Protest in Late Medieval Europe: Italy, France, and Flanders*. Manchester: Manchester University Press, 2004.

Cohn, Samuel K. *Lust for Liberty. The Politics of Social Revolt in Medieval Europe, 1200–1425*. Cambridge, MA: Harvard University Press, 2006.

Cohn, Samuel K. The Black Death and the Burning of Jews. *Past and Present* 196, 1 (2007), 3–36.

Cohn, Samuel K. *Cultures of Plague: Medical Thinking at the End of the Renaissance*. Oxford: Oxford University Press, 2010.

Cohn, Samuel K. Pandemics: Waves of Disease, Waves of Hate from the Plague of Athens to A.I.D.S. *Historical Research* 85, 230 (2012), 535–55.

Cohn, Samuel K. Renaissance Attachment to Things: Material Culture in Last Wills and Testaments. *Economic History Review* 65, 3 (2012), 984–1004.

Cohn, Samuel K. Plague Violence and Abandonment from the Black Death to the Early Modern Period. *Annales de démographie historique* 134, 2 (2017), 39–61.

Cohn, Samuel K. Cholera Revolts: A Class Struggle We May Not Like. *Social History* 42, 2 (2017), 162–80.

Cohn, Samuel K. *Epidemics: Hate and Compassion from the Plague of Athens to AIDS*. Oxford: Oxford University Press, 2018.

Cohn, Samuel K. Fear and the Corpse: Cholera and Plague Riots Compared. In: Christos Lynteris and Nicholas H.A. Evans, eds., *Histories of Post-Mortem Contagion: Infectious Corpses and Contested Burials*, 55–81. New York: Palgrave Macmillan, 2018.

Cohn, Samuel K., and Guido Alfani. Households and Plague in Early Modern Italy. *Journal of Interdisciplinary History* 38, 2 (2007), 177–205.

Cohn, Samuel K., and Ruth Kutalek. Historical Parallels, Ebola Virus Disease and Cholera: Understanding Community Distrust and Social Violence with Epidemics. *PLoS Currents Outbreaks* 8 (2016), 1–8.

Coomans, Janna. Varkens van de werf: Stadsreiniging in laatmiddeleeuws Utrecht. *Tijdschrift Oud-Utrecht* 85 (2012), 60–6.

Coomans, Janna. Policing Female Food Vendors in the Late Medieval Netherlands. *Yearbook of Women's History* 36 (2016), 97–113.

Coomans, Janna. Food Offenders: Public Health and the Marketplace in the Late Medieval Low Countries. In: Carole Rawcliffe and Claire Weeda, eds., *Policing the Urban Environment in Premodern Europe*, 121–48. Amsterdam: Amsterdam University Press, 2019.

Coomans, Janna. *Community, Urban Health and Environment in the Late Medieval Low Countries*. Cambridge: Cambridge University Press, 2021.

Coomans, Janna. Making Good and Breaking Bad: Materiality and Community in Netherlandish Cities, 1380–1520. *English Historical Review* 137, 587 (2022), 1053–81.

Coomans, Janna. Policing Itinerant Poor in the Northern Low Countries, 1450–1750: Making Vagrants. *BMGN: Low Countries Historical Review* 138, 2 (2023), 3–31.

Coomans, Janna and Guy Geltner. On the Street and in the Bathhouse. Medieval Galenism in Action? *Anuario de estudios medievales* 43, 1 (2013), 53–82.

Coomans, Janna, Léa Hermenault, Rogier van Kooten, and Claire Weeda. Plague, Religion and Urban Space in Sixteenth-Century Antwerp. *Social History of Medicine* 37, 3 (2024), 583–610.

Cooper, John P. Patterns of Inheritance and Settlement by Great Landowners from the Fifteenth to the Eighteenth Centuries. In: Jack Goody, Joan Thirsk, and Edward P. Thompson, eds., *Family and Inheritance: Rural Society in Western Europe 1200–1800*, 192–327. Cambridge: Cambridge University Press, 1978.

Coopmans, J.P.A. *De rechtstoestand van de godshuizen te 's-Hertogenbosch vóór 1629*. PhD Thesis: Radboud Universiteit Nijmegen, 1964.

Corporaal, Marguérite, and Lotte Jensen. Famine and "Hongersnood" as Transnational Memory: Literary Legacies of the 1840s Food Crises in Ireland and the Netherlands. *Memory Studies* 18, 6 (2024), 1365–80.

Coumans, Virginie. Notes sur l'ergotisme en Brabant au Moyen Âge, particulièrement à Oplinter. *Revue belge de philologie et d'histoire* 80, 4 (2002), 1125–41.

Craig, Heidi. "Villanies of that Damnd Kéeper": Caregiving, Criminality, and Contagion in Early Modern England. *Early Modern Women: An Interdisciplinary Journal* 16, 1 (2021), 72–81.

Criado Perez, Caroline. *Invisible Women: Exposing Data Bias in a World Designed for Men*. New York: Random House, 2019.

Cristoferi, Davide, ed., *Socio-Economic Inequalities during the Conjuncture of the Fourteenth Century: Sources and Methods, Dynamics and Representations (Italy and Europe, c. 1270 –c. 1350)*. Florence: Firenze University Press, 2025.

Crosby, Alfred W. *The Columbian Exchange: Biological and Cultural Consequences of 1492*. Westport, CO: Greenwood Press, 1972.

Cummins, Neil. Marital Fertility and Wealth during the Fertility Transition: Rural France, 1750–1850. *Economic History Review* 66, 2 (2013), 449–76.

Cummins, Neil. Lifespans of the European Elite, 800–1800. *Journal of Economic History* 77, 2 (2017), 406–39.

Cummins, Neil, Morgan Kelly, and Cormac Ó Gráda. Living Standards and Plague in London, 1560–1665. *Economic History Review* 69, 1 (2016), 3–34.

Curtis, Daniel R. The Impact of Land Accumulation and Consolidation on Population Trends in the Pre-Industrial Period: Two Contrasting Cases in the Low Countries. *Historical Research* 87, 236 (2014), 194–228.

Curtis, Daniel R. *Coping with Crisis: The Resilience and Vulnerability of Pre-Industrial Settlements*. Farnham: Ashgate, 2014.

Curtis, Daniel R. An Agro-Town Bias? Re-Examining the Micro-Demographic Model for Southern Italy in the Eighteenth Century. *Journal of Social History* 48, 3 (2015), 685–713.

Curtis, Daniel R. Was Plague an Exclusively Urban Phenomenon? Plague Mortality in the Seventeenth-Century Low Countries. *Journal of Interdisciplinary History* 47, 2 (2016), 139–70.

Curtis, Daniel R. Danger and Displacement in the Dollard: The 1509 Flooding of the Dollard Sea (Groningen) and its Impact on Long-Term Inequality in the Distribution of Property. *Environment and History* 22, 1 (2016), 103–35.

Curtis, Daniel R. Did the Commons Make Medieval and Early Modern Rural Societies More Equitable? A Survey of Evidence from across Western Europe, 1300–1800. *Journal of Agrarian Change* 16, 4 (2016), 646–64.

Curtis, Daniel R. Preserving the Ordinary: Social Resistance during Second Pandemic Plagues in the Low Countries. In: Christopher M. Gerrard, Paolo Forlin, and Peter J. Brown, eds., *Waiting for the Ends of the World: Perceptions of Disaster and Risk in Medieval Europe*, 280–97. London: Routledge, 2020.

Curtis, Daniel R. All Equal in the Presence of Death? Epidemics and Redistribution in the Pre-Industrial Period. In: Guido Alfani and Erik Thoen, eds., *Inequality in Rural Europe (Late Middle Ages – 18th Century)*, 123–42. Turnhout: Brepols, 2020.

Curtis, Daniel R. From One Mortality Regime to Another? Mortality Crises in Late Medieval Haarlem, Holland, in Perspective. *Speculum* 96, 1 (2021), 127–55.

Curtis, Daniel R. The Female Experience of Epidemics in the Early Modern Low Countries. *Dutch Crossing: Journal of Low Countries Studies* 45, 1 (2021), 3–20.

Curtis, Daniel R. Reduction in Grain Pollen Indicates Population Decline, but not Necessarily Black Death Mortality. *Nature Ecology & Evolution* 6 (2022), 1626–7.

Curtis, Daniel R. The Erasmian Way? Integrating Historical Analysis with Contemporary Challenges. *History Collective* 1, 1 (2023), 79–84.

Curtis, Daniel R. Trade, Production, and Disease in the Middle Ages. In: Hannele Klemettilä and Victoria McAlister, eds., *Routledge Medieval Encyclopedia*, 1–8. London: Routledge, 2024.

Curtis, Daniel R. Plague and Epidemic Disease in the Northern Parts of the Low Countries, 1349–1450: Evidence, Limitations, and Implications. *TSEG: Low Countries Journal of Social and Economic History* 21, 2 (2024), 75–104.

Curtis, Daniel R. Disasters. In: Tim Soens, ed., *A Cultural History of the Environment: Oceanic Age (1200CE – 1550CE)*, III. London: Bloomsbury, 2026.

Curtis, Daniel R. Where's the Disaster in Disaster Studies? Temporal and Spatial Complexities in Assessing Impact. *Journal of Disaster Studies* 2, 2 (2025), 33–61.

Curtis, Daniel R. In One Hand and Out the Other? Women's Ownership and Access to Land in a Seventeenth-Century Rural Community, Oudenbosch (West Brabant, Netherlands). *Working Paper, Rural History Conference, Coimbra, September 2025.*

Curtis, Daniel R. *The Impact of Epidemics on Women: A Long-Run History.* Cambridge: Cambridge University Press, 2026.

Curtis, Daniel R., and Bram van Besouw. Lifecycle Land Decumulation Strategies in a Seventeenth-Century Rural Community. *Economic History Review* 78, 4 (2025), 1088–117.

Curtis, Daniel R., Bram van Besouw, and Bram Hilkens. Household, Family, and Community Responses to the Direct Costs of Epidemics. *The History of the Family* 30, 3 (2025), 329–39.

Curtis, Daniel R., and Jessica Dijkman. The Escape from Famine in the Northern Netherlands: A Reconsideration Using the 1690s Harvest Failures and a Broader Northwest European Perspective. *The Seventeenth Century* 34, 2 (2019), 229–58.

Curtis, Daniel R., Jessica Dijkman, Thijs Lambrecht, and Eric Vanhaute. Low Countries. In: Guido Alfani and Cormac Ó Gráda, eds., *Famine in European History*, 119–40. Cambridge: Cambridge University Press, 2017.

Curtis, Daniel R., and Joris Roosen. On the Importance of History. *Inference* 4, 2 (2018).

Curtis, Daniel R., and Joris Roosen. The Sex-Selective Impact of the Black Death and Recurring Plagues in the Southern Netherlands, 1349–1450. *American Journal of Physical Anthropology* 164, 2 (2017), 246–59.

Curtis, Daniel R., and Qijun Han. The Female Mortality Advantage in the Seventeenth-Century Rural Low Countries. *Gender and History* 33, 1 (2021), 50–74.

Daelemans, Frank. Leiden 1581: Een sociodemografisch onderzoek. *AAG Bijdragen* 19 (1975), 137–215.

Daelemans, Frank. Tithe Revenues in Rural South Western Brabant, Fifteenth to Eighteenth Century. In: Herman Van der Wee and Eddy H.G. van Cauwenberghe, eds., *Productivity of Land and Agricultural Innovation in the Low Countries (1250–1800)*, 25–41. Louvain: Publications du centre belge d'histoire rurale, 1978.

Dale, J.H. van. De pest te Sluis, in de eerste helft der zeventiende eeuw. *Bijdragen tot de Oudheidkunde en Geschiedenis, inzonderheid van Zeeuwsch Vlaanderen* 3 (1858), 180–9.

Dam, Petra van. The Fight Against Cholera in Amsterdam in the Nineteenth Century: Clean Drinking Water as a New Weapon Against Disease. *Codex Historiae* 41, 2 (2020), 50–4.

Davies, Sara E., and Belinda Bennett. A Gendered Human Rights Analysis of Ebola and Zika: Locating Gender in Global Health Emergencies. *International Affairs* 92, 5 (2016), 1041–60.

Dean, Katharine, R., Fabienne Krauer, Lars Walløe, Lingjaerde, Ole Christian, Barbara Bramanti, Nils C. Stenseth, and Boris V. Schmid. Human Ectoparasites and the Spread of Plague in Europe during the Second Pandemic. *Proceedings of the National Academy of Sciences* 115, 6 (2018), 1304–9.

Dean, Trevor. Plague and Crime: Bologna, 1348–1351. *Continuity and Change* 30, 3 (2015), 367–93.

De Backer, Christian. Maatregelen tegen de pest te Diest in de vijftiende en zestiende eeuw. In: Anon., ed., *De pest in de Nederlanden. Medisch-historische beschouwingen 650 jaar na de Zwarte Dood*, 183–209. Brussels: Koninklijke Academie voor Geneeskunde van België, 1999.

De Blécourt, Willem, Willem Frijhoff, and Marijke Gijswijt-Hofstra, eds., *Grenzen van genezing: Gezondheid, ziekte en genezen in Nederland, zestiende tot begin twintigste eeuw.* Hilversum: Verloren, 1993.

De Boer, Dick E.H. *Graaf en grafiek. Sociale en economische ontwikkelingen in het middeleeuwse "Noordholland" tussen ± 1345 en ± 1415*. Leiden: New Rhine Publishers, 1978.

De Brouwer, Luud. "De aenclevende sieckte": De pest in Tilburg voor 1630. *Tilburg: Tijdschrift voor Geschiedenis, Monumenten en Cultuur* 13, 1 (1995), 3–13.

De Brouwer, Luud. Erfenisperikelen ten tijde van pest. *De Brabantse Leeuw* 49, 2 (2000), 74–83.

De Cupere, Bea, Lien Speleers, Piers D. Mitchell, Ann Degraeve, Marc Meganck, Emma Bennion-Pedley, et al. A Multidisciplinary Analysis of Cesspits from Late Medieval and Post-Medieval Brussels, Belgium: Diet and Health in the Fourteenth to Seventeenth Centuries. *International Journal of Historical Archaeology* 26 (2022), 531–72.

De Cuyper, Jan. Egied van der Hoye, deken van de Kortrijkse kapittelkerk, bestrijder van de beweging der Flagellanten (-1348–+-1361). *Handelingen van het Genootschap voor Geschiedenis* 108, 3/4 (1971), 174–91.

Deforce, Koen, Marie-Laure Van Hove, and Didier Willems. Analysis of Pollen and Intestinal Parasite Eggs from Medieval Graves from Nivelles, Belgium: Taphonomy of the Burial Ritual. *Journal of Archaeological Science: Reports* 4 (2015), 596–604.

De Graaf, Beatrice. "Dat een ieder zich beijvert zijn zwakke krachten in te spannen". Veerkracht en cholera in de negentiende eeuw. *De Moderne Tijd* 6, 4 (2022), 272–98.

De Graaf, Beatrice, Lotte Jensen, Rina Knoeff, and Catrien Santing. Dancing with Death. A Historical Perspective on Coping with Covid-19. *Risks, Hazards, & Crisis in Public Policy* 12, 3 (2021), 346–67.

Degroot, Dagomar. *The Frigid Golden Age: Climate Change, the Little Ice Age, and the Dutch Republic, 1560–1720*. Cambridge: Cambridge University Press, 2018.

De Haan, H.J., and Peter C.M Hoppenbrouwers. Intergenerational Transfer of Rural Property in the Netherlands. Law, Moral Code and Practice (16th–20th Centuries). *Mélanges de l'école française de Rome* 110, 1 (1988), 339–55.

De Hellinga, G. Amsterdamsche pesthuizen. *Nederlandse Tijdschrift voor Geneeskunde* 72 (1928), 5912–38.

De Herdt, René. La peste bovine et le cheptel de la châtellenie de Warneton au XVIIIe siècle. *Mémoires de la société d'histoire de Comines, Warneton et de la région* 6 (1976), 289–307.

De Iongh, S. De ontwrichtende pest? *Skript* 11 (1989), 109–11.

De Jager, H. Bijdrage tot de geschiedenis van het klooster van St. Andries te Rugge en van de kloosters der Cellezusters en Cellebroeders te Brielle. *Bijdragen voor Vaderlandsche Geschiedenis en Oudheidkunde* 3, 1 (1882), 119–75.

De Keyzer, Maïka. *Inclusive Commons and the Sustainability of Peasant Communities in the Medieval Low Countries*. Routledge: New York, 2018.

De Keyzer, Maïka. Access Versus Influence: Peasants in Court in the Late Medieval Low Countries. In: Miriam Müller, ed., *The Routledge Handbook of Medieval Rural Life*, 113–37. London: Routledge, 2021.

De Keyzer, Maïka, Tim Soens, and Christophe Verbruggen, eds., *Mens en natuur: Een geschiedenis*. Ghent: Academia Press, 2024.

Dekker, Rudolph. *Holland in beroering: Oproeren in de 17de en 18de eeuw*. Ambo: Baarn, 1982.

Dekker, Rudolph. Women in Revolt: Popular Protest and its Social Basis in Holland in the Seventeenth and Eighteenth Centuries. *Theory and Society* 16, 3 (1987), 337–62.

Dekker, Theo. God's Invisible Particles as an Explanation for the Rinderpest Outbreak (1713–1714): The Reception of Medical Knowledge in the Dutch

Republic. *European Journal for the History of Medicine and Health* 79, 1 (2022), 152–68.

Dekker, Theo. Coping with Epidemics in Early Modern Chronicles, The Low Countries, 1500–1800. In: Hanneke van Asperen and Lotte Jensen, eds., *Dealing with Disasters from Early Modern to Modern Times: Cultural Responses to Catastrophes*, 229–48. Amsterdam: Amsterdam University Press, 2023.

De Kwant, Art-Jan. "Waer datmen gingh/stont/ofte sach/ Het overal met dooden lach". De pestepidemie te Leiden, 1635. *Leids Jaarboekje voor Geschiedenis en Oudheidkunde van Leiden en Omstreken* 113 (2021), 28–45.

Delafaille, Frans Edward. *Hongersnooden en volksziekten: Episoden uit de geschiedenis van Mechelen*. Mechelen: Drukkerij H. Dierickx-Beke Zonen, 1870.

Delmaire, Bernard. Contribution à l'étude de la peste au bas Moyen Âge. Un fragment de compte inédit de l'abbaye de Saint-Bertin pour Bas-Warneton. *Mémoires de la société d'histoire de Comines, Warneton et de la région* 11 (1981), 35–50.

Delumeau, Jean. *La peur en occident, XIVe–XVIIIe siècle. Une cité assiégée*. Paris: Fayard, 1978.

Demets, Lisa. Spies, Instigators, and Troublemakers: Gendered Perceptions of Rebellious Women in Late Medieval Flemish Chronicles. *Journal of Women's History* 33, 2 (2021), 12–34.

De Meyere, Jos. Sint Sebastiaan op enkele schilderijen van Utrechtse caravaggisten. *Jaarboek Oud Utrecht* (2020), 179–99.

De Moor, Geertruida. Adriana Stoffelsdr. uit Gorinchem, helpster tijdens het optreden van de zweetziekte in het klooster Leeuwenhorst bij Noordwijkerhout in het jaar 1529/30. *Oud-Gorcum-Varia* 4 (1985), 5–9.

De Moor, Tine. Common Land and Common Rights in Flanders. In: Tine De Moor, Leigh Shaw-Taylor, and Paul Warde, eds., *The Management of Common land in Northwest Europe, c. 1500–1850*, 113–42. Turnhout: Brepols, 2002.

De Moor, Tine. The Silent Revolution: A New Perspective on the Emergence of Commons, Guilds, and Other Forms of Corporate Collective Action in Western Europe. *International Review of Social History* 53, 16 (2008), 179–212.

De Moor, Tine. *The Dilemma of the Commoners: Understanding the Use of Common-Pool Resources in Long-Term Perspective*. Cambridge: Cambridge University Press, 2015.

De Moor, Tine. Dare to Dig! More History is Needed to Take Historical Demography a Few Steps Further... In: Koen Matthijs, Saskia Hin, Jan Kok, and Hideko Matsuo, eds., *The Future of Historical Demography: Upside Down and Inside Out*, 16–18. Louvain: Acco, 2016.

De Moor, Tine, and Jan Luiten van Zanden. "Every Woman Counts": A Gender-Analysis of Numeracy in the Low Countries during the Early Modern Period. *Journal of Interdisciplinary History* 41, 2 (2010), 179–208.

De Moor, Tine, and Jan Luiten van Zanden. Girl Power: The European Marriage Pattern and Labour Markets in the North Sea Region in the Late Medieval and Early Modern Period. *Economic History Review* 63, 1 (2010), 1–33.

De Moreau de Gerbehaye, Claude. Une dépêche cryptée adressée au gouverneur luxembourgeois de la forteresse de Montmédy (1637). *Bulletin de la commission royale d'histoire* 175 (2009), 413–46.

Den Boer, Pim. Naar een geschiedenis van de dood. Mogelijkheden tot onderzoek naar de houding ten opzichte van de dode en de dood ten tijde van de Republiek. *Tijdschrift voor Geschiedenis* 89, 2 (1976), 161–201.

Deneweth, Heidi, and Patrick Wallis. Households, Consumption and the Development of Medical Care in the Netherlands, 1650–1900. *Journal of Social History* 49, 3 (2016), 532–57.

Dennison, Tracy, and Sheilagh Ogilvie. Does the European Marriage Pattern Explain Economic Growth? *Journal of Economic History* 74, 3 (2014), 651–93.

Depauw, Ewout, and Deborah Oxley. Toddlers, Teenagers, and Terminal Heights: The Importance of Puberty for Male Adult Stature, Flanders, 1800–76. *Economic History Review* 72, 3 (2019), 925–52.

De Pleijt, Alexandra, and Jan Luiten van Zanden. Two Worlds of Female Labour: Gender Wage Inequality in Western Europe, 1300–1900. *Economic History Review* 74, 3 (2021), 611–38.

De Potter, Frans. *Geschiedenis der stad Kortrijk*. Ghent: Drukkerij C. Annoot-Braeckman, 1874.

Deregnaucourt, Jean-Pierre. Le testament. Un reflet de la conjoncture sanitaire, individuelle et collective. L'exemple de Douai au bas Moyen Âge. *Revue du Terroir* 24 (1985), 117–29.

Deregnaucourt, Jean-Pierre. *Autour de la mort à Douai: Attitudes pratiques et croyances, 1200–1500*. PhD Thesis: Université Lille 3 Charles-de-Gaulle, 1992.

Derville, Alain. L'hôpital Saint-Julien de Cambrai au XIVe siècle. Étude économique. *Revue du Nord* 70, 277 (1988), 285–318.

Derville, Alain. La population du Nord au Moyen Age. I: Avant 1384. *Revue du Nord* 80, 326/7 (1998), 501–30.

Derville, Alain. *Les villes de Flandre et d'Artois (900–1500)*. Villeneuve d'Ascq: Presses universitaires du septentrion, 2002.

Der Weduwe, Arthur. *State Communication and Public Politics in the Dutch Golden Age*. Oxford: Oxford University Press, 2023.

Desierto, Desiree, and Mark Koyama. The Political Economy of Status Competition: Sumptuary Laws in Preindustrial Europe. *Journal of Economic History* 84, 2 (2024), 479–516.

Desportes, Pierre. Réceptions et inscriptions à la bourgeoisie de Lille aux XIVème et XVème siècles. *Revue du Nord* 62, 246 (1980), 541–71.

Despy, Georges. La "grande peste noire de 1348". A-t-elle touché le roman pays de Brabant? In: Anon., ed., *Centenaire du séminaire d'histoire médiévale de l'Université Libre de Bruxelles 1876–1976*, 195–217. Brussels: La renaissance du livre, 1977.

De Vos, A.G. *Het Heilige Geest- en Pesthuis ter Nieuwerkerk binnen Dordrecht*. Dordrecht: H.R. van Elk, 1869.

De Vos, Gustaaf. *"Onser Liever Vrouwe" hospitaal van Geeraardsbergen, van zijne stichting af tot na de Fransche omwenteling*. Geraardsbergen: Van Nieuwenhove, 1903.

Devos, Isabelle. *Allemaal beestjes: Mortaliteit en morbiditeit in Vlaanderen, 18de–20ste eeuw*. Ghent: Academia Press, 2006.

Devos, Isabelle, and Tine Van Rossem. Oud, ouder, oudst. Regionale en lokale verschillen in sterfte in het graafschap Vlaanderen tijdens de zeventiende en achttiende eeuw. *De Zeventiende Eeuw* 33 (2017), 39–53.

Devos, Isabelle, Angélique Janssens, Mayra Murkens, and Tim Riswick. Navigeren door de complexiteit van de coronapandemie: Perspectieven vanuit de historische demografie. *Tijdschrift voor Geschiedenis* 137, 2 (2024), 183–93.

Devos, Isabelle, Mélanie Bourguignon, Emmanuel Debruyne, Yoann Doignon, Thierry Eggerickx, Hilde Greefs, et al. The Spanish Flu in Belgium, 1918–1919. A State of the Art. *Historical Social Research / Historische Sozialforschung* 33S (2021), 251–83.

De Vries, Jan. An Inquiry into the Behaviour of Wages in the Dutch Republic and the Southern Netherlands, 1580–1800. In: I. Schöffer, ed., *Acta Historiae Neerlandicae: Studies on the History of the Netherlands*, X, 79–97. The Hague: Martinus Nijhoff, 1978.

De Vries, Jan. *Barges and Capitalism. Passenger Transportation in the Dutch Economy, 1632–1839*. Wageningen: AAG Bijdragen, 1978.

De Vries, Jan. The Economic Crisis of the Seventeenth Century After Fifty Years. *Journal of Interdisciplinary History* 40, 2 (2009), 151–94.

De Vries, Jan, and Ad. van der Woude. *The First Modern Economy: Success, Failure, and Perseverance of the Dutch Economy, 1500–1815*. Cambridge: Cambridge University Press, 1997.

Devriese, Luc. Dood en begraven. Deel 3: Reeuwers in tijden van pest (15de–17de eeuw). *Van Mensen en Dingen* 6, 3/4 (2008), 222–8.

Devriese, Luc, and Griet Maréchal. Kraakhuis in de Gentse Bijloke: Pesthuis. *Ghendtsche Tydinghen* 48, 4 (2019), 310–17.

De Waardt, Hans. *Toverij en samenleving: Holland 1500–1800*. The Hague: Stichting Hollandse Historische Reeks, 1991.

De Waele, Tom. Subjects' Strategies Against Lordship in Burgundian and Habsburg Flanders. *Rural History* 35, 2 (2024), 314–41.

DeWitte, Sharon. Age Patterns of Mortality during the Black Death in London, A.D. 1349–1350. *Journal of Archaeological Science* 37, 12 (2010), 3394–400.

DeWitte, Sharon, and James W. Wood. Selectivity of Black Death Mortality with Respect to Pre-Existing Health. *Proceedings of the National Academy of Sciences* 105, 5 (2008), 1436–41.

DeWitte, Sharon, and Gail Hughes-Morey. Stature and Frailty during the Black Death: The Effect of Stature on Risks of Epidemic Mortality in London, A.D. 1348–1350. *Journal of Archaeological Science* 39, 5 (2012), 1412–19.

DeWitte, Sharon, and Samantha L. Yaussy. Sex Differences in Adult Famine Mortality in Medieval London. *American Journal of Physical Anthropology* 171, 1 (2019), 164–69.

De Zwart, Pim, Daniel Gallardo-Albarrán, and Auke Rijpma. The Demographic Effects of Colonialism: Forced Labor and Mortality in Java, 1834–1879. *Journal of Economic History* 82, 1 (2022), 211–49.

Dhérent, Catherine. *Histoire sociale de la bourgeoisie de Douai, 1280–1350*, I. PhD Thesis: École nationale des chartes, Paris, 1981.

Dhérent, Catherine. *Abondance et crises: Douai, ville frontière, 1200–1375*, I. PhD Thesis: Université de Paris, 1992.

Diamond, Jared M. *Guns, Germs, and Steel: A Short History of Everybody for the Last 13,000 Years*. New York: W.W. Norton, 1997.

Didelot, Xavier, and Charles M. Evans. London Parochial Burial Records from 1563 to 1665 Indicate Higher Plague Death Rates for Males than Females: Some Possible Demographic and Social Explanations. *PLoS ONE* 17, 8 (2022), e0272278.

Diederen, J. Schinnen driemaal geplaagde door een dysenterie-epidemie. *Historie Schinnen Jaarboek* 5 (1992), 4–12.

Diegerick, I. La peste à Ypres (1316 et 1317). *Annales de la société historique, archéologique et littéraire de la ville d'Ypres et de l'ancienne West-Flandre* 1 (1861), 322–6.

Dijkman, Jessica. Bread for the Poor: Poor Relief and the Mitigation of the Food Crises of the 1590s and the 1690s in Berkel, Holland. In: Dominik Collet and Maximilian Schuh, eds., *Famines during the "Little Ice Age" (1300–1800)*, 171–93. Cham: Springer, 2018.

Dijkman, Jessica. Managing Food Crises: Urban Relief Stocks in Pre-Industrial Holland. *Past and Present* 251, 1 (2021), 41–74.

Dincecco, Mark, and Massimiliano Gaetano Onorato. Military Conflict and the Rise of Europe. *Journal of Economic Growth* 21, 3 (2016), 259–82.

Dincecco, Mark, and Massimiliano Gaetano Onorato. *From Warfare to Wealth*. Cambridge: Cambridge University Press, 2017.

Dings, M.P.H.M. Een dysenterie epidemie in 1702. *Tijdschrift voor de Geschiedenis der Geneeskunde, Natuurwetenschappen, Wiskunde en Techniek* 9, 1 (1986), 1–9.

Dings, M.P.H.M. Een dysenterie-epidemie in Limburg, 1676. *De Maasgouw: Tijdschrift voor Limburgse Geschiedenis en Oudheidkunde* 105, 3 (1986), 105–14.

Dippel, Regina. Kanttekening bij Jan van Scorel's Lochorst-Triptiek. *Oud-Holland* 55 (1938), 253–6.

Ditrich, Hans. The Transmission of the Black Death to Western Europe: A Critical Review of the Existing Evidence. *Mediterranean Historical Review* 32, 1 (2017), 25–39.

Dittmar, Jenna M., Piers D. Mitchell, Sarah A. Inskip, Craig Cessford, and John E. Robb. Tuberculosis Before and After the Black Death (1346–1353 CE) in the Hospital of St John the Evangelist in Cambridge, England. *Tuberculosis* 143 (2023), 102401.

Di Tullio, Matteo. Cooperating in Time of Crisis: War, Commons, and Inequality in Renaissance Lombardy. *Economic History Review* 71, 1 (2018), 82–105.

Dixhoorn, Arjan van. The Grain Issue of 1565–1566. Policy Making, Public Opinion, and the Common Good in the Habsburg Netherlands. In: Élodie Lecuppre-Desjardin and Anne-Laure Van Bruaene, eds., *De Bono Communi. The Discourse and Practice of the Common Good in the European City* (13th–16th C.), 171–204. Turnhout: Brepols, 2010.

Dobson, Mary. *Contours of Death and Disease in Early Modern England.* Cambridge: Cambridge University Press, 1997.

Doig, Andrew. *This Mortal Coil: A History of Death.* London: Bloomsbury, 2022.

Dombrecht, Kristof. "Edel, arm en rijk, maakt de dood gelijk?" Sociale ongelijkheid (post mortem) in plattelandsgemeenschappen ten noorden van Brugge (1500–1579). *Revue belge de philologie et d'histoire* 91, 2 (2013), 257–87.

Dombrecht, Kristof, and Wouter Ryckbosch. Wealth Inequality in a Time of Transition: Coastal Flanders in the Sixteenth Century. *TSEG: Low Countries Journal of Social and Economic History* 14, 2 (2017), 63–84.

Dommerholt, Charlotte. "O heere, de plage is dan alzoo in onze stad". Religie in dagboeken tijdens de cholera-epidemie van 1832 in Nederland. *Groniek Historisch Tijdschrift* 227 (2021), 188–95.

Doran, Áine, Christopher L. Colvin, and Eoin McLaughlin. What Can We Learn from Historical Pandemics? A Systematic Review of the Literature. *Social Science and Medicine* 342 (2023), 116534.

Drelichman, Mauricio, and David González Agudo. Housing and the Cost of Living in Early Modern Toledo. *Explorations in Economic History* 54 (2014), 27–47.

Drelichman, Mauricio, and David González Agudo. The Gender Wage Gap in Early Modern Toledo, 1550–1650. *Journal of Economic History* 80, 2 (2020), 351–85.

Dresen-Coenders, Lène. *Het verbond van heks en duivel: Een waandenkbeeld aan het begin van de moderne tijd als symptoom van een veranderende situatie van de vrouw en als middel tot hervorming der zeden.* Baarn: Ambo, 1983.

Driest, Frans van den. Hondenbaan: Hondenslagers op Walcheren. *Heemkundige Kring Walcheren* 38, 1 (2009), 39–44.

Dröge, Jan F. De bouwgeschiedenis van het pesthuis te Leiden. *Leids Jaarboekje voor Geschiedenis en Oudheidkunde van Leiden en Omstreken* 91 (2000), 75–96.

Druwé, Wouter. Pest en recht. Over het contractenrecht, de voedselmarkt en de ziekenzorg tijdens een epidemie. *Revue de droit commercial belge* 10 (2020), 1272–83.

Duiveman, Adriaan. Praying for (the) Community: Disasters, Ritual and Solidarity in the Eighteenth-Century Dutch Republic. *Cultural and Social History* 16, 5 (2019), 543–60.

Duiveman, Adriaan. Breaking the Cycles of Catastrophe: Disaster, Time, and Nation in Dutch Flood Commemoration Books, 1757–1800. In: Hanneke van Asperen and Lotte Jensen, eds., *Dealing with Disasters from Early Modern to Modern Times: Cultural Responses to Catastrophes*, 293–314. Amsterdam: Amsterdam University Press, 2023.

Duiveman, Adriaan. *Nature Triumphed: Disasters, Solidarity, and Identity in the Eighteenth-Century Dutch Republic*. PhD Thesis: Radboud Universiteit Nijmegen, 2023.

Dumolyn, Jan, and Jelle Haemers. Patterns of Urban Rebellion in Medieval Flanders. *Journal of Medieval History* 31, 4 (2005), 369–93.

Dupont, Wannes. "Sie eens 't verzwakte volk". De bestrijding van pest in Antwerpen tijdens de vijftiende en de zestiende eeuw. *Stadsgeschiedenis* 2 (2007), 85–104.

Dyer, Alan. The English Sweating Sickness of 1551: An Epidemic Anatomized. *Medical History* 41, 3 (1997), 362–84.

Dyer, Christopher. *Standards of Living in the Later Middle Ages: Social Change in England, c.1200–1520*. Cambridge: Cambridge University Press, 1998 [1989].

Dyer, Christopher, and Richard Jones, eds., *Deserted Villages Revisited*. Hatfield: University of Hertfordshire Press, 2010.

Edgerton-Tarpley, Kathryn. Family and Gender in Famine: Cultural Responses to Disaster in North China, 1876–1879. *Journal of Women's History* 16, 4 (2004), 119–47.

Eerenbeemt, H.F.J.M. van den. De "rode dood" in stad en meierij van 's-Hertogenbosch: Een dysenterie-epidemie in de jaren 1779–1783. *Economisch-en Sociaal-Historisch Jaarboek* 36 (1973), 75–101.

Eichenberger, Laura. SARS and New York's Chinatown: The Politics of Risk and Blame during an Epidemic of Fear. *Social Science and Medicine* 65, 6 (2007), 1284–95.

Einbinder, Susan L. *After the Black Death: Plague and Commemoration among Iberian Jews*. Philadelphia, PE: University of Pennsylvania Press, 2018.

Eisner, Manuel. Long-Term Historical Trends in Violent Crime. *Crime and Justice* 30 (2003), 83–142.

Ekamper, Peter. De summiere staat van Holland: Een volkstelling van 400 jaar geleden. *Demos: Bulletin over Bevolking en Samenleving* 38 (2022), 1–4.

Engelen, Theo, and Marloes Schoonheim. Mortality in the Netherlands: General Development and Regional Differences. In: Theo Engelen, John R. Shephard, and Yang Wen-shan, eds., *Death at the Opposite Ends of the Eurasian Continent: Mortality Trends in Taiwan and the Netherlands 1850–1945*, 81–98. Amsterdam: Amsterdam University Press, 2011.

Enschedé, Adriaan Justus. *Verslag over de geschiedenis en den eigendom van het St. Elizabeths of Groote Gasthuis, uitgebragt aan den gemeente-raad der stad Haarlem, den 11den Januarij 1860*. Haarlem: Joh. Enschedé & Zonen, 1860.

Epstein, S.R. Cities, Regions and the Late Medieval Crisis: Sicily and Tuscany Compared. *Past and Present* 130, 1 (1991), 3–50.

Epurescu-Pascovici, Ionuț. Facing the Pandemic in the Savoyard Heartlands: Local Communities and the Comital Administration, 1348–1356. *Journal of Medieval History* 51, 1 (2025), 1–24.

Erickson, Amy Louise. Afterword. In: Amanda L. Capan, Briony McDonagh, and Jennifer Aston, eds., *Women and the Land, 1500–1900*, 267–76. Woodbridge: The Boydell Press, 2019.

Ermus, Cindy. *The Great Plague Scare of 1720: Disaster and Diplomacy in the Eighteenth-Century Atlantic World*. Cambridge: Cambridge University Press, 2023.

Espeel, Stef. *Prices and Crises: The Grain Economy in Fourteenth-Century Flanders.* PhD Thesis: University of Antwerp, 2021.

Espeel, Stef. Plague and Hunger. Epidemic-Induced Pressures on Household Purchasing Power in Fourteenth-Century Flanders. *The History of the Family* 30, 3 (2025), 340–70.

Evans, Richard J. *Death in Hamburg. Society and Politics in the Cholera Years, 1830–1910.* Oxford: Clarendon Press, 1987.

Evans, Richard J. Epidemics and Revolutions: Cholera in Nineteenth-Century Europe. *Past and Present* 120, 1 (1988), 123–46.

Eversen, H.P.H. *Over de inlijving van de Nieuwstad bij Maastricht.* Roermond: J.J. Romen en Zonen, 1877.

Faber, J.A. Cattle-Plague in the Netherlands during the Eighteenth Century. *Mededelingen van de Landbouwhogeschool te Wageningen, Nederland* 62, 11 (1962), 1–7.

Faber, J.A. *Dure tijden en hongersnoden in pre-industrieel Nederland.* Amsterdam: Rodopi, 1976.

Feci, Simona. Trame di donne all'indomani della peste romana del 1656. La vicenda dell' «acqua tofana». *Mélanges de l'école française de Rome* 132, 1 (2020), 59–71.

Fertig, Christine, Richard Paping, and Henry French. Introduction. In: Christine Fertig, Richard Paping, and Henry French, eds., *Landless Households in Rural Europe, 1600–1900*, 1–11. Woodbridge: The Boydell Press, 2022.

Finley, Theresa, and Mark Koyama. Plague, Politics, and Pogroms: The Black Death, the Rule of Law, and the Persecution of Jews in the Holy Roman Empire. *Journal of Law and Economics* 61, 2 (2018), 253–77.

Fochesato, Mattia. Origins of Europe's North-South Divide: Population Changes, Real Wages and the "Little Divergence" in Early Modern Europe. *Explorations in Economic History* 70 (2018), 91–131.

Fokker, Adriaan Abraham. *Onderzoek naar den aard van de epidemische en contagieuse ziekten, die vroeger in Zeeland geheerscht hebben.* Middelburg: J.C. & W. Altorffer, 1860.

Foncke, Marianne E. *Water's Worth: Urban Society and Subsidiarity in Seventeenth-Century Holland.* PhD Thesis: University of Amsterdam, 2021.

Foucault, Michel. *Discipline and Punish: The Birth of the Prison.* New York: Vintage Books, 1995 [1975].

Frandsen, Karl-Erik. *The Last Plague in the Baltic Region, 1709–1713.* Copenhagen: Museum Tusculanum Press, 2010.

Francke, Marc, and Matthijs Korevaar. Housing Markets in a Pandemic: Evidence from Historical Outbreaks. *Journal of Urban Economics* 123 (2021), 103333.

Franken, Martien. De uitbarsting van de Patriottenbeweging in Arnhem door de bril van Willem Anne Schimmelpenninck van der Oije (december 1782–augustus 1783). In: B.G.J. Elias, W. Smit-Buit, H.A.M. Ummels, and A.C. van Woerden, eds., *Veluwse en andere geschiedenissen: Liber amicorum drs. R.M. Kemperink*, 141–58. Hilversum: Verloren, 2010.

Franklin, Peter. Peasant Widows' "Liberation" and Remarriage Before the Black Death. *Economic History Review* 39, 2 (1986), 186–204.

Friis, A. An Inquiry into the Relations between Economic and Financial Factors in the Sixteenth and Seventeenth Centuries. I: The Two Crises in the Netherlands in 1557. *Scandinavian Economic History Review* 1, 2 (1953), 193–217.

Frijhoff, Willem T.M. Satan en het magisch universum. Raakvlakken, wisselwerking, reminiscenties in Oost-Gelderland sedert de zestiende eeuw. *Tijdschrift voor Geschiedenis* 97, 3 (1984), 382–406.

Frijhoff, Willem T.M. Gods gave afgewezen: Op zoek naar genezing van de pest: Nijmegen, 1635–1636. *Volkskundig Bulletin* 17, 2 (1991), 143–70.

Fritschy, Wantje. *Public Finance of the Dutch Republic in Comparative Perspective: The Viability of an Early Modern Federal State (1570s–1795)*. Leiden: Brill, 2017.

Furió, Antoni. Economic Inequalities and Transformations of the Rural World in the Iberian Peninsula Before and After the Black Death. In: Davide Cristoferi, ed., *Socio-Economic Inequalities during the Conjuncture of the Fourteenth Century: Sources and Methods, Dynamics and Representations (Italy and Europe, c. 1270 –c. 1350)*, 315–38. Florence: Firenze University Press, 2025.

Fusco, Idamaria. The Importance of Prevention and Institutions. Governing the Emergency in the 1690–92 Plague Epidemic in the Kingdom of Naples. *Annales de démographie historique* 134, 2 (2017), 95–123.

Galanaud, Pierre, Anne Galanaud, and Patrick Giraudoux. Historical Epidemics Cartography Generated by Spatial Analysis: Mapping the Heterogeneity of Three Medieval "Plagues" in Dijon. *PLoS ONE* 10, 12 (2015), e0143866.

Gasquet, Francis Aidan. *The Black Death of 1348 and 1349*. London: George Bell and Sons, 1908.

Geens, Sam. The Great Famine in the County of Flanders (1315–17): The Complex Interaction between Weather, Warfare, and Property Rights. *Economic History Review* 71, 4 (2018), 1048–72.

Geens, Sam. *A Golden Age for Labour? Income and Wealth Before and After the Black Death in the Southern Low Countries and the Republic of Florence 1275–1550*. PhD Thesis: University of Antwerp, 2023.

Geens, Sam, and Bruno Blondé. An Apology for Unreal Wages: Building Labourers and Living Standards in the Southern Low Countries (1290–1560). *International Review of Social History* 70, S33 (2025), 21–49.

Gelderblom, Oscar. *Cities of Commerce: The Institutional Foundations of International Trade in the Low Countries, 1250–1650*. Princeton, NJ: Princeton University Press, 2013.

Geldhof, Jozef. De pestepidemie in Brugge 1665–1667. *Biekorf* 75, 3/4 (1974), 305–28.

Geltner, Guy. *Roads to Health: Infrastructure and Urban Wellbeing in Later Medieval Italy*. Philadelphia, PE: University of Pennsylvania Press, 2019.

Geltner, Guy. In the Camp and on the March: Military Manuals as Sources for Studying Premodern Public Health. *Medical History* 63, 1 (2019), 44–60.

Geltner, Guy. The Path to Pistoia: Urban Hygiene Before the Black Death. *Past and Present* 246, 1 (2020), 3–33.

Geltner, Guy. Rural Policing in the Long Trecento: An Urban Project and Its Obstruction. *English Historical Review* 137, 584 (2022), 47–79.

Geltner, Guy, and Claire Weeda. Underground and Over the Sea: More Community Prophylactics in Europe, 1100–1600. *Journal of the History of Medicine and Allied Sciences* 76, 2 (2021), 123–46.

Gemert, Lia van. The Power of the Weaker Vessels: Simon Schama and Johan van Beverwijck on Women. In: Els Kloek, Nicole Teeuwen, and Marijke Huisman, eds., *Women of the Golden Age: An International Debate on Women in Seventeenth-Century Holland, England and Italy*, 39–50. Hilversum: Verloren, 1994.

Génicot, Léopold. Formorture et mortemain dans le comté de Namur après 1431. In: Joseph Balon, ed., *Études d'histoire et d'archéologie Namuroises dédiées à Ferdinand Courtoy*, II, 499–517. Namur: Publication extraordinaire de la société archéologique de Namur, 1962.

Geremia, Claudia Stella Valeria. Plague and Superstition in the Canary Islands: Inquisitorial Trials (1523–1532). *RIVAR (Santiago)* 9, 25 (2022), 77–92.

Gessler, Jan. Remediën tegen de pest te Hasselt in 1598 opgeteekend. *Nederlandsch Tijdschrift voor Volkskunde* 33, 1 (1928), 65–9.

Gijswijt-Hofstra, Marijke. Inleiding. In: Willem de Blécourt, Willem Frijhoff, and Marijke Gijswijt-Hofstra, eds., *Grenzen van genezing: Gezondheid, ziekte en genezen in Nederland, zestiende tot begin twintigste eeuw*, 9–16. Hilversum: Verloren, 1993.

Gill, Geoffrey, Sean Burrell, and Jody Brown. Fear and Frustration—The Liverpool Cholera Riots of 1832. *The Lancet* 358, 9277 (2001), 233–7.

Gingerich, Daniel W., and Jan P. Vogler. Pandemics and Political Development: The Electoral Legacy of the Black Death in Germany. *World Politics* 73, 3 (2021), 393–440.

Gómez, José M., and Miguel Verdú. Network Theory May Explain the Vulnerability of Medieval Human Settlements to the Black Death Pandemic. *Scientific Reports* 7 (2017), 43467.

Gómez, Pablo F. COVID-19 Beyond Euro-American Historicism. *American Historical Review* 127, 3 (2022), 1348–54.

Goorts, Roeland. *War, State and Society in Liège: How a Small State of the Holy Roman Empire Survived the Nine Years' War (1688–1697)*. Louvain: Leuven University Press, 2019.

Gooskens, F.A. Pestepidemieën in Breda tijdens de middeleeuwen (1382–1535). *Jaarboek De Oranjeboom* 39 (1986), 18–54.

Goubert, Pierre. *Beauvais et le Beauvaisis de 1600 à 1730*. Paris: S.E.V.P.E.N., 1960.

Goubert, Pierre. Historical Demography and the Reinterpretation of Early Modern French History: A Research Review. *Journal of Interdisciplinary History* 1, 1 (1970), 37–48.

Govaerts, Sander. *Armies and Ecosystems in Premodern Europe: The Meuse Region, 1250–1850*. York: ARC Humanities Press, 2021.

Goyarts, C.B. De pest te Roosendaal. *Jaarboek Ghulden Roos* 18 (1958), 29–36.

Graff, Anna A., Emma Bennion-Pedley, Ariadin K. Jones, Marissa L. Ledger, Koen Deforce, Ann Degraeve, et al. A Comparative Study of Parasites in Three Latrines from Medieval and Renaissance Brussels, Belgium (14th–17th Centuries). *Parasitology* 147, 13 (2020), 1443–51.

Graas, Tim. De verbeelding van epidemieën en geneesheiligen. Kunst en erfgoed in Nederlandse kerken en kloosters. *Ex Tempore* 104 (2020), 171–95.

Green, Monica H. Women's Medical Practice and Health Care in Medieval Europe. *Signs* 14, 2 (1989), 434–73.

Green, Monica H. The Four Black Deaths. *American Historical Review* 125, 5 (2020), 1601–31.

Green, Monica H. Out of the East (or North or South): A Response to Philip Slavin. *Past and Present* 256, 1 (2022), 283–323.

Green, Monica H. A New Definition of the Black Death: Genetic Findings and Historical Interpretations. *De Medio Aevo* 11, 2 (2022), 139–55.

Green, Monica H., Kathleen Walker-Meikle, and Wolfgang P. Müller. Diagnosis of a "Plague" Image: A Digital Cautionary Tale. *The Medieval Globe* 1, 1 (2015), 310–26.

Grell, Ole Peter. Conflicting Duties: Plague and the Obligations of Early Modern Physicians Towards Patients and Commonwealth in England and The Netherlands. In: Andrew Wear, Johanna Geyer-Kordesch, and Roger French, eds., *Doctors and Ethics: The Historical Setting of Professional Ethics*, 131–52. Leiden: Brill, 1993.

Greve, Timo, and Joris Roosen. Complottheorieën en misinformatie tijdens de coronapandemie: Nieuw fenomeen of herhaalt de geschiedenis zich? *Tijdschrift voor Geschiedenis* 137, 2 (2024), 170–82.

Griffin, Emma. *Bread Winner: An Intimate History of the Victorian Economy*. Padstow: Yale University Press, 2020.

Grijp, Tessel. *Het gasthuis archeologisch onderzocht: Ruimtelijke ontwikkelingen van opgegraven gasthuizen in Nederland van de middeleeuwen tot de Reformatie, en het Joostengasthuis te Utrecht in het bijzonder*. MA Thesis: University of Amsterdam, 2021.

Groenendijk, Henny, and Remi van Schaïk. Isolated and Backward Westerwolde (Groningen, The Netherlands)? *Palaeohistoria* 61/2 (2021), 273–344.

Groenendijk, Leendert F., Fred A. van Lieburg, and John Exalto. "Away with All My Pleasant Things in the World..." Model Death-Bed Accounts of Two Young Victims of the Plague of 1664 in the Dutch Town of Leyden. *Paedagogica Historica* 46, 3 (2010), 271–88.

Gutmann, Myron P. Why They Stayed: The Problem of Wartime Population Loss. *Tijdschrift voor Geschiedenis* 91, 3 (1978), 407–28.

Gutmann, Myron P. *War and Rural Life in the Early Modern Low Countries*. Princeton, NJ: Princeton University Press, 1980.

Guzowski, Piotr. Did the Black Death Reach the Kingdom of Poland in the Mid-Fourteenth Century? *Journal of Interdisciplinary History* 53, 2 (2022), 193–223.

Habermehl, N.D.B. Leven in de schaduw van de dood. In: Paul H.A.M. Abels, Koen Goudriaan, N.D.B. Habermehl, and J.H. Kompagnie, eds., *Duizend jaar Gouda: Een stadsgeschiedenis*, 296–307. Hilversum: Verloren, 2002.

Hachez, Félix. Les fondations charitables de Mons. Chapitre II, Les hôpitaux de malades. Section IIe. Les hôpitaux de Pestiférés. *Annales du cercle archéologique de Mons* 1 (1837), 187–91.

Haensch, Stephanie, Raffaella Bianucci, Michel Signoli, Minoarisoa Rajerison, Michael Schultz, Sacha Kacki, et al. Distinct Clones of *Yersinia pestis* Caused the Black Death. *PLOS Pathogens* 6, 10 (2010), e1001134.

Hager, Anselm, and Hanno Hilbig. Do Inheritance Customs Affect Political and Social Inequality? *American Journal of Political Science* 63, 4 (2019), 758–73.

Haldon, John, Lee Mordechai, Andrew Dugmore, Merle Eisenberg, Georgina Endfield, Adam Izdebski, et al. Past Answers to Present Concerns. The Relevance of the Premodern Past for 21st Century Policy Planners: Comments on the State of the Field. *WIREs Climate Change* 16, 1 (2025), e923.

Hallema, A. Geschiedenis van een militair hospitaal te Breda 1640–1798. *Het Ziekenhuiswezen* 25 (1952), 154–8.

Hallema, A. Uit de geschiedenis van het St. Catharinen-gasthuis, Pesthuis en Stadsziekenhuis. Hoe Kampen zijn Engelenberg-Stichting kreeg. *Kamper Almanak* 25 (1957/8), 193–237.

Ham, Willem A. van. *Macht en gezag in het Markiezaat. Een politiek-institutionele studie over stad en land van Bergen op Zoom (1477–1583)*. Hilversum: Verloren, 2000.

Hamans, Camiel. The Observations of a Voyager Stephanus Hanewinckel on the Dialects of the Meijerij. *Voortgang: Jaarboek voor de Neerlandistiek* 30 (2012), 223–50.

Hamlin, Christopher. "Cholera Forcing": The Myth of the Good Epidemic and the Coming of Good Water. *American Journal of Public Health* 99, 11 (2009), 1946–54.

Han, Qijun, and Daniel R. Curtis. The Female Burden Visualized: Cinematic Representation of Women during Epidemics. *Journal of Popular Culture* 54, 5 (2021), 1116–42.

Han, Qijun, and Daniel R. Curtis. Cinematic Representation of Early Modern Women and Epidemics. *Early Modern Women: An Interdisciplinary Journal* 16, 1 (2021), 123–34.

Han, Qijun, and Daniel R. Curtis. *Infectious Inequalities: Epidemics, Trust, and Social Vulnerabilities in Cinema*. London: Routledge, 2022.

Haneca, Kristof, Vincent Debonne, and Patrick Hoffsummer. The Ups and Downs of the Building Trade in a Medieval City: Tree-Ring Data as Proxies for Economic, Social and Demographic Dynamics in Bruges (c. 1200–1500). *Dendrochronologia* 64 (2020), 125773.

Hanus, Jord. Real Inequality in the Early Modern Low Countries: The City of 's-Hertogenbosch, 1500–1660. *Economic History Review* 66, 3 (2013), 733–56.

Hardin, Garrett. The Tragedy of the Commons. *Science* 162, 3859 (1968), 1243–8.

Harding, Vanessa. Burial of the Plague Dead in Early Modern London. In: J.A.I. Champion, ed., *Epidemic Disease in London*, 53–64. London: Centre for Metropolitan History Working Paper Series, 1993.

Harding, Vanessa. *The Dead and the Living in Paris and London, 1500–1670.* Cambridge: Cambridge University Press, 2002.

Harkness, Deborah E. A View from the Streets: Women and Medical Work in Elizabethan London. *Bulletin of the History of Medicine* 82, 1 (2008), 52–85.

Harman, Sophie. Ebola, Gender and Conspicuously Invisible Women in Global Health Governance. *Third World Quarterly* 37, 3 (2016), 524–41.

Harper, Kristin N., Molly K. Zuckerman, Megan L. Harper, John D. Kingston, and George J. Armelagos. The Origin and Antiquity of Syphilis Revisited: An Appraisal of Old World Pre-Columbian Evidence for Treponemal Infection. *Yearbook of Physical Anthropology* 54 (2011), 99–133.

Harper, Kyle. *The Fate of Rome: Climate, Disease, and the End of an Empire.* Princeton, NJ: Princeton University Press, 2017.

Harper, Kyle. Germs, Genomes, and Global History in the Time of COVID-19. *Journal of Global History* 15, 3 (2020), 350–62.

Harper, Kyle. *Plagues upon the Earth: Disease and the Course of Human History.* Princeton, NJ: Princeton University Press, 2021.

Harrison, Mark. *Contagion: How Commerce Has Spread Disease.* New Haven, CT: Yale University Press, 2012.

Harrison, Mark. Pandemics. In: Mark Jackon, ed., *The Routledge History of Disease*, 129–46. Abingdon: Routledge, 2017.

Hart, Marjolein 't. *The Making of a Bourgeois State: War, Politics and Finance during the Dutch Revolt.* Manchester: Manchester University Press, 1993.

Hart, Marjolein 't. *Oorlog en ongelijkheid. Een inclusieve geschiedenis van de Gouden Eeuw.* Amsterdam: Boom, 2022.

Hart, Paul 't, *Utrecht en de cholera, 1832–1910.* Utrecht: De Walburg Pers, 1990.

Hart, Paul 't, G.J.C. Pouw, and Ronald Rommes. *Gepokt en gemazeld. Gids voor historisch onderzoek naar ziekte en gezondheid in de provincie Utrecht.* Utrecht: Het Utrechts Archief, 2002.

Harvey, Barbara. *Living and Dying in England, 1100–1540: The Monastic Experience.* Oxford: Oxford University Press, 1993.

Hatcher, John. *Plague, Population, and the English Economy, 1348–1530.* Basingstoke: Palgrave, 1977.

Hatcher, John. Mortality in the Fifteenth Century: Some New Evidence. *Economic History Review* 39, 1 (1986), 19–38.

Hatcher, John. England in the Aftermath of the Black Death. *Past and Present* 144, 1 (1994), 3–35.

Hatcher, John. The Great Slump of the Mid-Fifteenth Century. In: Richard Britnell and John Hatcher, eds., *Progress and Problems in Medieval England: Essays in Honour of Edward Miller*, 237–72. Cambridge: Cambridge University Press, 1996.

Hatcher, John, A.J. Piper, and David Stone. Monastic Mortality: Durham Priory, 1395–1529. *Economic History Review* 59, 4 (2006), 667–87.

Hatcher, John, and Judy Stephenson, eds., *Seven Centuries of Unreal Wages: The Unreliable Data, Sources and Methods That Have Been Used for Measuring Standards of Living in the Past.* Cham: Palgrave Macmillan, 2018.

Healey, Jonathan. Famine and the Female Mortality Advantage: Sex, Gender and Mortality in Northwest England, c. 1590–1630. *Continuity and Change* 30, 2 (2015), 153–92.

Hee, Robrecht Van, ed., *Ziek of gezond ten tijde van Keizer Karel. Vesalius en de gezondheidszorg in de 16*de *eeuw*. Ghent: Academia Press, 2000.

Hélin, Etienne. Les recherches sur la mortalité dans le région liégeoise (XVe–XIXe siècles). In: Paul Harsin and Etienne Hélin, eds., *Actes de colloque international de démographie historique*, 155–85. Liège: Université de Liège, 1965.

Helmers, Helmer J., and Geert H. Janssen, eds., *The Cambridge Companion to the Dutch Golden Age.* Cambridge: Cambridge University Press, 2018.

Henderson, John S. Charity and Welfare in Early Modern Tuscany. In: Ole Peter Grell, Andrew Cunningham, and Jon Arrizabalaga, eds., *Health Care and Poor Relief in Counter-Reformation Europe*, 56–86. London: Routledge, 1999.

Henderson, John S. *The Renaissance Hospital: Healing the Body and Healing the Soul.* New Haven, CT: Yale University Press, 2006.

Henderson, John S. Coping with Epidemics in Renaissance Italy: Plague and the Great Pox. In: Linda Clark and Carole Rawcliffe, eds., The *Fifteenth Century: Society in an Age of Plague*, XII, 175–94. Woodbridge: Boydell and Brewer, 2013.

Henderson, John S. Plague and the Social Order in Early Modern Italy: Tuscany, 1630–1633. In: Irena Benyovsky Latin, Martina Stercken, and Tonija Andrić, eds., *Protagonists of Urban Order from the Middle Ages to the Present: Actions, Ideas, Concepts*, 149–64. Amsterdam: Amsterdam University Press, 2025.

Herlihy, David. *Medieval and Renaissance Pistoia: The Social History of an Italian Town.* New Haven, CT: Yale University Press, 1967.

Herlihy, David. Santa Maria Impruneta: A Rural Commune in the Late Middle Ages. In: Nicolai Rubinstein, ed., *Florentine Studies: Politics and Society in Renaissance Florence*, 242–76. London: Faber & Faber, 1968.

Herlihy, David. *The Black Death and the Transformation of the West*, ed. Samuel K. Cohn. Cambridge, MA: Harvard University Press, 1997.

Heuvel, Danielle van den. *Women and Entrepreneurship. Female Traders in the Northern Netherlands, c. 1580–1815.* Amsterdam: Askant, 2007.

Heuvel, Danielle van den. Gender in the Streets of the Premodern City. *Journal of Urban History* 45, 4 (2019), 693–710.

Heyning, Katie. *Turbulente tijden: Zorg en materiële cultuur in Zierikzee in de zestiende eeuw.* Hilversum: Verloren, 2017.

Hildebrand, P. Hollandsche Kapucijnen in de oude Belgische Provincie vóór 1600 geprofest. *Uni trinoque* 4, 6 (1934), 78–80, 98–101.

Hilkens, Bram. Mortality, Morcellation, and the Market: The Impact of Epidemic Disease on Land Distribution in a Seventeenth-Century Holland Village. *The History of the Family* 30, 3 (2025), 413–41.

Hilkens, Bram. Verschillende ongelijkheden? The New History of Old Inequality en *Oorlog en ongelijkheid. TSEG: Low Countries Journal of Social and Economic History* 22, 1 (2025), 75–90.

Hilkens, Bram. *Living Off the Land: Land Inequality in Early Modern Holland.* PhD Thesis: Erasmus University Rotterdam, 2026.

Hilkens, Bram, Bram van Besouw, and Daniel R. Curtis. A Modern Rendition of a Pre-Modern Scenario: Imperfect Institutions and Obscured Vulnerabilities. *Journal for the History of Environment and Society* 5 (2020), 211–21.

Hilton, Rodney. Reasons for Inequality Among Medieval Peasants. *Journal of Peasant Studies* 5, 3 (1978), 271–84.

Hofman, Beno. *Sint Anthony Gasthuis Groningen, 1517–2017: Vijf eeuwen geborgenheid.* Groningen: In Boekvorm, 2017.

Hofstee, E.W. *Korte demografische geschiedenis van Nederland van 1800 tot heden.* Haarlem: Fibula-Van Dishoeck, 1981.

Höhl, Monika. *Die Pest in Hildesheim. Krankheit als Krisenfaktor im städtischen Leben des Mittelalters und der Frühen Neuzeit (1350–1750).* Hildesheim: Stadtarchiv, 2002.

Holleville, Marion, Dominique Castex, Marie-France Deguilloux, and Sacha Kacki. Nouvelles données sur un assemblage ostéoarchéologique en lien avec la première pandémie de peste historique: La nécropole tardoantique du "Clos des Cordeliers" à Sens (Yonne, France). *Bulletins et mémoires de la société d'anthropologie de Paris* 36, 2 (2024), 1–17.

Hollewand, K.E. *Funeral Consumption and Social Distinction in the Early Modern Netherlands.* MA Thesis: Utrecht University, 2011.

Honacker, Karin Van. Résistance locale et émeutes dans les chef-villes brabançonnes aux XVIIe et XVIIIe siècles. *Revue d'histoire moderne et contemporaine* 47, 1 (2000), 37–68.

Hoppenbrouwers, Peter C.M. *Een middeleeuwse samenleving. Het Land van Heusden, ca. 1360 – ca. 1515*, I–II. Wageningen: AAG Bijdragen, 1992.

Hoppenbrouwers, Peter C.M. Doorgifte van erfgoed op het laatmiddeleeuwse platteland. *Madoc* 4 (1994), 88–98.

Hoppenbrouwers, Peter C.M. The Use and Management of Commons in the Netherlands: An Overview. In: Tine De Moor, Leigh Shaw-Taylor, and Paul Warde, eds., *The Management of Common land in Northwest Europe, c. 1500–1850*, 88–112. Turnhout: Brepols, 2002.

Horrell, Sara, Jane Humphries, and Jacob Weisdorf. Malthus's Missing Women and Children: Demography and Wages in Historical Perspective, England 1280–1850. *European Economic Review* 129 (2020), 103534.

Houlbrooke, Ralph. *Death, Religion, and the Family in England, 1480–1750.* Oxford: Oxford University Press, 2000.

Howell, Martha C. *Women, Production, and Patriarchy in Late Medieval Cities.* Chicago, IL: Chicago University Press, 1986.

Howell, Martha C. The Problem of Women's Agency in Late Medieval and Early Modern Europe. In: Sarah Joan Moran and Amanda C. Pipkin, eds., *Women and Gender in the Early Modern Low Countries, 1500–1750*, 21–31. Brill: Leiden, 2019.

Huffmeijer, Jos. Op weg naar Moermont. *De Waterschans* 40 (2010), 35–9.

Huisman, Frank. *Stadsbelang en standsbesef: Gezondheidszorg en medisch beroep in Groningen 1500–1730.* Rotterdam: Erasmus Publishing, 1992.

Huisman, Frank. De maatschappelijke reacties op ziekte. In: Harry Hillen, Eddy Houwaart, and Frank Huisman, eds., *Leerboek medische geschiedenis*, 19–33. Houten: Bohn Stafleu Van Loghum, 2018.

Huiting, Jan. *Domeinen in beweging: Samenleving, bezit en exploitatie in het West-Utrechtse landschap tot in de Nieuwe Tijd.* PhD Thesis: University of Groningen, 2020.

Huizinga, Johan. *The Waning of the Middle Ages: A Study of the Forms of Life, Thought and Art in France and the Netherlands in the XIVth and XVth Centuries.* London: E. Arnold & Company, 1924.

Hulshof, M.H., ed., Gebed en voorschriften tegen pest in een Utrechtsch getijdenboekje uit 1440. *Nederlandse Tijdschrift voor Geneeskunde* 83, 1 (1939), 533–5.

Humphries, Jane, and Jacob Weisdorf. The Wages of Women in England, 1260–1850. *Journal of Economic History* 75, 2 (2015), 405–47.

Hurwich, Judith J. Inheritance Practices in Early Modern Germany. *Journal of Interdisciplinary History* 23, 4 (1993), 699–718.

Hutton, Shennan. Women, Men, and Markets: The Gendering of Market Space in Late Medieval Ghent. In: Albrecht Claessen, ed., *Urban Space in the Middle Ages and the Early Modern Age*, 409–31. Berlin: De Gruyter, 2009.

Huyghebaert, J. Reeuwers in Vlaanderen in 1468. *Biekorf* 68 (1967), 97–104.

Indekeu, Bruno. Van de "rode dood" verlos ons Heer! (Over een dysenterie-epidemie te Lommel, anno 1779). *Te Lomelle op die Campine: Driemaandelijks Tijdschrift van Heemkundige Kring Lommel* 11, 4 (1985), 104–10.

Ingholt, Mathias Mølbak. The Last Hunger Years? The 1826–1832 Mortality Crisis in Denmark. *Scandinavian Journal of History* 48, 4 (2023), 480–502.

Ingholt, Mathias Mølbak, Maarten van Wijhe, Lone Simonsen, and Daniel M. Weinberger. The Disappearance of Malaria from Denmark, 1862–1900. *Economic History Review* (2025), early view.

Israel, Jonathan I. *The Dutch Republic and the Hispanic World, 1606–1661*. Oxford: Oxford University Press, 1982.

Israel, Jonathan I. *The Dutch Republic: Its Rise, Greatness, and Fall, 1477–1806*. New York: Oxford Clarendon Press, 1995.

Israel, Jonathan I. *Conflict of Empires: Spain, the Low Countries and the Struggle for World Supremacy, 1585–1713*. London: The Hambledon Press, 1997.

Izdebski, Adam, Piotr Guzowski, R. Poniat, Lucrezia Masci, J. Palli, C. Vignola, et al. Palaeoecological Data Indicates Land-Use Changes across Europe Linked to Spatial Heterogeneity in Mortality during the Black Death Pandemic. *Nature Ecology & Evolution* 6 (2022), 297–306.

Izdebski, Adam, Martin Bauch, Piotr Guzowski, Scott Mensing, Anna Maria Mercuri, Timothy Newfield, et al. Reply to "Reduction in Grain Pollen Indicates Population Decline, but not Necessarily Black Death Mortality". *Nature Ecology & Evolution* 6 (2022), 1628–9.

Jacquet-Ladrier, Françoise. Les épidémies de peste aux XVIe–XVIIe siècles: L'exemple de Namur. *Cahiers de Sambre et Meuse* 83, 4 (2007), 122–41.

Janse, Antheun. *Ridderschap in Holland: Portret van een adellijke elite in de late middeleeuwen*. Hilversum: Verloren, 2001.

Jansen-Sieben, Ria. Ooggetuigen en flagellanten anno 1349. In: Anon., ed., *De pest in de Nederlanden: Medisch historische beschouwingen 650 jaar na de Zwarte Dood*, 175–98. Brussels: Koninklijke Academie voor Geneeskunde van België, 1999.

Janssens, Angélique, and Tim Riswick. What was Killing Babies in Amsterdam? A Study of Infant Mortality Patterns Using Individual-Level Cause of Death Data, 1856–1904. *Historical Life Course Studies* 13 (2023), 235–64.

Janssens, Paul A., and Walter Van den Branden. De pest in het algemeen en in het bijzonder te Poederlee, Lille, Gierle en Wechelderzande in de zeventiende eeuw. *Jaarboek van de Heemkundige Kring Norbert de Vrijter* 3 (1985), 5–99.

Jedwab, Remi, Amjad M. Khan, Jason Russ, and Esha D. Zaveri. Epidemics, Pandemics, and Social Conflict: Lessons from the Past and Possible Scenarios for COVID-19. *World Development* 147 (2021), 105629.

Jedwab, Remi, Noel D. Johnson, and Mark Koyama. The Economic Impact of the Black Death. *Journal of Economic Literature* 60, 1 (2022), 132–78.

Jedwab, Remi, Noel D. Johnson, and Mark Koyama. Negative Shocks and Mass Persecutions: Evidence from the Black Death. *Journal of Economic Growth* 24 (2019), 345–95.

Jenner, Mark. Death, Decomposition and Dechristianisation? Public Health and Church Burial in Eighteenth-Century England. *English Historical Review* 120, 487 (2005), 615–32.

Jensen, Lotte. "Disaster upon Disaster Inflicted on the Dutch". Singing about Disasters in the Netherlands, 1600–1900. *BMGN: Low Countries Historical Review* 134, 2 (2019), 45–70.

Jensen, Lotte. Cultural Resilience during Nineteenth-Century Cholera Outbreaks in the Netherlands. In: Hanneke van Asperen and Lotte Jensen, eds., *Dealing with Disasters from Early Modern to Modern Times: Cultural Responses to Catastrophes*, 121–36. Amsterdam: Amsterdam University Press, 2023.

Jensen, Lotte. Remembered and Forgotten: The Nineteenth-Century Flemish and Dutch Famine in Cultural Memory. *Dutch Crossing: Journal of Low Countries Studies* 49, 1 (2025), 1–15.

Jensma, Goffe, and Mart van Lieburg. *Het "doktersboek" van Douwe Ales. De medische aantekeningen en recepten van een Friese boer uit 1699*. Rotterdam: Erasmus Publishing, 2011.

Jervis, Ben, Chris Briggs, Alice Forward, Tomasz Gromelski, and Matthew Tompkins. *The Material Culture of English Rural Households c. 1250–1600*. Cardiff: Cardiff University Press, 2023.

Jirková, Pavla. Plague Year 1680 in Central Europe: Using Czech Plague Registers to Monitor Epidemic Progression. In: A.T. Brown, Andy Burn, and Rob Doherty, eds., *Crises in Economic and Social History: A Comparative Perspective*, 213–34. Woodbridge: The Boydell Press, 2015.

Johnson, Bethany L. The Johnes of Glasgow: Searching, Plague and Early Modern Municipal Power. *Social History of Medicine* 35, 4 (2022), 1162–82.

Jones, Lori. *From Diseased Bodies to Disordered Bodies Politic: Rereading Medical Writing on the Plague in England and France, 14th–18th Centuries*. PhD Thesis: University of Ottawa, 2017.

Jones, Lori. Apostumes, Carbuncles, and Botches: Visualizing the Plague in Late Medieval and Early Modern Medical Treatises. In: Rinaldo Fernando Canalis and Massimo Ciavolella, eds., *Disease and Disability in Medieval and Early Modern Art and Literature*, 173–200. Turnhout: Brepols, 2021.

Jordà, Òscar, Sanjay R. Singh, and Alan M. Taylor. Longer-Run Economic Consequences of Pandemics. *Review of Economics and Statistics* 104, 1 (2022), 166–75.

Jordan, William Chester. *The Great Famine: Northern Europe in the Early Fourteenth Century*. Princeton, NJ: Princeton University Press, 1996.

Juch, A. *Voorkomen is beter. Gemeentelijke gezondheidszorg in Arnhem*. Utrecht: Matrijs, 1996.

Kaal, Harm, and Jelle van Lottum. Applied History. Past, Present, and Future. *Journal of Applied History* 3 (2021), 135–54.

Kacki, Sacha. Digging Up the Victims of the Black Death. A Bioarchaeological Perspective on the Second Plague Pandemic. In: Christopher M. Gerrard, Paolo Forlin, and Peter J. Brown, eds., *Waiting for the Ends of the World: Perceptions of Disaster and Risk in Medieval Europe*, 259–79. London: Routledge, 2020.

Kaniewski, David, and Nick Marriner. Conflicts and the Spread of Plagues in Pre-Industrial Europe. *Humanities & Social Sciences Communications* 7 (2020), no. 162.

Kappelhof, Ton C.M. Pest en rode loop in de Baronie van Breda in de tweede helft van de 17e eeuw. *De Oranjeboom* 26 (1973), 75–90.

Kappelhof, Ton C.M. Verzorging van pestlijders op het Brabantse platteland in 1582. *Zorggeschiedenis* 7 (2009), 1–3.

Kappner, Kalle. Did Cholera "Force" the Reform of Urban Water Infrastructure? Lessons from Nineteenth-Century Berlin. *Journal of Urban History* 51, 3 (2024), 545–66.

Karlsson, Martin, Therese Nilsson, and Stefan Pichler. The Impact of the 1918 Spanish Flu Epidemic on Economic Performance in Sweden: An Investigation into the Consequences of an Extraordinary Mortality Shock. *Journal of Health Economics* 36 (2014), 1–19.

Kay, Janet E., István Koncz, Jordan Wilson, Rachel Singer, Merle Eisenberg, Lee Mordechai, et al. Burial Archaeology and the First Plague Pandemic. *Speculum* 100, 2 (2025), 321–64.

Kayser, Edouard M. Le phénomène épidémique dans le duché de Luxembourg à la fin du régime autrichien. *Medizinhistorisches Journal* 24, 1/2 (1989), 65–78.

Kelleher, Margaret. *The Feminization of Famine: Expressions of the Inexpressible?* Durham, NC: Duke University Press, 1997.

Keller, Marcel, Maria A. Spyrou, Christiana L. Scheib, Gunnar U. Neumann, Andrea Kröpelin, Brigitte Haas-Gebhard, et al. Ancient *Yersinia pestis* Genomes from Across Western Europe Reveal Early Diversification during the First Pandemic (541–750). *Proceedings of the National Academy of Sciences* 116, 25 (2019), 12363–72.

Keller, Marcel, Meriam Guellil, Philip Slavin, Lehti Saag, Kadri Irdt, Helja Niinemäe, et al. A Refined Phylochronology of the Second Plague Pandemic in Western Eurasia. *bioRxiv* (2023), 1–30.

Kelly, Morgan, and Cormac Ó Gráda. Living Standards and Mortality Since the Middle Ages. *Economic History Review* 67, 2 (2014), 358–81.

Kelly Wray, Shona. *Communities and Crisis: Bologna during the Black Death.* Leiden: Brill, 2009.

Kerkhoff, A.H.M. *Per imperatief plakkaat: Overheid en pestbestrijding in de Republiek der Zeven Verenigde Nederlanden.* Hilversum: Verloren, 2020.

Kis, Oksana. Defying Death: Women's Experience of the Holodomor, 1932–1933. *Aspasia* 7, 1 (2013), 42–67.

Klein-Hamming, Gea. Van burenplicht tot begrafenisvereniging De Laatste Eer, tijdens het leven van Jacob Mooi. *Op de Hòògte* 23, 1 (2011), 22–7.

Klinkenberg, J. Th. "Dye quade siecte". De pest in Maastricht in de zestiende en zeventiende eeuw. *Tijdschrift voor Sociale Geschiedenis* 16, 3 (1990), 267–86.

Knegtel, Jacob, and Jos Cuijpers, eds., *Rampjaar of jubeljaar? Brabant in 1672–74.* Woudrichem: Pictures Publishers, 2022.

Knibbe, Merijn. Enkele Friese lonen, 1697–1824. *Historia Agriculturae* 38 (2009), 99–110.

Knottnerus, Otto S. Malaria Around the North Sea: A Survey. In: Gerold Wefer, Wolfgang H. Berger, Karl-Ernst Behre, and Eynstein Jansen, eds., *Climate Development and History of the North Atlantic Realm*, 339–53. Berlin: Springer, 2002.

Knottnerus, Otto S. Yeomen and Farmers in the Wadden Sea Coastal Marshes, c. 1500–c. 1900. In: Bas J.P. van Bavel and Peter C.M. Hoppenbrouwers, eds., *Landholding and Land Transfer in the North Sea Area (Late Middle Ages – 19th Century)*, 149–86. Turnhout: Brepols, 2004.

Koene, Bert. *De Caeskopers: Een Zaanse koopmansfamilie in de Gouden Eeuw.* Hilversum: Verloren, 2011.

Kohle, Hubertus. The Road from Rome to Paris: The Birth of a Modern Neoclassicism. In: Dorothy Johnson, ed., *Jacques-Louis David: New Perspectives*, 71–80. Newark, DE: University of Delaware Press, 2006.

Koslofsky, Craig M. *The Reformation of the Dead. Death and Ritual in Early Modern Germany, 1450–1700.* New York: St. Martin's Press, 2000.

Kool-Blokland, Johanna Louise. *De zorg gewogen: Zeven eeuwen godshuizen in Middelburg.* Middelburg: Koninklijk Zeeuwsch Genootschap der Wetenschappen, 1990.

Kooten, Rogier van. Levelling through Space? The Redistributive Capacity of Demographic Decline in Antwerp's Darkest Hour (1584–1586). In: Bruno Blondé, Sam Geens, Hilde Greefs, Wouter Ryckbosch, Tim Soens, and Peter Stabel, eds.,

Inequality and the City in the Low Countries (1200–2020), 231–49. Turnhout: Brepols, 2020.

Kooystra, Ulco. Een ramp voor de stad, maar ook een zegen voor de mensheid. *Historisch Jaarboek Groningen* (2018), 70–87.

Korst, J.K. van der. *Om lijf te leven. Gezondheidszorg en geneeskunst in Nederland circa 1200–1960*. Utrecht: Bohn, Scheltema & Holkema, 1988.

Krauer, Fabienne, and Boris V. Schmid. Mapping the Plague through Natural Language Processing. *Epidemics* 41 (2022), 100656.

Krauer, Fabienne, Hildegunn Viljugreinm, and Katharine R. Dean. The Influence of Temperature on the Seasonality of Historical Plague Outbreaks. *Proceedings of the Royal Society B* 288 (2021), 20202725.

Kuijpers, Erika. *Migrantenstad: Immigratie en sociale verhoudingen in 17ᵉ-eeuwse Amsterdam*. Hilversum: Verloren, 2005.

Kumon, Yuzuru. Adoption, Inheritance, and Wealth Inequality in Pre-Industrial Japan and Western Europe. *Journal of Economic History* 85, 1 (2025), 250–86.

Kuttner, Erich. *Het hongerjaar 1566*. Amsterdam: N.V. Amsterdamsche Boek- en Courantmaatschappij, 1949.

Labbé, Thomas. Aux origines des politiques compassionnelles: Émergence de la sensibilité envers les victimes de catastrophes à la fin du Moyen Âge. *Annales. Histoire, sciences sociales* 74, 1 (2019), 45–71.

Lachenal, Guillaume, and Gaëtan Thomas. Epidemics Have Lost the Plot. *Bulletin of the History of Medicine* 94, 4 (2020), 670–89.

Lachiver, Marcel. *Les années de misère. La famine au temps du Grand Roi*. Paris: Fayard, 1991.

Ladan, Rudolph. De Engelse zweetziekte in Leiden. *Leids Jaarboekje voor Geschiedenis en Oudheidkunde van Leiden en Omstreken* 85 (1993), 51–5.

Ladan, Rudolph. *Gezondheidszorg in Leiden in de late middeleeuwen*. Hilversum: Verloren, 2012.

Ladan, Rudolph. *De pest tijdens het beleg van Leiden*. Leiden: Primavera Pers, 2021.

Lagerlöf, Nils-Petter. From Malthus to Modern Growth: Can Epidemics Explain the Three Regimes? *International Economic Review* 44, 2 (2003), 755–77.

Lambrecht, Thijs. Geboorte, huwelijk en dood: Parochieregisters als bron voor je historisch artikel. *Bladwijzer* 12 (2014), 15–26.

Lambrecht, Thijs, and Wouter Ryckbosch. Economic Inequality in the Rural Southern Low Countries during the Fifteenth Century: Sources, Data and Reflections. In: Giampiero Nigro, ed., *Disuguaglianza economica nelle società preindustriali: Cause ed effetti / Economic Inequality in Pre-Industrial Societies: Causes and Effects*, 205–29. Florence: Firenze University Press, 2020.

Lana Berasain, José Miguel. From Equilibrium to Equity. The Survival of the Commons in the Ebro Basin: Navarra from the 15th to the 20th Centuries. *International Journal of the Commons* 2, 2 (2008), 162–91.

Lauwerier, Roel C.G.M. Ratten in de Nederlandse archeologie. In: Bea De Cupere, Koen Deforce, Koen De Groote, and Kristof Haneca, eds., *Alle dieren groot ende clene: Studies over natuurwetenschappen en archeologie*, 33–44. Brussels: Onroerend Erfgoed, 2025.

Lebon, Pieter. *Een kijk op de hygiënische maatregels en het leefmilieu te Brugge aan de hand van de Brugse hallegeboden (1490–1513): Men beveilt eenighe vuullighede, mesh ofte andre onreynichede wech te doene*. MA Thesis: KU Leuven, 2014.

Leen, J. van der. *Geschiedenis van het pest- en dolhuis der gemeente Rotterdam*. Rotterdam: Gemeente Rotterdam, 1934.

Lejeune, Théophile. *Mémoire historique sur l'ancienne ville de Soignies*. Mons: Dequesne-Masquillier, 1870.

Lemaire, Lucien. *La peste de 1666 à Dunkerque: Étude médico-historique*. Dunkirk: Paul Michel, 1911.

Lenarduzzi, Carolina M., and Judith S. Pollmann. Bread and Stone: Catholic Memory in Post-Reformation Leiden. In: Brian Cummings, Ceri Law, Karis Riley, and Alexandra Walsham, eds., *Remembering the Reformation*, 61–77. New York: Routledge, 2020.

Leppink, Gerda B., and R.C.M. Wientjes. *Het Sint Catharinae Gasthuis in Arnhem in de eerste vier eeuwen van zijn bestaan (1246–1636)*. Hilversum: Verloren, 1996.

Le Roy Ladurie, Emmanuel. *Les paysans du Languedoc*, I. Paris: S.E.V.P.E.N., 1966.

Le Roy Ladurie, Emmanuel. Un concept. L'unification microbienne du monde (XVIe–XVIIe siècles). *Revue suisse d'histoire* 23, 4 (1973), 627–96.

Lesger, Clé. *Huur en conjunctuur. De woningmarkt in Amsterdam, 1550–1850*. Amsterdam: Historisch Seminarium van de Universiteit van Amsterdam, 1986.

Leuris, C.L.J. De pest in Hapert, Hoogeloon en Casteren (1656–1659). *Campinia: Driemaandelijks Blad van het Streekarchivariaat Noord-Kempenland* 3, 9 (1973), 176–7.

Lewis, Carenza. Disaster Recovery: New Archaeological Evidence for the Long-Term Impact of the "Calamitous" Fourteenth Century. *Antiquity* 90, 351 (2016), 777–97.

Lieburg, Fred van. Kinderziekten en kindergeneeskunde in de journalen van Constantijn Huygens (1595–1687). *Tijdschrift voor Kindergeneeskunde* 56 (1988), 154–61.

Lieburg, Fred van. Revisiting the History of Religious Resistance to Vaccination in the Netherlands. *NTT Journal for Theology and the Study of Religion* 76, 3 (2022), 215–39.

Lieburg, M.J. van. Het dagboek (1679–1703) van Jan Brouwer, binnenvader van het Rotterdamse dolhuis. *Rotterdamse Jaarboekje* 8, 9 (1981), 243–59.

Ligtenberg, Christina. *De armezorg te Leiden tot het einde van de 16e eeuw*. The Hague: Martinus Nijhoff, 1908.

Lipscomb, Suzannah. How Can We Recover the Lost Lives of Women? In: Helen Carr and Suzannah Lipscomb, eds., *What Is History, Now? How the Past and the Present Speak to Each Other*, 178–96. London: Weidenfeld & Nicolson, 2022 [2021].

Lis, Catharina, and Hugo Soly. *Poverty and Capitalism in Pre-Industrial Europe*. Atlantic Highlands, NJ: Humanities Press, 1979.

Liu, Ziang. Wages, Labour Markets, and Living Standards in China, 1530–1840. *Explorations in Economic History* 92 (2024), 101569.

Lonsain, B. Een oproer in het pestjaar 1623. *Groningsche Volksalmanak* (1918), 54–9.

Lopez, Bianca M. *Queen of Sorrows: Plague, Piety, and Power in Late Medieval Italy*. Ithaca, NY: Cornell University Press, 2024.

Lord, Graham M., Giuseppe Matarese, Jane K. Howard, Richard J. Baker, Stephen R. Bloom, and Robert I. Lechler. Leptin Modulates T-Cell Immune Response and Reverse Starvation Induced Immunosuppression. *Nature* 394 (1998), 897–901.

Loschky, David, and Ben D. Childers. Early English Mortality. *Journal of Interdisciplinary History* 24, 1 (1993), 85–97.

Lummel, Hendrik Bastiaan van. *Noviomagum: Herinneringen aan Nijmegen's geschiedenis*. Nijmegen: P.J. Milborn, 1883.

Lust, Kersti. Prospering Despite the Adverse Terms of Emancipation? Accumulation of Wealth by Peasant Farmers in the Tsarist Russian Province of Livonia, 1853–1913. *Rural History* 35, 2 (2024), 294–313.

Lynn, John A. *Giant of the Grand Siècle: The French Army, 1610–1715*. Cambridge: Cambridge University Press, 1997.

Lynn, John A. *The Wars of Louis XIV, 1667–1714*. Routledge: Abingdon, 2013 [1999].

Lynteris, Christos. *Visual Plague: The Emergence of Epidemic Photography*. Cambridge, MA: The MIT Press, 2022.

Maanen, Rudi C.J. van. De grote epidemie van 1669–1670. *Leids Jaarboekje voor Geschiedenis en Oudheidkunde van Leiden en Omstreken* 113 (2021), 67–85.

Macintyre, Kate. Famine and the Female Mortality Advantage. In: Tim Dyson and Cormac Ó Gráda, eds., *Famine Demography: Perspectives from the Past and Present*, 240–59. Oxford: Oxford University Press, 2002.

Macrì, Geltrude. Quarantena e isolamento domiciliare. Palermo durante la peste del 1624. *Rivista dell'Istituto di Storia dell'Europa Mediterranea* 9, 3 (2021), 195–222.

Maillard-Luypaert, Monique. La tradition historiographique d'une procession exceptionnelle pendant l'épidémie de peste noire (1349). In: Jacques Deveseleer, Philippe Desmette, and Monique Maillard-Luypaert, eds., *Reliques et châsses de la collégiale de Soignies. Objets, cultes et traditions*, 93–108. Soignies: Musée du chapitre, 2001.

Malenstein, M.M. van. Het Sint-Petersgasthuis te Culemborg: Een archief-studie vanuit medisch-historisch oogpunt. *Tijdschrift voor de Geschiedenis der Geneeskunde, Natuurwetenschappen, Wiskunde en Techniek* 5 (1982), 65–77.

Mansholt, W.H. Ziekenhuizen te Groningen in het verleden. *Nederlandse Tijdschrift voor Geneeskunde* (1926), 987–8.

Mardaga, Pierre, ed., *La Patrimoine monumental de la Belgique: Wallonie. Province du Luxembourg, Virton*. Liège: Editions Mardaga, 1995.

Maréchal, Griet. De Zwarte Dood te Brugge (1349–1351). *Biekorf* 80 (1980), 377–92.

Mareel, Samuel. Urban Literary Patronage in the Early Modern Low Countries: Public Festive Culture and Individual Authorship. *Renaissance Quarterly* 64, 1 (2011), 50–78.

Margerison, Beverley J., and Christopher J. Knüsel. Paleodemographic Comparison of a Catastrophic and an Attritional Death Assemblage. *American Journal of Physical Anthropology* 119, 2 (2002), 134–43.

Marsilje, Jannis Willem. Aangelijnd in middeleeuws Leiden. De houding van de magistraat ten opzichte van de hond in de periode tot 1573. *Leids Jaarboekje voor Geschiedenis en Oudheidkunde van Leiden en Omstreken* 83 (1991), 51–68.

Martin, Philippe. *La Guerre de trente ans en Lorraine, 1631–1661*. Metz: Serpenoise, 2002.

Martinez-Galarraga, Julio, and Marc Prat. Inequality in Rural Catalonia in the Early Eighteenth Century. *Cliometrica* 19 (2025), 195–247.

Martyn, George, and Fred Stevens. Testamenten van pestlijders in de Zuidelijke Nederlanden. In: Geert Van Reyn, ed., *De pest te Leuven, 1634–1636. De kapucijnen en de zorg om de mens*, 33–5. Louvain: KU Leuven, 2016.

Massong, Natalie. The Mobile Woman: Getting Around during the 1630 Plague in Bologna. *Connections: A Journal of Language, Media and Culture* 2, 1 (2021), 42–54.

Mathijsen, Marita. *De gemaskerde eeuw*. Amsterdam: Querido, 2002.

McCants, Anne E.C. Inequality Among the Poor of Eighteenth Century Amsterdam. *Explorations in Economic History* 44, 1 (2007), 1–21.

McCormick, Michael. Rats, Communications, and Plague: Toward an Ecological History. *Journal of Interdisciplinary History* 34, 1 (2003), 1–25.

McKinley, Alan. Foucault, Plague, Defoe. *Culture and Organization* 15, 2 (2009), 167–84.

McMichael, Anthony J. Insights from Past Millennia into Climatic Impacts on Human Health and Survival. *Proceedings of the National Academy of Sciences* 109, 13 (2012), 4730–7.

McNeill, William H. *Plagues and Peoples*. New York: Anchor Books, 2010 [1976].

McNeill, William H. *Mosquito Empires: Ecology and War in the Greater Caribbean, 1620–1914*. Cambridge: Cambridge University Press, 2010.

Meert, Caroline. Bruxelles sous l'Emprise de la dysenterie, 1779–1783. *Brusselse Cahiers. Tijdschrift voor Stadsgeschiedenis* 40 (2008/9), 69–103.

Meier, Mischa. The "Justinianic Plague": An "Inconsequential Pandemic"? A Reply. *Medizinhistorisches Journal* 55, 2 (2020), 172–99.

Meinsma, K.O. *De Zwarte Dood*. Zutphen: W.J. Thieme & Cie, 1924.

Meloni, Maurizio. An Unproblematized Truth: Foucault, Biopolitics, and the Making of a Sociological Canon. *Social Theory & Health* 21 (2023), 99–119.

Mengel, D.C. A Plague on Bohemia? Mapping the Black Death. *Past and Present* 211, 1 (2011), 3–34.

Mentink, G.J. De rode loop in Gelderland. De dysenterie epidemie in de jaren 1778–1779 en 1782–1783. *Bijdragen en Mededelingen Gelre* 64 (1970), 124–44; and 65 (1971), 29–38.

Mentink, G.J., and Ad. van der Woude. *De demografische ontwikkeling te Rotterdam en Cool in de 17e en 18e eeuw: Een methodisch en analyserend onderzoek van de retroacta van de burgerlijke stand van Rotterdam en Cool*. Rotterdam: Gemeentearchief, 1965.

Mercier, Franck. *La vauderie d'Arras: Une chasse aux sorcières à l'automne du Moyen Âge*. Rennes: Presses universitaires de Rennes, 2006.

Mertens, Jozef. Oorlog, epidemie en emigratie: Stagnatie van het Loonse platteland. In: Julien Daenen and Jozef Mertens, eds., *Limburg in 't geweer. Oorlogsleed in het Land van Loon van Alva tot Napoleon*, 127–37. Bilzen: Landcommanderij Alden Biezen, 2008.

Meeteren, Aries van. *Op hoop van akkoord: Instrumenteel forumgebruik bij geschilbeslechting in Leiden in de zeventiende eeuw*. Hilversum: Verloren, 2006.

Meulemans, A. Dysenterie te Leuven in de XVIIe en de XVIIIe eeuw. *Kring voor de Geschiedenis van de Pharmacie in Benelux* 60 (1980), 35–46.

Michel, Megan, Eirini Skourtanioti, Federica Pierini, Evelyn K. Guevara, Angela Mötsch, Arthur Kocher, et al. Ancient Plasmodium Genomes Shed Light on the History of Human Malaria. *Nature* 631 (2024), 125–33.

Minnen, Bart. *"Den heyligen Sant al in Brabant". De Sint-Martinuskerk van Wezemaal en de cultus van Sint-Job 1000–2000*. PhD Thesis: Radboud University Nijmegen, 2011.

Miquel Milian, Laura, and Jordi Morelló Baget. Economic Inequalities in an Iberian Urban Society: Tortosa Before and After the Black Death. In: Davide Cristoferi, ed., *Socio-Economic Inequalities during the Conjuncture of the Fourteenth Century: Sources and Methods, Dynamics and Representations (Italy and Europe, c. 1270 –c. 1350)*, 129–52. Florence: Firenze University Press, 2025.

Mitchell, Piers D. Historical Sources, Historiography, and Paleopathology. In: Anne L. Grauer, ed., *The Routledge Handbook of Paleopathology*, 180–91. Abingdon: Routledge, 2023.

Miyanaga, Kentaro, and Daisaku Shimada. "The Tragedy of the Commons" by Underuse: Toward a Comparative Framework Based on Ecosystem Services and Satoyama Perspective. *International Journal of the Commons* 12, 1 (2018), 332–51.

Mohr, James C. *Plague and Fire: Battling Black Death and the 1900 Burning of Honolulu's Chinatown*. New York: Oxford University Press, 2005.

Molinder, Jakob, and Christopher Pihl. Women's Work and Wages in the Sixteenth Century and Sweden's Position in the "Little Divergence". *Economic History Review* 76, 1 (2023), 145–68.

Monballyu, Jos. Schadelijke toverij te Brugge en te Ieper in de 15[de] eeuw. *Handelingen van het Genootschap voor Geschiedenis* 121, 3/4 (1984), 265–9.

Monballyu, Jos. *Van hekserij beschuldigd: Heksenprocessen in Vlaanderen tijdens de 16de en 17de eeuw*. Heule: UGA, 1996.

Monecke, Stefan, Hannelore Monecke, and Jochen Monecke. Modelling the Black Death: A Historical Case Study and Implications for the Epidemiology of Bubonic Plague. *International Journal of Medical Microbiology* 299, 8 (2009), 582–93.

Monter, E. William. *Witchcraft in France and Switzerland: The Borderlands during the Reformation*. Ithaca, NY: Cornell University Press, 1976.

Moquette, H.C.H. Pestepidemieën in Rotterdam. *Rotterdamsch Jaarboekje* 3 (1925), 10–52.

Moran, Sarah Joan, and Amanda C. Pipkin, eds., *Women and Gender in the Early Modern Low Countries, 1500–1750*. Brill: Leiden, 2019.

Mordechai, Lee, and Eisenberg, Merle. Rejecting Catastrophe: The Case of the Justinianic Plague. *Past and Present* 244, 1 (2019), 3–50.

Mordechai, Lee, Merle Eisenberg, Timothy P. Newfield, Adam Izdebski, Janet E. Kay, and Hendrik Poinar. The Justinianic Plague: An Inconsequential Pandemic? *Proceedings of the National Academy of Sciences* 116, 51 (2019), 25546–54.

Munkhoff, Richelle. Searchers of the Dead: Authority, Marginality, and the Interpretation of Plague in England, 1574–1665. *Gender and History* 11, 1 (1999), 1–29.

Munkhoff, Richelle. Poor Women and Parish Public Health in Sixteenth-Century London. *Renaissance Studies* 28, 4 (2014), 579–96.

Murkens, Mayra, Ben Pelzer, and Angélique Janssens. Transitory Inequalities: How Individual-Level Cause-Specific Death Data Can Unravel Socioeconomic Inequalities in Infant Mortality in Maastricht, the Netherlands, 1864–1955. *The History of the Family* 28, 1 (2023), 95–131.

Murphy, Neil. Plague Ordinances and the Management of Infectious diseases in Northern French Towns, c.1450–c.1560. In: Linda Clark and Carole Rawcliffe, eds., *The Fifteenth Century Plague: Society in an Age of Plague*, XII, 139–60. Woodbridge: The Boydell Press, 2014.

Murphy, Neil. Plague Hospitals, Poverty and the Provision of Medical Care in France, c.1450–c.1650. *Journal of Social History* 55, 4 (2022), 825–53.

Murphy, Neil. Plague Hospitals and Poor Relief in Late Medieval and Early Modern France. *Social History* 47, no. 4 (2022), 349–71.

Murphy, Neil. *Plague, Towns and Monarchy in Early Modern France*. Cambridge: Cambridge University Press, 2024.

Muurling, Sanne, Jeannette Kamp, and Ariadne Schmidt. Unwed Mothers, Urban Institutions and Female Agency in Early Modern Dutch, German and Italian Towns. *The History of the Family* 26, 1 (2021), 11–28.

Muurling, Sanne, and Peter Ekamper. A World of (In)Difference? Social Inequalities Among Infants' Causes of Death in Mid-Nineteenth-Century Amsterdam. *Social History of Medicine* 38, 2 (2025), 291–322.

Muurling, Sanne, Tim Riswick, and Katalin Buzasi. The Last Nationwide Smallpox Epidemic in the Netherlands: Infectious Disease and Social Inequalities in Amsterdam, 1870–1872. *Social Science History* 47, 2 (2023), 189–216.

Naaktgeboren, Patrick. Policing the Environment of Late Medieval Dordrecht. In: Carole Rawcliffe and Claire Weeda, eds., *Policing the Urban Environment in Premodern Europe*, 149–78. Amsterdam: Amsterdam University Press, 2019.

Namouchi, Amine, Meriam Guellil, Oliver Kersten, Stephanie Hänsch, Claudio Ottoni, Boris V. Schmid, et al. Integrative Approach Using *Yersinia pestis* Genomes to Revisit the Historical Landscape of Plague during the Medieval Period. *Proceedings of the National Academy of Sciences* 115, 50 (2018), e11790–7.

Naphy, William G. *Plagues, Poisons, and Potions. Plague-Spreading Conspiracies in the Western Alps c. 1530–1640*. Manchester: Manchester University Press, 2002.

Naphy, William G., and Andrew Spicer. *The Black Death: A History of Plagues, 1345–1730*. Stroud: Tempus, 2001.

Naphy, William G., and Andrew Spicer. *Plague: Black Death and Pestilence in Europe*. Stroud: Tempus, 2004.

Nederveen Meerkerk, Elise van. Creatief met het archief. Over het opsporen van economische activiteiten van Leidse vrouwen in de vroegmoderne tijd. *Leids Jaarboekje voor Geschiedenis en Oudheidkunde van Leiden en Omstreken* 102 (2010), 19–40.

Nederveen Meerkerk, Elise van. Market Wage or Discrimination? The Remuneration of Male and Female Wool Spinners in the Seventeenth-Century Dutch Republic. *Economic History Review* 63, 1 (2010), 165–86.

Neumayer, Eric, and Thomas Plümper. The Gendered Nature of Natural Disasters: The Impact of Catastrophic Events on the Gender Gap in Life Expectancy, 1981–2002. *Annals of the American Association of Geographers* 97, 3 (2007), 551–66.

Neveux, Hugues. La mortalité des pauvres à Cambrai (1377–1473). *Annales de démographie historique* (1968), 73–97.

Newman, Kira L.S. Shutt Up: Bubonic Plague and Quarantine in Early Modern England. *Journal of Social History* 45, 3 (2012), 809–34.

Newfield, Timothy P. A Cattle Panzootic in Early Fourteenth-Century Europe. *Agricultural History Review* 57, 2 (2009), 155–90.

Nicholas, David. *The Metamorphosis of a Medieval City: Ghent in the Age of the Arteveldes, 1302–1390*. Leiden: Brill, 1987.

Nicholas, David. *Medieval Flanders*. London: Longman Group, 1992.

Nierop, H.F.K. van. *Het verraad van het Noorderkwartier. Oorlog, terreur en recht in de Nederlandse Opstand*. Amsterdam: Bert Bakker, 1999.

Nightingale, Pamela. Some New Evidence of Crises and Trends of Mortality in Late Medieval England. *Past and Present* 187, 1 (2005), 33–68.

Nijboer, Harm. De Slaande Ingel gie om de Aldehou. Eat oer de pest yn Ljouwert. *De Vrije Fries* 75 (1995), 61–78.

Nijssen, Rombout. Zo ging dat in Herk-de-Stad: Aanstelling van een pestmeester in 1623 en 1624. *Heemkunde Limburg* 2 (2020), 49–52.

Nimwegen, Olaf van. *The Dutch Army and the Military Revolutions, 1588–1688*. Woodbridge: Boydell & Brewer, 2010.

Nirenberg, David. *Communities of Violence: Persecution of Minorities in the Middle Ages*. Princeton, NJ: Princeton University Press, 1996.

Noël, René. Première attaque de la peste en Lorraine du Nord: De la ville à la campagne? In: Jean-Marie Duvosquel and Erik Thoen, eds., *Peasants and Townsmen in Medieval Europe. Studia in honorem Adriaan Verhulst*, 739–51. Ghent: Snoeck-Ducaju & Zoon, 1995.

Noordegraaf, Leo. Dearth, Plague, and Trade: Economy and Politics in the Northern Netherlands, Fifteenth to Nineteenth Centuries. *Economic and Social History in the Netherlands* 1 (1989), 49–66.

Noordegraaf, Leo. Calvinism and the Plague in the Seventeenth-Century Dutch Republic. In: Rudolf Dekker, ed., *Curing and Insuring: Essays in Illness in Past Times*, 21–31. Rotterdam: Erasmus Publishing, 1992.

Noordegraaf, Leo. Zacharias Heyns' Pest-Spieghel uit 1602. In: Willem de Blécourt, Willem Frijhoff, and Marijke Gijswijt-Hofstra, eds., *Grenzen van genezing:*

Gezondheid, ziekte en genezen in Nederland, zestiende tot begin twintigste eeuw, 155–71. Hilversum: Verloren, 1993.

Noordegraaf, Leo, and Gerrit Valk. *De Gave Gods: De pest in Holland vanaf de late middeleeuwen*. Bergen: Octavo, 1988.

Noordegraaf, Leo, and Gerrit Valk. Rotterdam in de zeventiende eeuw: De navel van de wereld? *Skript* 11 (1989), 174–7.

Nusteling, Hubert P.H. La population d'Amsterdam de la fin du XVIe siècle au début du XIXe siècle. Une méthode de reconstitution. *Population* 41, 6 (1986), 961–77.

Oakes, Rebecca. Adolescent Mortality at Winchester College, 1393–1540: New Evidence for Medieval Mortality and Methodological Considerations for Historical Demography. *Local Population Studies* 88 (2012), 12–32.

Oerle, Hugo Anthonius van. *Leiden, binnen en buiten de stadsvesten: De geschiedenis van de stedebouwkundige ontwikkeling binnen het Leidse rechtsgebied tot aan het einde van de gouden eeuw*, I–II. Leiden: Brill, 1975.

Ogilvie, Sheilagh. *Controlling Contagion: Epidemics and Institutions from the Black Death to COVID*. Princeton, NJ: Princeton University Press, 2025.

Ó Gráda, Cormac. *Famine: A Short History*. Princeton, NJ: Princeton University Press, 2009.

Olivarius, Kathryn. *Necropolis: Disease, Power, and Capitalism in the Cotton Kingdom*. Cambridge, MA: Harvard University Press, 2022.

Onacker, Eline Van. Bedrijvige boeren? Peasants en de land-en kredietmarkt in de vijftiende en zestiende-eeuwse Kempen. *TSEG: Low Countries Journal of Social and Economic History* 10, 1 (2013), 40–70.

Onacker, Eline Van, and Hadewijch Masure. Unity in Diversity: Rural Poor Relief in the Sixteenth-Century Southern Low Countries. *TSEG: Low Countries Journal of Social and Economic History* 12, 4 (2015), 59–88.

Onacker, Eline Van. Social Vulnerability, Social Structures and Household Grain Shortages in Sixteenth-Century Inland Flanders. *Continuity and Change* 34, 1 (2019), 91–115.

Oosten, Roos van. The "Great Sanitary Awakening" Questioned: Is There a Solid Argument in Favour of the "Filthy Medieval City" Hypothesis? *Medieval and Modern Matters* 5 (2014), 95–116.

Oosten, Roos van. *De stad, het vuil en de beerput. De opkomst, verbreiding en neergang van de beerput in stedelijke context*. Leiden: Sidestone Press, 2015.

Oosten, Roos van. The Dutch Great Stink: The End of the Cesspit Era in the Pre-Industrial Towns of Leiden and Haarlem. *European Journal of Archaeology* 19, 4 (2016), 704–27.

Oosten, Roos van. The Cursed Side. A Folk Belief Evidenced by Documentary Records in 's-Hertogenbosch (1782–1858). In: Roos van Ooosten, Rachel Schats, and Kerry Fast, eds., *Osteoarchaeology in Historical Context. Cemetery Research from the Low Countries*, 151–61. Leiden: Sidestone Press, 2019.

Oosthuizen, Susan. *Tradition and Transformation in Anglo-Saxon England: Archaeology, Common Rights and Landscape*. London: Bloomsbury, 2013.

Ostherr, Kirsten. *Cinematic Prophylaxis: Globalization and Contagion in the Discourse of World Health*. Durham, NC: Duke University Press, 2005.

Ostrom, Elinor. *Governing the Commons: The Evolution of Institutions for Collective Action*. Cambridge: Cambridge University Press, 1990.

Outram, Quentin. The Demographic Impact of Early Modern Warfare. *Social Science History* 26, 2 (2002), 245–72.

Pamuk, Şevket. The Black Death and the Origins of the "Great Divergence" across Europe, 1300–1600. *European Review of Economic History* 11, 3 (2007), 289–317.

Pamuk, Şevket, and Maya Shatzmiller. Plagues, Wages, and Economic Change in the Islamic Middle East, 700–1500. *Journal of Economic History* 74, 1 (2014), 196–229.

Pannier, Stan. From Crisis Management towards a Mediterranean Model? Maritime Quarantine in the Austrian Netherlands, c. 1720–1795. *BMGN: Low Countries Historical Review* 138, 2 (2023), 32–74.

Paping, Richard F.J., and Erwin Karel. The Rural Succession Myth: Occupational Careers and Household Formation of Peasants' and Farmers' Offspring Around 1800. *TSEG: Low Countries Journal of Social and Economic History* 8, 4 (2011), 44–75.

Paping, Richard F.J., and Vincent Tassenaar. The Consequences of the Potato Disease in the Netherlands 1845–1860: A Regional Approach. In: Cormac Ó Gráda, Richard F.J. Paping, and Eric Vanhaute, eds., *When the Potato Failed: Causes and Effects of the "Last" European Subsistence Crisis, 1845–1850*, 149–83. Turnhout: Brepols, 2007.

Parker, Cody E., Alina N. Hiss, Maria A. Spyrou, Gunnar U. Neumann, Philip Slavin, Elizabeth A. Nelson, et al. 14th Century *Yersinia pestis* Genomes Support Emergence of *pestis secunda* Within Europe. *PLoS Pathogens* 19, 7 (2023), e1011404.

Parker, Geoffrey. *The Army of Flanders and the Spanish Road, 1567–1659: The Logistics of Spanish Victory and Defeat in the Low Countries' Wars*. Cambridge: Cambridge University Press, 1972.

Parker, Geoffrey. *The Thirty Years' War*. London: Routledge, 2006 [1997].

Parker, Geoffrey. *Global Crisis: War, Climate Change, and Catastrophe in the Seventeenth Century*. New Haven, CT: University of Yale Press, 2013.

Parrott, David. *Richelieu's Army: War, Government and Society in France, 1624–1642*. Cambridge: Cambridge University Press, 2001.

Pauly, Michel. Pestepidemien in Luxemburg (14.–18. Jahrhundert). In: Georg Mein and Johannes Pause, eds., *Self and Society in the Corona Crisis: Perspectives from the Humanities and Social Sciences*, 55–74. Esch-sur-Alzette: Melusina Press, 2021.

Peckham, Robert. *Fear: An Alternative History of the World*. London: Profile Books, 2023.

Peeters, L. Mariken van Nieumeghen en de Antwerpse volksboekcultuur. *Spiegel der Letteren: Tijdschrift voor Nederlandse Literatuurgeschiedenis en voor Literatuurwetenschap* 25, 1 (1983), 81–97.

Pelling, Margaret. *The Common Lot: Sickness, Medical Occupations, and the Urban Poor in Early Modern England*. Abingdon: Routledge, 2013 [1998].

Pelling, Margaret. "Bosom Vipers": Endemic Versus Epidemic Disease. *Centaurus* 62, 2 (2020), 294–301.

Pelling, Margaret. Epidemics in Nineteenth-Century British Towns: How Important was Cholera? *Journal of Victorian Culture* 27, 2 (2022), 346–55.

Penning, C.P.J. Het vroegere pesthuis te Harderwijk. *Nederlandse Tijdschrift voor Geneeskunde* 73 (1929), 3569–71.

Perk, Godelinde Gertrude. Adapting Saints: Memory, Imagination, and the Liturgy of St. Agnes of Rome in the Diepenveen Sister-Book. *Ons Geestelijk Erf* 94 (2025), 183–215.

Person, Bobbie, Francisco Sy, Kelly Holton, Barbara Govert, Arthur Liang, Brenda Garza, et al. Fear and Stigma: The Epidemic within the SARS Outbreak. *Emerging Infectious Diseases* 10, 2 (2004), 358–63.

Pettegree, Andrew, and Arthur der Weduwen. News, Neighbours, and Commerce: Newspaper Advertising in the Information Culture of the Dutch Republic. *Early Modern Low Countries* 2, 1 (2018), 103–18.

Pfeffer, Michelle. Astrology, Plague, and Prognostication in Early Modern England: A Forgotten Chapter in the History of Public Health. *Past and Present* 263, 1 (2024), 81–124.

Pfister, Christian. When Europe was Burning: The Multi-Season Mega-Drought of 1540 and Arsonist Paranoia. In: Gerrit Jasper Schenk, ed., *Historical Disaster Experiences: Towards a Comparative and Transcultural History of Disasters across Asia and Europe*, 155–85. Berlin: Springer, 2017.

Pfister, Ulrich. Economic Inequality in Germany, 1500–1800. In: Giampiero Nigro, ed., *Disuguaglianza economica nelle società preindustriali: Cause ed effetti / Economic Inequality in Pre-Industrial Societies: Causes and Effects*, 301–24. Florence: Firenze University Press, 2020.

Piccardt, Rixtinus Arnoldus Soetbrood. *Bijzonderheden uit de geschiedenis der stad Goes*. Goes: P. Kleeuwens & Zoon, 1864.

Pol, Lotte van de, and Erika Kuijpers. Poor Women's Migration to the City. The Attraction of Amsterdam Health Care and Social Assistance in Early Modern Times. *Journal of Urban History* 32, 1 (2005), 44–60.

Polak-de-Booy, E.P. Dansen op de doodkist. *Maandblad van Oud Utrecht* 43 (1970), 23–4.

Pollmann, Judith. Iconoclasts Anonymous: Why Did it Take Historians So Long to Identify the Image-Breakers of 1566? *BMGN: Low Countries Historical Review* 131, 1 (2016), 155–76.

Pollmann, Judith. Hunger Tales: Remembering Famine in Sixteenth-Century Leiden. In: Claire Weeda, Robert Stein, and Louis Sicking, eds., *Communities, Environment and Regulation in the Premodern World*, 121–34. Turnhout: Brepols, 2022.

Poppel, Frans van, Dirk J. van de Kaa, and Govert E. Bijwaard. Life Expectancy of Artists in the Low Countries from the Fifteenth to the Twentieth Century. *Population Studies* 67, 3 (2013), 275–92.

Poppel, Frans van, Govert Bijwaard, Mart van Lieburg, Fred van Lieburg, Rik Hoekstra, and Frans Verkade. The Life Expectancy of Medical Professionals in the Netherlands, Sixteenth to Twentieth Centuries. *Population* 71, 4 (2016), 619–40.

Poppel, Frans van, Govert Bijwaard, Mart van Lieburg, Fred van Lieburg, Rik Hoekstra, and Frans Verkade. Medische opleiding gaf geen overlevingsvoordeel: Levensverwachting van Nederlandse medici geboren in 1550–1909. *Nederlandse Tijdschrift voor Geneeskunde* 162, 29 (2018), 1–8.

Poppel, Frans van, Jona Schellekens, and Aart C. Liefbroer. Religious Differentials in Infant and Child Mortality in Holland, 1855–1912. *Population Studies* 56, 3 (2002), 277–89.

Poppel, Frans van, Marianne Jonker, and Kees Mandemakers. Differential Infant and Child Mortality in Three Dutch regions, 1812–1909. *Economic History Review* 58, 2 (2005), 272–309.

Postan, M.M. *Essays on Medieval Agriculture and General Problems of the Medieval Economy*. Cambridge: Cambridge University Press, 1973.

Pot, G. Peter. M. *Arm Leiden. Levensstandaard, bedeling en bedeelden, 1750–1854*. Hilversum: Verloren, 1994.

Prak, Maarten. *Gezeten burgers: De elite in een Hollandse stad, Leiden 1700–1780*. De Amsterdam: Bataafsche Leeuw, 1985.

Prak, Maarten. *The Dutch Republic in the Seventeenth Century*. Cambridge: Cambridge University Press, 2005.

Prak, Maarten, Catharina Lis, Jan Lucassen, and Hugo Soly, eds., *Craft Guilds in the Early Modern Low Countries: Work, Power, and Representation*. Aldershot: Ashgate, 2006.

Prak, Maarten, and Jan Luiten van Zanden. Demographic Change and Migration Flows in Holland, 1500–1800. In: Marcel van der Linden and Leo Lucassen, eds., *Working on Labor: Essays in Honor of Jan Lucassen*, 237–45. Leiden: Brill, 2012.

Prak, Maarten, and Jan Luiten van Zanden. *Pioneers of Capitalism: The Netherlands 1000–1800*. Princeton, NJ: Princeton University Press, 2022.

Price, J.L. *The Dutch Republic in the Seventeenth Century*. New York: St. Martin's Press, 1998.

Pullan, Brian. Plague and Perception of the Poor in Early Modern Italy. In: Terence Ranger and Paul Slack, eds., *Epidemics and Ideas: Essays on the Historical Perception of Pestilence*, 101–23. Cambridge: Cambridge University Press, 1992.

Quanjer, Björn. Height and the Disease Environment of Children: The Association Between Mortality and Height in the Netherlands 1850–1940. *Economic History Review* 77, 2 (2024), 391–415.

Rabinow, Sophie, Koen Deforce, and Piers D. Mitchell. Continuity in Intestinal Parasite Infection in Aalst (Belgium) from the Medieval to Early Modern Period (12th–17th Centuries). *International Journal of Paleopathology* 41 (2023), 43–9.

Rabinow, Sophie, Tianyi Wang, Roos van Oosten, Yolande Meijer, and Piers D. Mitchell. Intestinal Parasite Infection and Sanitation in Medieval Leiden, the Low Countries. *Antiquity* 98, 400 (2024), 1006–22.

Raftis, J.A. *Tenure and Mobility: Studies in the Social History of the Medieval English Village*. Toronto: Pontifical Institute of Medieval Studies, 1964.

Rawcliffe, Carole. *Medicine and Society in Later Medieval England*. Stroud: Sutton, 1999.

Rawcliffe, Carole. *Medicine for the Soul: The Life, Death and Resurrection of an English Medieval Hospital, St. Giles's, Norwich, c.1249–1550*. Stroud: Sutton, 1999.

Rawcliffe, Carole. *Urban Bodies: Communal Health in Late Medieval English Towns and Cities*. Woodbridge: The Boydell Press, 2013.

Read, Sara. "Thy Righteousness is but a Menstrual Clout": Sanitary Practices and Prejudice in Early Modern England. *Early Modern Women: An Interdisciplinary Journal* 3 (2008), 1–25.

Reilingh, Harm. *Geschiedkundig-geneeskundige beschouwing der in de provincie Groningen epidemisch geheerscht hebbende tusschenpoozende koortsen sedert de elfde eeuw*, I. Groningen: Barghoorn, 1858.

Reimann, Christina. Hospitality and Securitization in Times of Cholera: Eastern European Migrants in Rotterdam and Antwerp, 1880–1914. In: Sari Nauman, Wojtek Jezierski, Christina Reimann, and Leif Runevelt, eds., *Baltic Hospitality from the Middle Ages to the Twentieth Century: Receiving Strangers in Northeastern Europe*, 359–86. Cham: Palgrave Macmillan, 2022.

Reinhardt, Renzo. *Plague Workers and Sorcerers in the Duchy of Brabant and the County of Flanders (1347–1550)*. MA Thesis: Leiden University, 2024.

Reis, Jaime. Deviant Behaviour? Inequality in Portugal 1565–1770. *Cliometrica* 11, 3 (2017), 297–319.

Reynolds, Susan. *Kingdoms and Communities in Western Europe, 900–1300*. Oxford: Oxford University Press, 1997 [1984].

Rigby, S.H. Gendering the Black Death: Women in Later Medieval England. *Gender and History* 12, 3 (2000), 745–54.

Riguelle, William. Que la peste soit de l'animal! La législation à l'encontre des animaux en période d'épidémies dans les villes des Pays-Bas méridionaux et de la principauté de Liège (1600–1670). In: Rémi Luglia, ed., *Sales bêtes! Mauvaises herbes! "Nuisible", une notion en débat*, 109–24. Rennes: Presses universitaires de Rennes, 2018.

Riguelle, William. La police des animaux dans les Pays-Bas et la principauté de Liège (XVIIe–XVIIIe siècles). *Revue belge de philologie et d'histoire* 97, 2 (2019), 159–83.

Rijpma, Auke, Ingrid K. van Dijk, Ruben Schalk, Richard L. Zijdeman, and Rick J. Mourits. Unequal Excess Mortality during the Spanish Flu Pandemic in the Netherlands. *Economics & Human Biology* 47 (2022), 101179.

Riswick, Tim, Sanne Muurling, and Katalin Buzasi. Exploring the Mortality Advantage of Jewish Neighbourhoods in Mid-Nineteenth-Century Amsterdam. *Demographic Research* 46, 25 (2022), 723–36.

Rivers, Joan P.W. Women and Children Last: An Essay on Sex Discrimination in Disasters. *Disasters* 6, 4 (1982), 256–67.

Rocha, Gino Chaves da, Stephanie Harter-Lailheugue, Matthieu Le Bailly, Adauto Araújo, Luiz Fernando Ferreira, Nicolau Maués da Serra-Freire, et al. Paleoparasitological Remains Revealed by Seven Historic Contexts from "Place d'Armes", Namur, Belgium. *Memórias do Instituto Oswaldo Cruz* 101, 2 (2006), 43–52.

Roelens, Jonas. Visible Women: Female Sodomy in the Late Medieval and Early Modern Southern Netherlands (1400–1550). *BMGN: Low Countries Historical Review* 130, 3 (2015), 3–24.

Roelens, Jonas. Het sodom van het Noorden. Mogelijke verklaringen voor de sodomierepressie in Brugge (ca. 1400–1700). *Handelingen van het Genootschap voor Geschiedenis* 157, 2 (2020), 185–234.

Rogghé, Paul. De Zwarte Dood in de Zuidelijke Nederlanden. *Revue Belge de philologie et d'histoire* 30, 3–4 (1952), 834–7.

Rohr, Christian. Disaster Memory and "Banished Memory": General Considerations and Case Studies from Europe and the United States (19th–21st Centuries). In: Hanneke van Asperen and Lotte Jensen, eds., *Dealing with Disasters from Early Modern to Modern Times: Cultural Responses to Catastrophes*, 315–37. Amsterdam: Amsterdam University Press, 2023.

Roitman, Janet. *Anti-Crisis*. Durham, NC: Duke University Press, 2013.

Rombach, F.J.C. Zenuwzinkingkoorts in Montfoort en omgeving: Een hardnekkige epidemie eind 1817 en in het jaar 1818. *Heemtijdinghen: Orgaan van de Stichts-Hollandse Vereniging* 21, 1 (1985), 10–30.

Rommes, Ronald. Pest in perspectief: Aspecten van een gevreesde ziekte in de vroeg-moderne tijd. *Tijdschrift voor Sociale Geschiedenis* 16, 3 (1990), 244–67.

Rommes, Ronald. Op het spoor van de dood: De pest in en rond Utrecht. *Jaarboek Oud-Utrecht* (1991), 93–120.

Rommes, Ronald. "Geen vrolijk geloei der melkzwaare koeijen": Runderpest in Utrecht in de achttiende eeuw. *Jaarboek Oud-Utrecht* (2001), 87–136.

Rommes, Ronald. Plague in Northwestern Europe. The Dutch Experience, 1350–1670. *Popolazione e Storia* 15, 1 (2015), 47–71.

Rooden, Peter van. God en de pest. *NRC-Handelsblad* [7/1/1989; 14/1/1989].

Roosbroeck, Filip Van. Experts, Experiments, and the Fight against Rinderpest in the Austrian Netherlands, 1769–1785. *Tijdschrift voor Geschiedenis* 128, 1 (2015), 23–43.

Roosbroeck, Filip Van. Caring for Cows in a Time of Rinderpest: Non-Academic Veterinary Practitioners in the County of Flanders, 1769–1785. *Social History of Medicine* 32, 3 (2019), 502–22.

Roosen, Joris. Severity and Selectivity of the Black Death and Recurring Plague in the Southern Netherlands (1349–1450). *TSEG: Low Countries Journal of Social and Economic History* 14, 4 (2017), 25–55.

Roosen, Joris. *The Black Death and Recurring Plague during the Late Middle Ages in the County of Hainaut*. PhD Thesis: Utrecht University, 2020.

Roosen, Joris. The Black Death: Window of Opportunity or Disaster? Demographic Growth, Stagnation and Decline in the County of Hainaut (1349–1541). *De Medio Aevo* 11, 2 (2022), 157–73.

Roosen, Joris, and Daniel R. Curtis. Dangers of Noncritical Use of Historical Plague Data. *Emerging Infectious Diseases* 24, 1 (2018), 103–10.

Roosen, Joris, and Daniel R. Curtis. The "Light Touch" of the Black Death in the Southern Netherlands: An Urban Trick? *Economic History Review* 72, 1 (2019), 32–56.

Rose, Colin. Plague and Violence in Early Modern Italy. *Renaissance Quarterly* 71, 3 (2018), 1000–35.

Rosenthal, Jean-Laurent, and Roy Bin Wong. *Before and Beyond Divergence: The Politics of Economic Change in China and Europe.* Cambridge, MA: Harvard University Press, 2011.

Ross, Eric B. Syphilis, Misogyny and Witchcraft in 16th-Century Europe. *Current Anthropology* 36, 2 (1995), 333–7.

Rota, Mauro, and Jacob Weisdorf. Italy and the Little Divergence in Wages and Prices: New Data, New Results. *Journal of Economic History* 80, 4 (2020), 931–60.

Ruggles, Steven. The Revival of Quantification: Reflections on Old New Histories. *Social Science History* 45, 1 (2021), 1–25.

Rutten, Willibrord. In de schaduw van de pest. Reacties op pokkenepidemieën in de zeventiende en achttiende eeuw. In: Willem de Blécourt, Willem Frijhoff, and Marijke Gijswijt-Hofstra, eds., *Grenzen van genezing: Gezondheid, ziekte en genezen in Nederland, zestiende tot begin twintigste eeuw*, 172–202. Hilversum: Verloren, 1993.

Rutten, Willibrord. Smallpox, Subfecundity, and Sterility: A Case Study from a Nineteenth-Century Dutch Municipality. *Social History of Medicine* 6, 1 (1993), 85–99.

Rutten, Willibrord. *"De vreselijkste aller harpijen". Pokkenepidemieën en pokkenbestrijding in Nederland in de achttiende en negentiende eeuw: Een sociaal-historische en historisch-demografische studie.* Wageningen: AAG Bijdragen, 1997.

Ryckbosch, Wouter. Economic Inequality and Growth Before the Industrial Revolution: The Case of the Low Countries (Fourteenth to Nineteenth Centuries). *European Review of Economic History* 20, 1 (2016), 1–22.

Sabean, David. *Property, Production, and Family in Neckarhausen, 1700–1870.* Cambridge: Cambridge University Press, 1990.

Sales i Favà, Lluís. Leasing, Fattening and Guarding Livestock in Times of Crises: North-Eastern Catalonia, c.1330–70. *Agricultural History Review* 69, 2 (2021), 169–91.

Salomé, Karine. Le massacre des "empoisonneurs" à Paris au temps du choléra (1832). *Revue historique* 317, 673 (2015), 103–24.

Sarris, Peter. New Approaches to the "Plague of Justinian". *Past and Present* 254, 1 (2022), 315–46.

Sas, Benedict. Die Swaerigheyt des levens te Gierle tijdens de miserabele tweede helft van de 17de eeuw. *Heemkundige Kring – Norbert De Vrijter – Lille* 26 (2008), 105–34.

Sasse van Ysselt, A.F.O. van, ed., *Chronologisch overzicht van de geschiedenis van Geertruidenberg.* Geertruidenberg: Antoine, 1938.

Satterfield, George. *Princes, Posts and Partisans: The Army of Louis XIV and Partisan Warfare in the Netherlands (1673–1678).* Leiden: Brill, 2003.

Schaïk, Remi van. *Belasting, bevolking en bezit in Gelre en Zutphen (1350–1550).* Hilversum: Verloren, 1987.

Schaïk, Remi van. De teloorgang van de kerk van Lutjewolde. *Groninger Kerken* 39, 2 (2022), 6–15.

Schäfer, Regina. Land Transactions Within Rural Society in the Middle Rhine Valley (ca. 1400–1535). *The History of the Family* 27, 1 (2022), 37–53.

Schaff, Felix S.F. Warfare and Economic Inequality: Evidence from Preindustrial Germany (c. 1400–1800). *Explorations in Economic History* 89 (2023), 101495.

Schama, Simon. *The Embarrassment of Riches: An Interpretation of Dutch Culture in the Golden Age*. Berkeley, CA: University of California Press, 1988 [1987].

Schama, Simon. *Foreign Bodies: Pandemics, Vaccines and the Health of Nations*. London: Simon & Schuster, 2023.

Schats, Rachel, and Michael Klomp. In Sickness and in Health: An Archaeological and Osteoarchaeological Analysis of St. Gertrude's Infirmary in Kampen (1382–c. 1611). In: Roos van Oosten, Rachel Schats, and Kerry Fast, eds., *Osteoarchaeology in Historical Context: Cemetery Research from the Low Countries*, 105–19. Leiden: Sidestone Press, 2019.

Scheidel, Walter. *The Great Leveler: Violence and the History of Inequality from the Stone Age to the Twenty-First Century*. Princeton, NJ: Princeton University Press, 2017.

Schellekens, Jona. Mortality and Socio-Economic Status in Two Eighteenth-Century Villages. *Population Studies* 43, 3 (1989), 391–404.

Schevensteen, A.F.C. Van. Les traités de pestilence publiés à Anvers. Essai de bibliographie. *De Gulden Passer* 9 (1931), 101–95.

Schevensteen, A.F.C. Van. Over pestepidemiën te Antwerpen in vroeger tijden. *Verslagen en Mededelingen van de Koninklijke Vlaamse Academie voor Taal- en Letterkunde* (1932), 1055–92.

Schevensteen, A.F.C. Van. Un traité anversois sur la Suette Anglaise. *De Gulden Passer* 10 (1932), 51–71.

Schmid, Boris, Ulf Büntgen, W. Ryan Easterday, Christian Ginzler, Lars Walløe, Barbara Bramanti, et al. Climate-Driven Introduction of the Black Death and Successive Plague Reintroductions into Europe. *Proceedings of the National Academy of Sciences* 112, 10 (2015), 3020–5.

Schmidt, Ariadne. Generous Provisions or Legitimate Shares? Widows and the Transfer of Property in 17th-Century Holland. *The History of the Family* 15, 1 (2010), 13–24.

Schmidt, Ariadne. Women and Work in the Dutch Republic. *Early Modern Low Countries* 9, 1 (2025), 14–33.

Schmidt, Ariadne, and Elise van Nederveen Meerkerk. Reconsidering The "First Male-Breadwinner Economy": Women's Labor Force Participation in the Netherlands, 1600–1900. *Feminist Economics* 18, 4 (2012), 69–96.

Schmidt, Ariadne, and Manon van der Heijden. Women Alone in Early Modern Dutch Towns: Opportunities and Strategies to Survive. *Journal of Urban History* 42, 1 (2016), 21–38.

Schmitz, H. Schiedam en de pest. *Historisch Tijdschrift Holland* 3, 5 (1971), 125–37.

Schofield, Roger. The Last Visitation of the Plague in Sweden: The Case of Bräkne-Hoby in 1710–11. *Economic History Review* 69, 2 (2016), 600–26.

Schroor, Meindert. *Rurale metropool. Bevolking, migratie en financiën van de stad Groningen ten tijde van de Republiek (1595–1795)*. Groningen: Nederlands Agronomisch Historisch Instituut, 2014.

Schulten, J.W.M. Het beleg van Breda in 1637. *Jaarboek De Oranjeboom* 41 (1988), 156–67.

Schulz, Wiebke, Ineke Maas, and Marco H.D. van Leeuwen. When Women Disappear from the Labour Market: Occupational Status of Dutch Women at Marriage in a Modernizing Society, 1865–1922. *The History of the Family* 19, 4 (2014), 426–46.

Schurer, Andrew P., Gabriele C. Hegerl, Jürg Luterbacher, Stefan Brönnimann, Tim Cowan, Simon F.B. Tett, et al. Disentangling the Causes of the 1816 European Year Without a Summer. *Environmental Research* 14, 9 (2019), 094019.

Seebohm, Frederic. The Black Death and its Place in English History. *Fortnightly Review* 2 (1865), 268–79.

Segers, Yves. *Armenzorg op het platteland tijdens graancrisissen: Onderzoek naar de efficiëntie van armendissen tijdens de graanduurtes van 1556 en 1565*. PhD Thesis: University of Antwerp, 2014.

Séguy, Isabelle, S. Pennec, Stéfan Tzortzis, and Michel Signoli. Modélisation de l'impact de la peste à travers l'exemple de Martigues (Bouches-du-Rhône). In: L. Buchet, C. Dauphin, and I. Séguy, eds., *La paléodémographie. Mémoire d'os, mémoire d'hommes*, 323–31. Antibes: Editions APDCA, 2006.

Sellers-García, Sylvia. A Hidden Plague: Violence and Public Health in Colonial Guatemala City. *Medical History Journal* 25, 1 (2022), 7–31.

Semih Akçomak, İ., Dinand Webbink, and Bas ter Weel. Why Did the Netherlands Develop So Early? The Legacy of the Brethren of the Common Life. *The Economic Journal* 126, 593 (2016), 821–60.

Sen, Amartya. *Poverty and Famines: An Essay on Entitlement and Deprivation*. Oxford: Clarendon Press, 1981.

Servaas van Rooijen, A.J. Toen en nu. Sint Anthonius-kapel. "Siekhuis". Pesthuis. Dolhuis. Verbeteringhuis. Krankzinnigengesticht. *De Huisvriend* 2 (1900), 238–9.

Seth, Susan. *Difference and Disease: Medicine, Race, and the Eighteenth-Century British Empire*. Cambridge: Cambridge University Press, 2018.

Sharp, Buchanan. *Famine and Scarcity in Late Medieval and Early Modern England: The Regulation of Grain Marketing, 1256–1631*. Cambridge: Cambridge University Press, 2016.

Sharpe, Jim A. Quantification and the History of Crime in Early Modern England: Problems and Results. *Historical Social Research / Historische Sozialforschung* 15, 4 (1990), 17–32.

Shirk, Melanie V. The Black Death in Aragon, 1348–1351. *Journal of Medieval History* 7, 4 (1981), 357–67.

Shirk, Melanie V. Violence and the Plague in Aragón, 1348–1351. *Journal of the Rocky Mountain Medieval and Renaissance Association* 5 (1984), 31–9.

Siena, Kevin. Searchers of the Dead in Long Eighteenth Century London. In: Kim Kippen and Lori Woods, eds., *Worth and Repute: Valuing Gender in Late Medieval and Early Modern Europe: Essays in Honour of Barbara Todd*, 123–52. Toronto: Centre for Reformation and Renaissance Studies, 2011.

Siena, Kevin. Poor Bodies and Disease. In: David Hitchcock and Julia McClure, eds., *The Routledge History of Poverty, c.1450–1800*, 120–37. Abingdon: Routledge, 2021.

Simons, Walter. *Cities of Ladies: Beguine Communities in the Medieval Low Countries, 1200–1565*. Philadelphia, PA: University of Pennsylvania Press, 2001.

Singer, Julie. Hearing an Urban Plague Soundscape: Gilles li Muisis in Tournai, 1349–50. *Speculum* 99, 4 (2024), 1225–46.

Singer, Linda. *Erotic Welfare: Sexual Theory and Politics in the Age of Epidemic*. London: Routledge, 1993.

Sivéry, Gérard. La Hainaut et la Peste Noire. *Mémoires et publications de la société des sciences, des arts et des lettres du Hainaut* 79 (1965), 431–47.

Sivéry, Gérard. La peste noire et l'épidémie de 1400–1401 dans le Hainaut. Questions de méthodologie. *Annalen van de Belgische Vereniging voor Hospitaalgeschiedenis* 4 (1966), 51–65.

Siuda, Fabian, and Uwe Sunde. Disease and Demographic Development: The Legacy of the Plague. *Journal of Economic Growth* 26 (2021), 1–30.

Slack, Paul. *The Impact of Plague in Tudor and Stuart England.* London: Routledge, 1985.

Slack, Paul. *Plague: A Very Short Introduction.* Oxford: Oxford University Press, 2012.

Slack, Paul. Responses to Plague in Early Modern Europe: The Implications of Public Health. *Social Research* 87, 2 (2020), 409–28.

Slavin, Philip. Death by the Lake: Mortality Crisis in Early Fourteenth-Century Central Asia. *Journal of Interdisciplinary History* 50, 1 (2019), 59–90.

Slavin, Philip. The Birth of the Black Death: Biology, Climate, Environment, and the Beginnings of the Second Plague Pandemic in Early Fourteenth-Century Central Asia. *Environmental History* 28, 2 (2023), 300–34.

Slavin, Philip. Plague Strikes Back: The *Pestis Secunda* of 1361–62 and its Demographic Consequences in England and Wales. *Journal of Medieval and Early Modern Studies* 54, 3 (2024), 457–91.

Slicher van Bath, Bernard H. *Een samenleving onder spanning. Geschiedenis van het platteland in Overijssel.* Utrecht: HES, 1977 [1957].

Smail, Daniel Lord. Accommodating Plague in Medieval Marseille. *Continuity and Change* 11, 1 (1996), 11–41.

Smith, Julia. Overcoming the "Tyranny of the Urgent": Integrating Gender into Disease Outbreak Preparedness and Response. *Gender and Development* 27, 2 (2019), 355–69.

Smith, Richard M. Measuring Adult Mortality in an Age of Plague. In: Mark Bailey and Stephen Rigby, eds., *Measuring Adult Mortality in an Age of Plague: England, 1349–1540*, 43–85. Turnhout: Brepols, 2012.

Snowden, Frank M. Cholera in Barletta 1910. *Past and Present* 132, 1 (1991), 67–103.

Snowden, Frank M. Emerging and Reemerging Diseases: A Historical Perspective. *Immunological Review* 225, 1 (2008), 9–26.

Snowden, Frank M. *Epidemics and Society: From the Black Death to the Present.* New Haven, CT: Yale University Press, 2020.

Soens, Tim. *De spade in de dijk? Waterbeheer en rurale samenleving in de Vlaamse kustvlakte (1280–1580).* Ghent: Academia Press, 2009.

Soens, Tim. Resilient Societies, Vulnerable People. Coping with North Sea Floods Before 1800. *Past and Present* 241, 1 (2018), 143–77.

Soens, Tim. No Second Lord. Agriculture and Climatic Variability in the Late Medieval Low Countries. In: Claire Weeda, Robert Stein, and Louis Sicking, eds., *Communities, Environment and Regulation in the Premodern World: Essays in Honour of Peter Hoppenbrouwers*, 71–98. Turnhout: Brepols, 2022.

Soens, Tim. The Black Death and the Commoner: Tales of Crisis from the Urban Low Countries. *International Medieval Congress Keynote Lecture,* University of Leeds, 2024.

Soens, Tim, Dries Tys, and Erik Thoen. Landscape Transformation and Social Change in the North Sea Polders, the Example of Flanders (1000–1800 AD). *Siedlungsforschung. Archäologie – Geschichte – Geographie* 31 (2014), 133–60.

Soens, Tim, and Erik Thoen. Vegetarians or Carnivores? Standards of Living and Diet in Late Medieval Flanders. In: Simonetta Cavaciocchi, ed., *Le interazioni fra economia e ambiente biologico nell'Europa preindustriale secc. XII–XVIII*, 483–516. Florence: Firenze University Press, 2010.

Sogner, Sølvi, and Jelle van Lottum. An Immigrant Community? Norwegian Sailors and their Wives in 17th-Century Amsterdam. *The History of the Family* 12, 3 (2007), 153–68.

Sontag, Susan. *Illness as Metaphor and AIDS and its Metaphors.* New York: Picador, 2001 [1978/1988].

Spaans, Joke. *Armenzorg in Friesland 1500–1800: Publieke zorg en particuliere liefdadigheid in zes Friese steden Leeuwarden, Bolsward, Franeker, Sneek, Dokkum en Harlingen*. Hilversum: Verloren, 1997.

Spanhove, J. De pest te Bollebeek in de 17de eeuw. *Eigen Schoon en de Brabander* 76 (1993), 337–42.

Speakman, John R. Sex- and Age-Related Mortality Profiles during Famine: Testing the "Body Fat" Hypothesis. *Journal of Biosocial Science* 45, 6 (2013), 823–40.

Speecke, Mathijs, and Thijs Lambrecht. Social Inequalities and the Great Famine in the County of Flanders (1315–7). In: Davide Cristoferi, ed., *Socio-Economic Inequalities during the Conjuncture of the Fourteenth Century. Sources and Methods, Dynamics and Representations (Italy and Europe, c. 1270–c. 1350)*, 223–47. Florence: Firenze University Press, 2025.

Spinney, Laura. *Pale Rider: The Spanish Flu of 1918 and How it Changed the World*. London: Vintage, 2017.

Spyrou, Maria A., Marcel Keller, Rezeda I. Tukhbatova, Christiana L. Scheib, Elizabeth A. Nelson, Aida Andrades Valtueña, et al. Phylogeography of the Second Plague Pandemic Revealed through Analysis of Historical *Yersinia pestis* Genomes. *Nature Communications* 10, 4470 (2019), 1–13.

Spyrou, Maria A., Lyazzat Musralina, Guido A. Gnecchi Ruscone, Arthur Kocher, Pier-Giorgio Borbone, Valeri I. Khartanovich, et al. The Source of the Black Death in Fourteenth-Century Central Eurasia. *Nature* 606 (2022), 718–24.

Stalpers, Lukas J.A., Jan M.M. de Meere, and Edward L. Kaplan. De sterfte in Amsterdam van 1554 tot 2021. *Nederlandse Tijdschrift voor Geneeskunde* 165 (2021), D5962.

Stathakopoulos, Dionysios, Timothy P. Newfield, Elena Xoplaki, John Haldon, Marcel Keller, Neil Roberts, et al. The First Plague Pandemic in the Byzantine Empire – Toward a New Dynamic Consensus. *Human Ecology* (2025), 1–21.

Steendijk-Kuypers, J. *Volksgezondheidszorg in de 16e en 17e eeuw te Hoorn. Een bijdrage tot de beeldvorming van sociaal-geneeskundige structuren in een stedelijke samenleving*. Rotterdam: Erasmus Publishing, 1994.

Steensel, Arie van, Roos van Oosten, and Martin Hooymans. Housing Inequality and Social Segregation in Leiden, 1561–1606. *Urban History* first view (2025), 1–22.

Stein, Robert. An Urban Network in the Low Countries. A Cultural Approach. In: Robert Stein and Judith Pollmann, eds., *Networks, Regions and Nations: Shaping Identities in the Low Countries, 1300–1650*, 43–71. Leiden: Brill, 2010.

Steiner, Daria. Heroines of Hunger Relief: Challenging Feminization of Famine in Twenty-First Century Cultural Archive(s). *Diffractions* 4, 2 (2021), 33–55.

Steinhoff, Judith. Artistic Working Relationships After the Black Death: A Sienese "Compagnia", c. 1350–1363(?). *Renaissance Studies* 14, 1 (2000), 1–45.

Sundberg, Adam. *Natural Disaster at the Closing of the Dutch Golden Age: Floods, Worms, and Cattle Plague*. Cambridge: Cambridge University Press, 2022.

Sundberg, Adam. Building the Social Cascade: Connecting Culture, Disaster, and Persecution in the 1730s. *Journal for the History of Environment and Society* 8 (2024), 29–57.

Tamis, Rozemarijn. Ook zij slaat wel eens terug: Vrouwencriminaliteit in Leiden in de tweede helft van de vijftiende eeuw. *Leidschrift* 37 (2022), 81–98.

Tanis, Nelleke. *An Epidemic and its Aftermath: Cholera in Utrecht, 1866*. MA Thesis: Utrecht University, 2023.

Tanis, Nelleke. "To Think Seriously About the Relatives Left Behind". Charity and Widows' Financial Strategies in the Aftermath of Utrecht's Cholera Epidemic of 1866. *BMGN: Low Countries Historical Review* 139, 4 (2024), 60–84.

Teeuwen, Daniëlle. *Financing Poor Relief through Charitable Collections in Dutch Towns, c. 1600–1800*. Amsterdam: Amsterdam University Press, 2006.

Temminck, Jaap. Begraven in Haarlem tot 1800. *Haerlem Jaarboek 1999* (2000), 139–53.

Theilmann, John, and Frances Cate. A Problem of Plagues: The Problem of Plague Diagnosis in Medieval England. *Journal of Interdisciplinary History* 37, 3 (2007), 371–93.

Thoen, Erik. *Landbouwekonomie en bevolking in Vlaanderen gedurende de late middeleeuwen en het begin van de moderne tijden. Testregio: De kasselrijen van Oudenaarde en Aalst (eind 13de–eerste helft van de 16de eeuw)*, I–II. PhD Thesis: University of Ghent, 1988.

Thoen, Erik. Historical Demography in Late Medieval Rural Flanders: Recent Results and Hypotheses. In: Jean-Marie Duvosquel and Erik Thoen, eds., *Peasants and Townsmen in Medieval Europe: Studia in Honorem Adriaan Verhulst*, 573–82. Ghent: Snoeck-Ducaju, 1995.

Thoen, Erik. De twee gezichten van de Vlaamse landbouw en het probleem der "Wüstungen". Middeleeuwen – Modern Tijden. In: Jan Art and Luc François, eds., *Docendo discimus: Liber amicorum Romain Van Eenoo*, 75–84. Ghent: Academia Press, 1999.

Thoen, Erik. A "Commercial Survival Economy" in Evolution: The Flemish Countryside and the Transition to Capitalism (Middle Ages–19th Century). In: Peter C.M. Hoppenbrouwers and Jan Luiten van Zanden, eds., *Peasants into Farmers? The Transformation of Rural Economy and Society in the Low Countries (Middle Ages–19th Century) in Light of the Brenner Debate*, 102–57. Turnhout: Brepols, 2001.

Thoen, Erik. "Social Agrosystems" as an Economic Concept to Explain Regional Differences: An Essay Taking the Former County of Flanders as an Example (Middle Ages–19th Century). In: Bas van Bavel and Peter C.M. Hoppenbrouwers, eds., *Landholding and Land Transfer in the North Sea Area (Late Middle Ages–19th Century)*, 47–66. Turnhout: Brepols, 2004.

Thoen, Erik, and Isabel Devos. Pest in de Zuidelijke Nederlanden tijdens de middeleeuwen en de moderne tijden: Een status quaestionis over de ziekte in haar sociaal-economische context. In: Anon., ed., *De pest in de Nederlanden: Medisch historische beschouwingen 650 jaar na de Zwarte Dood*, 19–43. Brussels: Koninklijke Academie voor Geneeskunde van België, 1999.

Thoen, Erik, and Tim Soens. The Family or the Farm: A Sophie's Choice? The Late Medieval Crisis in the Former County of Flanders. In: John Drendel, ed., *Crisis in the Later Middle Ages: Beyond the Postan-Duby Paradigm*, 195–224. Turnhout: Brepols, 2015.

Thomas, Lynn M. Historicising Agency. *Gender and History* 28, 2 (2016), 324–39.

Thompson, Kristina, and Johan van Ophem. Re-Examining the Social Gradient in Health: A Study of Dutch Men, 1850–1984. *SSM – Population Health* 24 (2023), 101518.

Thorpe, Lara Elyse. *"In Middest of Death": Medical Responses to the Great Plague of 1665 with Special Reference to John Allin.* PhD Thesis: Royal Holloway University of London, 2018.

Tian, Huidong, Chuan Yan, Lei Xu, Ulf Büntgen, Nils C. Stenseth, and Zhibin Zhang. Scale-Dependent Climatic Drivers of Human Epidemics in Ancient China. *Proceedings of the National Academy of Sciences* 114, 39 (2017), 12970–5.

Tielhof, Milja van, and Petra van Dam. *Waterstaat in stedenland: Het hoogheemraadschap van Rijnland voor 1857*. Utrecht: Matrijs: 2006.

Timmers, J.J.M. *Symboliek en iconographie der christelijke kunst.* Roermond-Maaseik: J.J. Romen & Zonen, 1947.

Timmers, Olaf. Elisabeth Strouven: Hoe de pestziekte zich uitbreidt in Maastricht en de stedelijke regearing aan Elisabeth Strouven tijdens haar verblijf te Hoesselt een schrijven zendt. *Sint Franciscus: Maandschrift voor Leden der Derde Orde* 48, 3 (1933), 87–93.

Tramper, Ad. De pest in het Vlissingen van 1666. *Den Spiegel* 38, 3 (2020), 3–8.

Trénard, Louis. Roubaix, ville drapante entre Lille et Tournai (1469–1776). *Revue du Nord* 51, 201 (1969), 175–99.

Trio, Paul. De grote sterfte van 1438–39 in Ieper. Nieuwe inzichten op basis van een rekening van de O.L.V.-broederschap van Parijse scholieren. *Handelingen van het Genootschap voor Geschiedenis* 143, 1/2 (2006), 226–45.

Turner, Claire. Intersensory Experiences of the Plague in Seventeenth-Century London. *Social History of Medicine* 36, 1 (2023), 42–61.

Udale, Charlie. *The Plague and the State in Early Modern England, 1538–1667*. PhD Thesis: London School of Economics and Political Science, 2023.

Ufkes, Tonko. De verzorging van zieke en gewonde soldaten in Groningen en de Ommelanden, 1665 en 1672. *Gewina: Tijdschrift voor de Geschiedenis der Geneeskunde, Natuurwetenschappen, Wiskunde en Techniek* 17 (1994), 26–31.

Uytven, Raymond Van. *Stadsfinanciën en stadsekonomie te Leuven (van de XIIe tot het einde der XVIe eeuw)*. Brussels: Koninklijke Academie voor Wetenschappen, Letteren en Schone Kunsten van België, 1961.

Uytven, Raymond Van. De bevolking. In: Raymond Van Uytven, ed., *Leuven. "De beste stad van Brabant". De geschiedenis van het stadsgewest Leuven tot omstreeks 1600*, I, 113–28. Louvain: Stadsbestuur, 1980.

Valenti, Salvatore. From Plague to Cholera: Public Health and the Urban Poor in Nineteenth-Century Italy. *Social History* 50, 1 (2025), 35–62.

Vanbossele, José. Egidius Li Muisis over de pest, de Jodenvervolging, het zedenbederf en de flagellanten in 1349. *De Leiegouw* 54 (2012), 5–38.

Vandeburie, Jan. De Zwarte Dood te Brugge. Een status questionis en enkele nieuwe beschouwingen. *Handelingen van het Genootschap voor Geschiedenis* 147, 2 (2010), 269–309.

Vanden Bossche, Hugo. Een pest-antifoon uit de muziekcollectie van het Turnhoutse begijnhof. *Begijnhofkrant (Vrienden van het Begijnhof van Turnhout)* 22 (2008), 12–14.

Vandendriessche, Joris. Ophtalmia Crossing Borders. Belgian Army Doctors Between the Military and Civilian Society 1830–1860. *Journal of Belgian History* 46, 2 (2016), 48–71.

Vanduynhoven, Paul. De jaren 1637 en 1668 waren pestjaren te Meldert. *Hoegaards Erfgoed Vzw* 54, 5 (2017), no. 209.

Vanhaute, Eric, Richard Paping, and Cormac Ó Gráda. The Subsistence Crisis of 1845–1850. In: Eric Vanhaute, Richard Paping, and Cormac Ó Gráda, eds., *When the Potato Failed: Causes and Effects of the "Last" European Subsistence Crisis*, 15–40. Turnhout: Brepols, 2007.

Vanhaute, Eric, and Thijs Lambrecht. Famine, Exchange Networks, and the Village Community: A Comparative Analysis of the Subsistence Crises of the 1740s and the 1840s in Flanders. *Continuity and Change* 26, 2 (2011), 155–86.

Vargas, Michael. How a "Brood of Vipers" Survived the Black Death: Recovery and Dysfunction in the Fourteenth-Century Dominican Order. *Speculum* 86, 3 (2011), 688–714.

Various. Patiënt, ziekte en medische zorg in het verleden. Themanummer. *Tijdschrift voor Sociale Geschiedenis* 8 (1982), 91–223.

Varlik, Nükhet. *Plague and Empire in the Early Modern Mediterranean World: The Ottoman Experience, 1347–1600*. Cambridge: Cambridge University Press, 2015.

Veen, J.S. van. De pest en hare bestrijding in Gelderland, in het bijzonder te Arnhem. *Bijdragen en Mededelingen Gelre* 6 (1903), 1–66.

Vera, Hein. *...dat men het goed van den ongeboornen niet mag verkoopen. Gemene gronden in de Meierij van Den Bosch tussen hertog en hertgang, 1000–2000.* Woudrichem: Pictures Publishers, 2014.

Vermeer, Mark. Testamentary Practices and Village Courts in the Bailiwick of 's-Hertogenbosch (c. 1470–1550). *Tijdschrift voor Rechtsgeschiedenis* 91, 3/4 (2023), 471–524.

Vermeersch, Joren. *1349. Hoe de Zwarte Dood Vlaanderen en Europa veranderde.* Antwerp: Uitgeverij Vrijdag, 2019.

Vermeesch, Griet. *Oorlog, steden en staatsvorming: De grenssteden Gorinchem en Doesburg tijdens de geboorte-eeuw van de Republiek (1570–1680).* Amsterdam: Amsterdam University Press, 2006.

Vermunt, Marco. Onder de zoden... Enkele resultaten van de opgravingen op het Gouvernementsplein in 1999. *De Waterschans* 31, 2 (2001), 51–6.

Vermunt, Marco, and Alexander van der Kallen. *Opgravingen in Bergen op Zoom.* Utrecht: Matrijs, 2012.

Vervaeke, Ans, and Isabelle Devos. Much Ado about Nothing? Reconsidering the Smallpox Effect. Height in the Nineteenth-Century Town of Thielt, Belgium. *TSEG: Low Countries Journal of Social and Economic History* 14, 4 (2017), 56–83.

Vervaet, Lies. Women and Leasehold in Rural Flanders, c. 1290 to c. 1570. *Rural History* 30, 1 (2019), 1–15.

Vervaet, Lies. The Economic Opportunities of Rural Women in Late Medieval Flanders. In: Miriam Müller, ed., *The Routledge Handbook of Medieval Rural Life*, 282–300. Abingdon: Routledge, 2022.

Viaene, Antoon. Een woelige pestlijder te Nieuwpoort, 1609. *Biekorf* 50 (1949), 140.

Viaene, Antoon. Reeuwers. *Biekorf* 61 (1960), 177–9.

Viaene, Antoon. Reeuweghe. *Biekorf* 72 (1971), 316–17.

Viaene, Antoon. Smette. *Biekorf* 72 (1971), 317.

Viaene, Antoon. Smettelic. *Biekorf* 72 (1971), 318.

Viaene, Antoon. Judocus Clichtove van Nieuwpoort 1472–1543. Zijn sermoen over de pestziekte in dietse versie. *Biekorf* 73 (1972), 343–7.

Vijver, K. van de. Past Life and Death in a Flemish Town. An Archaeo-Anthropological Study of Burials from the Medieval and Post-Medieval St. Rombout's Cemetery in Mechelen, Belgium (10th–18th Centuries CE). *Journal of Archaeological Science* 20 (2018), 524–55.

Vis, G.N.M. *650 jaar ziekenzorg in Alkmaar, 1341–1991: Hoofdstukken uit de geschiedenis en voorgeschiedenis van de Alkmaarse zieken- en gezondheidszorg.* Hilversum: Verloren, 1991.

Vis, G.N.M. *Het weeshuis van Woerden: 400 jaar Stadsweeshuis en Gereformeerd wees- en oudeliedenhuis te Woerden 1595–1995.* Hilversum: Verloren, 1996.

Visscher, Henk. De Rotterdamse zorg om de cholera in 1866 en 1867: De Swaans theoretisch model van collectieve actie getoetst. *Sociologische Gids* 45, 4 (1998), 217–33.

Vlis, Ingrid van der. *Leven in armoede. Delftse bedeelden in de zeventiende eeuw.* Amsterdam: Prometheus/Bert Bakker, 2001.

Vogelzang, Fred. Et in arcadia ego? Kastelen en buitenplaatsen in tijden van pest. *Het Buiten* 5, 2 (2020), 22–6.

Voigtländer, Nico, and Hans-Joachim Voth, The Three Horsemen of Riches: Plague, War, and Urbanization in Early Modern Europe. *Review of Economic Studies* 80, 2 (2013), 774–811.

Waddington, Keir. "In Constant Fear of some Dire Epidemic Breaking Out": Rural Responses to Infectious and Epidemic Disease, 1870–1920. *Rural History* 35, 2 (2024), 211–32.

Wagenaar, F.P. *"Dat de regeringe niet en bestaet by het corpus van de magistraet van Den Hage alleen". De Sociëteit van 's-Gravenhage (1587–1802). Een onderzoek naar bureaucratisering*. Hilversum: Verloren, 1999.

Wald, Priscilla. *Contagious: Cultures, Carriers, and the Outbreak Narrative*. Durham, NC: Duke University Press, 2008.

Walhout, Eveline C. *An Infants' Graveyard? Region, Religion, and Infant Mortality in North Brabant, 1840–1940*. PhD Thesis: Tilburg University, 2019.

Walhout, Eveline C., and Erik Beekink. Just Another Crisis? Individual's Experiences and the Role of the Local Government and Church during the 1866 Cholera Epidemic in a Small Dutch Town. *Historical Social Research / Historische Sozialforschung* 33S (2021), 54–78.

Wan, Sim Hinman. Paradox of Isolation: Amsterdam's Pest Asylums and the City's Continual Modernization. *Change Over Time* 11, 1 (2022), 10–35.

Wang, Han, and Andrés Rodríguez-Pose. Local Institutions and Pandemics: City Autonomy and the Black Death. *Applied Geography* 136 (2021), 102582.

Wassink, J.F.A. *Van stad en buitenie: Een institutionele studie van rechtspraak en bestuur in Weert 1568–1795*. Hilversum: Verloren, 2005.

Watts, Sheldon J. *Epidemics and History: Disease, Power, and Imperialism*. New Haven, CT: Yale University Press, 1997.

Weeda, Claire. The Porous City: Dealing with Public Health Crises in Fifteenth-Century Sint-Truiden. In: Claire Weeda, Robert Stein, and Louis Sicking, eds., *Communities, Environment and Regulation in the Premodern World: Essays in Honour of Peter Hoppenbrouwers*, 99–120. Turnhout: Brepols, 2022.

Weeda, Claire. Doing the Dirty Work: Ribalds, Armies, and Public Health in the Southern Low Countries, 1100–1500. In: Els Rose, Robert Flierman, and Merel de Bruin-van de Beek, eds., *City, Citizen, Citizenship, 400–1500: A Comparative Approach*, 293–92. Cham: Palgrave-Macmillan, 2024.

Wegge, Simone A. Inheritance Institutions and Landholding Inequality in Nineteenth-Century Germany: Evidence from Hesse-Cassel Villages and Towns. *Journal of Economic History* 81, 3 (2021), 909–42.

Wendling, Miriam. Death and Burial in Late Medieval Women's Houses. *Mortality* 30, 1 (2025), 287–305.

Wenham, Clare, Julia Smith, and Rosemary Morgan. COVID-19: The Gendered Impacts of the Outbreak. *The Lancet* 395, 10227 (2020), 846–8.

Wenham, Clare, Julia Smith, Sara E. Davies, Huiyun Feng, Karen A. Grépin, Sophie Harman, Asha Herten-Crabb, and Rosemary Morgan. Women are Most Affected by Pandemics—Lessons from Past Outbreaks. *Nature* 583, 7815 (2020), 194–8.

Werveke, Hans Van. *De Zwarte Dood in de Zuidelijke Nederlanden (1349–1351)*. Brussels: Mededelingen van de Koninklijke Vlaamse Academie voor Wetenschappen, Letteren en Schone Kunsten van België, 1950.

Werveke, Hans Van. Nogmaals: De Zwarte Dood in de Nederlanden. *Bijdragen voor de Geschiedenis der Nederlanden* 8 (1953/4), 251–8.

Werveke, Hans Van. Bronnenmateriaal uit de Brugse stadsrekeningen betreffende de hongersnood van 1316. *Bulletin de la commission royale d'histoire* 125 (1959), 431–510.

Werveke, Hans Van. La famine de l'an 1316 en Flandre et dans les régions voisines. *Revue du Nord* 41, 161 (1959), 5–14.

Westerholt, Riemke. Genoeg voor een heel weeshuis? De voeding van kinderen in het Groene Weeshuis in Groningen, 1631–1830. *TSEG: Low Countries Journal of Social and Economic History* 4, 1 (2007), 89–116.

Westeringh, W. van de. De rode loop in het schoutambt Heteren 1783. *NGV Afdeling Betuwe* 6, 2 (2003), 6–11.

Westeringh, W. van de. De rode loop in Andelst 1783. *NGV Afdeling Betuwe* 7 (2004), 22–5.

Weyde, A.J. van der. Bijdrage tot de geschiedenis der pest te Utrecht. *Nederlandse Tijdschrift voor Geneeskunde* 71, 23 (1927), 3119–39.

Weyde, A.J. van der. Over begraafplaatsen en begraven in het bijzonder te Utrecht. *Jaarboekje van Oud-Utrecht* (1930), 85–113.

Whaley, Leigh Ann. *Women and the Practice of Medical Care in Early Modern Europe, 1400–1800*. Basingstoke: Palgrave Macmillan, 2011.

Whittle, Jane. Inheritance, Marriage, Widowhood and Remarriage: A Comparative Perspective on Women and Landholding in North-East Norfolk, 1440–1580. *Continuity and Change* 13, 1 (1998), 33–72.

Whittle, Jane. *The Development of Agrarian Capitalism: Land and Labour in Norfolk, 1440–1580*. Oxford: Oxford University Press, 2000.

Whittle, Jane. A Critique of Approaches to "Domestic Work": Women, Work and the Pre-Industrial Economy. *Past and Present* 243, 1 (2019), 35–70.

Whittles, Lilith K., and Xavier Didelot. Epidemiological Analysis of the Eyam Plague Outbreak of 1665–1666. *Proceedings of the Royal Society B* 283 (2016), 20160618.

Wiel, Kees van der, and Peter Ekamper. Kromme sikkel des doods, of de pest van 1624 in Delft. *Jaarboek Delfia Batavorum* 27 (2018), 75–95.

Wiersma, G. Observaties van Pieter van Foreest tijdens de pest in Delft (1557/'58). *Nederlandse Tijdschrift voor Geneeskunde* 138, 52 (1994), 2618–21.

Wiersum, E. Grafschriften uit de Prinsenkerk. *Rotterdamse Jaarboekje* 10 (1912), 7–52.

Williams, Samantha. Urban Governance, Public Health and the Impact of Plague on Everyday Life in Cambridge, 1625–1630. *Social History* 50, 1 (2025), 1–34.

Winer, Rebecca Lynn. The Enslaved Wet Nurse as Nanny: The Transition from Free to Slave Labor in Childcare in Barcelona after the Black Death (1348). *Slavery and Abolition* 38, 2 (2017), 303–19.

Winkelman, Henri Pierre. *Geschiedkundige plaatsbeschrijving van Vlissingen*, I. Vlissingen: P.G. De Veij Mestdagh, 1873.

Woude, Ad van der. Demografische ontwikkeling van de noordelijke Nederlanden 1500–1800. In: Dirk P. Blok, ed., *Algemene geschiedenis der Nederlanden*, V, 102–68. Haarlem: Fibula-Van Dishoeck, 1980.

Wrigley, E.A., and Roger S. Schofield. *The Population History of England, 1541–1871: A Reconstruction*. Cambridge: Cambridge University Press, 1981.

Wubs-Mrozewicz, Justyna. The Hanse in Medieval and Early Modern Europe: An Introduction. In: Justyna Wubs-Mrozewicz and Stuart Jenks, eds., *The Hanse in Medieval and Early Modern Europe*, 1–25. Leiden: Brill, 2013.

Yates, Margaret. Change and Continuities in Rural Society from the Later Middle Ages to the Sixteenth Century: The Contribution of West Berkshire. *Economic History Review* 52, 4 (1999), 617–46.

Yaussy, Samantha L., Sharon N. DeWitte, and Rebecca C. Redfern. Frailty and Famine: Patterns of Mortality and Physiological Stress among Victims of Famine in Medieval London. *American Journal of Biological Anthropology* 160, 2 (2016), 272–83.

Yue, Ricci P.H., and Harry Lee. Pre-Industrial Plague Transmission is Mediated by the Synergistic Effect of Temperature and Aridity Index. *BMC Infectious Diseases* 18, 1 (2018), 134.

Yue, Ricci P.H., Harry F. Lee, and Connor Y.H. Hu. Navigable Rivers Facilitated the Spread and Recurrence of Plague in Pre-Industrial Europe. *Scientific Reports* 6 (2016), 34867.

Yue, Ricci P.H., Harry F. Lee, and Connor Y.H. Hu. Trade Routes and Plague Transmission in Pre-Industrial Europe. *Scientific Reports* 7 (2017), 12973.

Zaidman-Mauer, Daniella. The Key Role of Maskiel El Dal and Dr. E.J. Goldsmit in the Smallpox Vaccination in Amsterdam. "Blessed is he that Considereth the Poor". *Studia Rosenthaliana* 48, 2 (2022), 139–73.

Zalinge-Sporen, Lia van. "Die contagieuse sieckte der peste is grasserende..." De pest in Helmond in 1636. *Vlasbloem* 14 (1994), 57–92.

Zalinge-Spooren, Lia van. *Gemeint en gemeenschap: Jaargeboden in Peelland, circa 1300–1795*. Hilversum: Verloren, 2018.

Zanden, Jan Luiten van. Tracing the Beginning of the Kuznets Curve: Western Europe during the Early Modern Period. *Economic History Review* 48, 4 (1995), 643–64.

Zanden, Jan Luiten van. The Paradox of the Marks. The Exploitation of Commons in the Eastern Netherlands, 1250–1850. *Agricultural History Review* 47, 2 (1999), 125–44.

Zanden, Jan Luiten van. A Third Road to Capitalism? Proto-Industrialisation and the Moderate Nature of the Late Medieval Crisis in Flanders and Holland, 1350–1550. In: Peter C.M. Hoppenbrouwers and Jan Luiten van Zanden, eds., *Peasants into Farmers? The Transformation of Rural Economy and Society in the Low Countries (Middle Ages–19th Century) in Light of the Brenner Debate*, 85–101. Turnhout: Brepols, 2001.

Zanden, Jan Luiten van. What Happened to the Standard of Living Before the Industrial Revolution? New Evidence from the Western Part of the Netherlands. In: Robert C. Allen, Tommy Bengtsson, and Martin Dribe, eds., *Living Standards in the Past: New Perspectives on Well-Being in Asia and Europe*, 173–94. Oxford: Oxford University Press, 2005.

Zanden, Jan Luiten van. *The Long Road to the Industrial Revolution: The European Economy in a Global Perspective, 1000–1800*. Leiden: Brill, 2009.

Zanden, Jan Luiten van, and Arthur van Riel. *The Strictures of Inheritance: The Dutch Economy in the Nineteenth Century*, trans. Ian Cressie. Princeton, NJ: Princeton University Press, 2004.

Zanden, Jan Luiten van, and Bas van Bavel. The Jump-Start of the Holland Economy during the Late-Medieval Crisis, c.1350–1500. *Economic History Review* 57, 3 (2004), 503–32.

Zanden, Jan Luiten van, and Lee Soltow. *Income and Wealth. Inequality in the Netherlands 1500–1990*. Amsterdam: Het Spinhuis, 1998.

Zanden, Jan Luiten van, Tine De Moor, and Sarah G. Carmichael. *Capital Women: The European Marriage Pattern, Female Empowerment and Economic Development in Western Europe 1300–1800*. Oxford: Oxford University Press, 2019.

Zapnik, Jörg. *Pest und Krieg im Ostseeraum. Der "Schwarze Tod" in Stralsund während des Großen Nordischen Krieges (1700–1721)*. Hamburg: Kovač, 2007.

Zarulli, Virginia, Julia A. Barthold Jones, Anna Oksyzyan, Rune Lindahl-Jacobsen, Kaare Christensen, and James W. Vaupel. Women Live Longer than Men Even during Severe Famines and Epidemics. *Proceedings of the National Academy of Sciences* 115, 4 (2018), e832–40.

Zazvonilová, Eliška, Hana Brzobohatá, Jan Frolík, Petr Velemínský, and Jaroslav Brůžek. Using Cementochronology to Assess the Seasonality of Catastrophic Events in Medieval Mass Graves (Kutná Hora-Sedlec, Czechia, 14th Century): Preliminary Results. *PLoS ONE* 18, 12 (2023), e0295757.

Zimmerman, Susan. Leprosy in the Medieval Imaginary. *Journal of Medieval and Early Modern Studies* 38, 3 (2008), 559–87.

Zuijderduijn, Jaco. Living la vita apostolica. Longevity of Nuns in Late Medieval Holland. *Age, Culture, Humanities* 9, 1 (2025), 1–29.

Zuijderduijn, Jaco. Grave Concerns: Entailment and Intergenerational Agency in Amsterdam (1600–1800). *The History of the Family* 16, 4 (2011), 343–53.
Zwaan, Abram de. *Zorg en de staat. Welzijn, onderwijs en gezondheidszorg in Europa en de Verenigde Staten in de nieuwe tijd*. Amsterdam: Bert Bakker, 2004 [1989].
Zwart-Kramer, A.G., and P.A.M. Zwart. *Van pest tot pokken. 5 eeuwen gezondheidszorg in Enkhuizen*. Schoorl: Vereniging Oud Enkhuizen, 1993.

Index

Page numbers in **bold** denote tables, those in *italic* denote figures.